Secondary Headache

Editor

RANDOLPH W. EVANS

NEUROLOGIC CLINICS

www.neurologic.theclinics.com

Consulting Editor
RANDOLPH W. EVANS

May 2014 • Volume 32 • Number 2

ELSEVIER

1600 John F. Kennedy Boulevard • Suite 1800 • Philadelphia, Pennsylvania, 19103-2899

http://www.theclinics.com

NEUROLOGIC CLINICS Volume 32, Number 2
May 2014 ISSN 0733-8619, ISBN-13: 978-0-323-29719-6

Editor: Joanne Husovski
Developmental editor: Donald Mumford

Neurologic Clinics (ISSN 0733-8619) is published quarterly by Elsevier Inc., 360 Park Avenue South, New York, NY 10010–1710. Months of issue are February, May, August, and November. Periodicals postage paid at New York, NY, and additional mailing offices. Subscription prices are $300.00 per year for US individuals, $517.00 per year for US institutions, $145.00 per year for US students, $375.00 per year for Canadian individuals, $627.00 per year for Canadian institutions, $415.00 per year for international individuals, $627.00 per year for international institutions, and $210.00 for Canadian and foreign students/residents. To receive student/resident rate, orders must be accompanied by name of affiliated institution, date of term, and the *signature* of program/residency coordinator on institution letterhead. Orders will be billed at individual rate until proof of status is received. Foreign air speed delivery is included in all *Clinics* subscription prices. All prices are subject to change without notice. **POSTMASTER:** Send address changes to *Neurologic Clinics*, Elsevier Health Sciences Division, Subscription Customer Service, 3251 Riverport Lane, Maryland Heights, MO 63043. **Customer Service: Telephone: 1-800-654-2452 (U.S. and Canada); 314-447-8871 (outside U.S. and Canada). Fax: 314-447-8029. E-mail: journalscustomerservice-usa@elsevier.com (for print support); journalsonlinesupport-usa@elsevier.com (for online support).**

Reprints. For copies of 100 or more of articles in this publication, please contact the Commercial Reprints Department, Elsevier Inc., 360 Park Avenue South, New York, New York, 10010-1710; Tel.: +1-212-633-3874; Fax: +1-212-633-3820, and E-mail: reprints@elsevier.com.

Neurologic Clinics is also published in Spanish by Nueva Editorial Interamericana S.A., Mexico City, Mexico.

Neurologic Clinics is covered in *Current Contents/Clinical Medicine, MEDLINE/PubMed (Index Medicus), EMBASE/Excerpta Medica,* and *PsycINFO,* and *ISI/BIOMED.*

Printed and bound by CPI Group (UK) Ltd, Croydon, CR0 4YY

Contributors

CONSULTING EDITOR

RANDOLPH W. EVANS, MD
Clinical Professor of Neurology, Baylor College of Medicine, Houston, Texas

EDITOR

RANDOLPH W. EVANS, MD
Clinical Professor of Neurology, Baylor College of Medicine, Houston, Texas

AUTHORS

NAGHAM AL-ZUBIDI, MD
Department of Ophthalmology, The Methodist Hospital, Houston, Texas

JENNIFER P. BASSIUR, DDS
Director, Center for Oral, Facial & Head Pain, Columbia University College of Dental Medicine; Assistant Professor of Dental Medicine at CUMC, New york, New York

HILARY A. BEAVER, MD
Department of Ophthalmology, The Methodist Hospital, Houston, Texas; Department of Ophthalmology, Weill Cornell Medical College, New York, New York

NIKOLAI BOGDUK, MD, PhD, DSc
Professor of Pain Medicine, University of Newcastle, and Director of Clinical Research, Newcastle Bone and Joint Institute, Royal Newcastle Centre, Newcastle, New South Wales, Australia

PAUL W. BRAZIS, MD
Departments of Ophthalmology and Neurology, Mayo Clinic, Jacksonville, Florida

F. MICHAEL CUTRER, MD
Associate Professor of Neurology, Headache Division Chair, Headache Section, Consultant, Department of Neurology, Mayo Medical School, Mayo Clinic, Rochester, Minnesota

JUSTIN DELANGE, DO
Headache Medicine Fellow, Department of Neurology, Mayo Clinic, Rochester, Minnesota

RANDOLPH W. EVANS, MD
Clinical Professor of Neurology, Baylor College of Medicine, Houston, Texas

DEBORAH I. FRIEDMAN, MD, MPH
Professor, Departments of Neurology and Neurotherapeutics and Ophthalmology, University of Texas Southwestern Medical Center, Dallas, Texas

JONATHAN GLADSTONE, MD, FRCPC
Director, Gladstone Headache Clinic; Headache Specialist, The Hospital for Sick Children; Toronto Rehabilitation Institute; Cleveland Clinic Canada; Sunnybrook Health Sciences Centre, Toronto, Ontario, Canada

STEVEN B. GRAFF-RADFORD, DDS
Director, the Program for headache and Orofacial Pain, Cedars Sinai Medical Center; Adjunct Professor, UCLA School of Dentistry, California

SARAH KIRBY, MD, FRCPC
Division of Neurology, Department of Medicine, QEII Health Sciences Centre, Dalhousie University, Halifax, Nova Scotia, Canada

ANA MARISSA LAGMAN-BARTOLOME, MD
Headache Medicine Clinical Fellow, Division of Pediatric Neurology, Hospital for Sick Children, Women's College Hospital, University of Toronto, Toronto, Ontario, Canada

ANDREW G. LEE, MD
Department of Ophthalmology, The Methodist Hospital, Houston, Texas; Departments of Ophthalmology, Neurology, and Neurosurgery, Weill Cornell Medical College, New York, New York; Clinical Professor, Department of Ophthalmology, The University of Texas Medical Branch, Galveston, Texas; Adjunct Professor, Department of Ophthalmology, The University of Iowa Hospitals and Clinics, Iowa City, Iowa; Adjunct Professor, Department of Ophthalmology, Baylor College of Medicine, Houston, Texas

MICHAEL J. MARMURA, MD
Thomas Jefferson University Hospital, Department of Neurology, Jefferson Headache Center, Philadelphia, Pennsylvania

BAHRAM MOKRI, MD
Professor of Neurology, Mayo Clinic College of Medicine, Rochester, Minnesota

R. ALLAN PURDY, MD, FRCPC, FACP, FAHS
Division of Neurology, Department of Medicine, QEII Health Sciences Centre, Dalhousie University, Halifax, Nova Scotia, Canada

GADDUM DUEMANI REDDY, MD, PhD
Neurosurgery Resident, Department of Neurosurgery, Baylor College of Medicine, Houston, Texas

JOHN F. ROTHROCK, MD
Professor and Chair, Department of Neurosciences, University of Nevada (Reno) School of Medicine; Director, Renown Neurosciences Institute, Reno, Nevada

STEPHEN D. SILBERSTEIN, MD
Thomas Jefferson University Hospital, Department of Neurology, Jefferson Headache Center, Philadelphia, Pennsylvania

ASHWIN VISWANATHAN, MD
Assistant Professor, Department of Neurosurgery, Baylor College of Medicine, Houston, Texas

DAVID S. YOUNGER, MD
Clinical Associate Professor of Neurology, New York University School of Medicine; Division of Neurology, Department of Medicine, Lenox Hill Hospital, New York, New York

Contents

no more than a diagnosis of probable cervicogenic headache. Definitive diagnosis requires evidence of a cervical source of pain. For most treatments, the evidence is limited or poor. Many patients with probable cervicogenic headache can be managed with exercise therapy, with or without manual therapy. Intractable cervicogenic headache can be investigated with controlled diagnostic blocks of the upper cervical joints and treated with thermal radiofrequency neurotomy. Other interventions are experimental or speculative.

An Update on Eye Pain for the Neurologist

Andrew G. Lee, Nagham Al-Zubidi, Hilary A. Beaver, and Paul W. Brazis

Pain in and around the eye with or without an associated headache is a common presenting complaint to the neurologist. Although the main causes for eye pain are easily diagnosed by simple examination techniques that are readily available to a neurologist, sometimes the etiology is not as obvious and may require a referral to an ophthalmologist. This article summarizes and updates our prior review in *Neurologic Clinics* on this topic and includes (1) ocular and orbital disorders that produce eye pain with a normal examination, (2) neurologic syndromes with predominantly ophthalmologic presentations, and (3) ophthalmologic presentations of selected headache syndromes.

Headaches Caused by Nasal and Paranasal Sinus Disease

Michael J. Marmura and Stephen D. Silberstein

Headache and rhinosinusitis are 2 of the most common conditions seen in clinical practice. In general, chronic and disabling headaches, especially if migraine features are present, are not due to sinus abnormalities. In suspected cases of bacterial sinusitis, computed tomography and magnetic resonance imaging are both effective in demonstrating the infection. Although most cases of sinusitis are fairly easy to diagnose, sphenoid sinusitis may be overlooked, and can present with progressive or thunderclap headache in adults. Contact-point headache should be considered in patients with focal headaches and a contact point on the lateral nasal wall.

Temporomandibular Disorders and Headaches

Steven B. Graff-Radford and Jennifer P. Bassiur

Headache and temporomandibular disorders should be treated together but separately. If there is marked limitation of opening, imaging of the joint may be necessary. The treatment should then include education regarding limiting jaw function, appliance therapy, instruction in jaw posture, and stretching exercises, as well as medications to reduce inflammation and relax the muscles. The use of physical therapies, such as spray and stretch and trigger point injections, is helpful if there is myofascial pain. Tricyclic antidepressants and the new-generation antiepileptic drugs are effective in muscle pain conditions. Arthrocentesis and/or arthroscopy may help to restore range of motion.

NEUROLOGIC CLINICS

RELATED INTEREST

Otolaryngologic Clinics of North America, April 2014 (Vol. 47, No. 2)
Headache in Otolaryngology: Rhinogenic and Beyond
Howard Levine and Michael Setzen, *Editors*

**DOWNLOAD
Free App!**

Review Articles
THE CLINICS

NOW AVAILABLE FOR YOUR iPhone and iPad

Preface

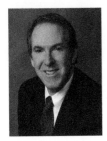

Randolph W. Evans, MD
Editor

Although an estimated 90% of headaches are of the primary type, the other 10% are secondary headache disorders, which are diverse and fascinating, at times potentially life-threatening, and sometimes challenging to diagnose. We update our well-received first issue on this topic, which appeared in February 2004.

This issue reviews 13 types and causes of the many secondary headache and facial pain disorders: posttraumatic; vascular disorders; vasculitis; pseudotumor cerebri syndrome; low cerebrospinal fluid volume syndromes; brain tumors; cough, exertional, and sex headaches; metabolic headaches; the neck; painful ophthalmologic disorders and eye pain; nasal and paranasal sinus disease; temporomandibular joint disorders and bruxism; and trigeminal neuralgia and glossopharyngeal neuralgia. These headaches range from the rare to the mundane and from the well established to the highly controversial. I hope this issue will stimulate further interest in the subspecialty of headache medicine.

I appreciate the outstanding contributions of our distinguished contributors. I thank Joanne Husovski, Senior Editor, *Neurologic Clinics;* Don Mumford, Senior Developmental Editor, Elsevier; and the production team at Elsevier for their great work.

Randolph W. Evans, MD
Clinical Professor of Neurology
Baylor College of Medicine
1200 Binz #1370
Houston, TX 77004, USA

E-mail address:
revansmd@gmail.com

Neurol Clin 32 (2014) xi
http://dx.doi.org/10.1016/j.ncl.2014.01.002
0733-8619/14/$ – see front matter © 2014 Published by Elsevier Inc.

Posttraumatic Headaches in Civilians, Soldiers, and Athletes

Randolph W. Evans, MD

KEYWORDS

- Headaches • Posttraumatic • Migraine • Tension-type • Occipital neuralgia
- Soldiers • Athletes

KEY POINTS

- Mild head injury accounts.
- Headache is the most common symptom of the postconcussion syndrome (PCS) and develops in more than 50% of those who sustain mild head injuries.
- Tension, migraine, and occipital neuralgia are the most common types.
- There are few randomized placebo-controlled trial for treatment.

Headaches as a result of head trauma are one of the most common secondary headache types. Because of the medicolegal aspects, posttraumatic headaches have been one of the most controversial headache topics, and, for many physicians, one of their least favorite types to treat. In the past decade, however, there has been increasing interest in posttraumatic headaches among physicians and the public because of the headaches occurring in US soldiers with blast trauma and in athletes with concussions. This article reviews the PCS and posttraumatic headaches.

THE POSTCONCUSSION SYNDROME

PCS refers to a large number of symptoms and signs that may occur alone or in combination, usually after mild head trauma.[1] Concussion is a clinical syndrome of biomechanically induced alteration of brain function, typically affecting memory and orientation, that may or may not involve loss of consciousness.[2] A patient's account of loss of consciousness and duration may not be reliable. Loss of consciousness does not have to occur for PCS to develop.

The following symptoms and signs are associated with PCS, which develops in more than 50% of patients who have mild head injuries: headaches, dizziness, vertigo, tinnitus, hearing loss, blurred vision, diplopia, convergence insufficiency, light and noise sensitivity, diminished taste and smell, irritability, anxiety, depression, personality

Baylor College of Medicine, 1200 Binz #1370, Houston, TX 77004, USA
E-mail address: revansmd@gmail.com

Neurol Clin 32 (2014) 283–303
http://dx.doi.org/10.1016/j.ncl.2013.11.010
0733-8619/14/$ – see front matter © 2014 Elsevier Inc. All rights reserved.

neurologic.theclinics.com

change, fatigue, sleep disturbance, decreased libido, decreased appetite, posttraumatic stress disorder, memory dysfunction, impaired concentration and attention, slowing of reaction time, and slowing of information processing speed (**Box 1**).[3] Headaches, dizziness, fatigue, irritability, anxiety, insomnia, loss of concentration and memory, and noise sensitivity are the most common complaints.[4]

In a study of 118 patients who sustained a mild traumatic brain injury (TBI), symptoms were reported 1 month after the injury in the following percentages of patients: fatigue, 91%; headaches, 78%; forgetfulness, 73%; sleep disturbance, 70%; anxiety, 63%; irritability, 62%; dizziness, 59%; noise sensitivity, 46%; and light sensitivity, 44%.[5] PCS may be subdivided into early PCS and late or persistent PCS, which is when symptoms and signs persist for more than 6 months.[6] Among 53 patients referred to a headache clinic with chronic posttraumatic headaches, approximately half had cognitive complaints, a quarter had psychological complaints, and 17% had an isolated complaint of headache.[7]

HISTORICAL ASPECTS OF POSTCONCUSSION SYNDROME

PCS has been controversial for more than 150 years.[8,9] Erichsen, a London surgeon, beginning with a series of lectures in 1866, opined that minor injuries to the head could result in severe disability as a result of "subacute cerebral meningitis and arachnitis."[10] Symptoms reported by these patients included headaches, memory complaints, nightmares, irritability, and light and noise sensitivity. Erichsen was defensive about these cases of cerebral concussion because many occurred after railway accidents in which litigation was involved. On the title page of his book, he quotes Montaigne, "Je raconte, je ne juge pas" ("I tell, I do not judge"). These injuries became known as "railway brain" and those of the spine as "railway spine." He pointed out that earlier investigators had described the same symptoms in the prerailway era. He also was concerned about misdiagnosing these cases as hysteria: "Hysteria is the disease for which I have more frequently seen concussion of the spine, followed by meningo-myelitis, mistaken, and it certainly has always appeared extraordinary to me that so great an error of diagnosis could so easily be made."

Railway spine and brain became topics of intense controversy. In 1879, Rigler[11] raised the important issue of compensation neurosis when he described the increased incidence of posttraumatic invalidism after a system of financial compensation was established for accidental injuries on the Prussian railways in 1871. In 1888, Strumpell discussed how the desire for compensation could lead to exaggeration. In 1889, Oppenheim popularized the concept of traumatic neurosis, in which a strong afferent stimulus resulted in impairment of function of the central nervous system. Charcot countered Oppenheim's work and suggested that the impairment described actually was the result of hysteria and neurasthenia.

PCS also was controversial throughout the twentieth century. Miller, in 1961, summarized the viewpoint of those who believed that PCS actually was a compensation neurosis: "The most consistent clinical feature is the subject's unshakable conviction of unfitness for work."[12] In 1962, Symonds took an equally strong opposing viewpoint: "It is, I think, questionable whether the effects of concussion, however slight, are ever completely reversible."[13]

In a survey performed among neurologists in the United States in 1992,[14] 25% believed that prolonged postconcussion symptoms were likely psychogenic in origin rather than due to any true pathology and 35% agreed that effective treatment of PCS was available. One respondent opined, "I am appalled at the number of groundless personal injury patients I see. Pain seems to occupy the position that

Box 1
Sequelae of mild head injury

Headaches
  Tension type
  Migraine with and without aura
  Medication overuse
  Trigeminal autonomic cephalalgias
  Hemicrania continua
  Occipital neuralgia
  C2-3 facet joint
  Cervicogenic
  Supraorbital and infraorbital neuralgia
  Scalp lacerations and local trauma
  Temporomandibular joint
  Subdural or epidural hematomas
  Low CSF pressure syndrome
  Hemorrhagic cortical contusions
  Carotid and vertebral artery dissections
  Cerebral venous thrombosis
  Carotid-cavernous fistula
Cranial nerve symptoms and signs
  Dizziness
  Vertigo
  Tinnitus
  Hearing loss
  Blurred vision
  Diplopia
  Convergence insufficiency
  Light and noise sensitivity
  Diminished taste and smell
Psychologic and somatic complaints
  Irritability
  Anxiety
  Depression
  Personality change
  Posttraumatic stress disorder
  Fatigue
  Sleep disturbance
  Decreased libido
  Decreased appetite

Initial nausea or vomiting

Cognitive impairment

Memory dysfunction

Impaired concentration and attention

Slowing of reaction time

Slowing of information processing speed

Rare sequelae

Subdural and epidural hematomas

Cerebral venous thrombosis

Second impact syndrome

Seizures

Nonepileptic posttraumatic seizures

Transient global amnesia

Tremor

Dystonia

From Evans RW. Post-concussion syndrome. In: Evans RW, Baskin DS, Yatsu FM, editors. Prognosis of neurologic disorders. 2nd edition. New York: Oxford University Press; 2000. p. 367; with permission.

hysteria did seventy years ago." Another, "Lawyers who focus in on these 'reported' injuries are causing a collapse in our medical and medico-legal systems."

EPIDEMIOLOGY OF TRAUMATIC BRAIN INJURY
Civilians

Traumatic brain injury is a cause of significant morbidity and mortality worldwide with approximately 54 to 60 million injuries annually.[15] Mild head injury accounts for 80% or more of all TBIs.[15] The Centers for Disease Control estimates that 1.4 to 3.8 million concussions occur per year in the United States,[16] resulting in more than 800,000 outpatient visits (most primary care) and 1.2 million emergency department visits for minor head injury or concussion.[17]

The annual incidence of mild head injury per 100,000 in the United States is between 100 and 300 (in a meta-analysis)[18] and 749 for New Zealand (95% of all brain injury cases).[15] The annual incidence may be as high as 600 per 100,000 in the United States[18] because many cases are unreported.[19] In addition, some patients may have hidden TBI, where they develop PCS but do not make the causal connection between the injury and its consequences.[20]

In an industrialized country, such as the United States, the relative causes of head trauma are approximately as follows: motor vehicle accidents, 45%; falls, 30%; occupational accidents, 10%; recreational accidents, 10%; and assaults, 5%.[21,22] Approximately one-half of all patients who have mild head injury are between the ages of 15 and 34. Motor vehicle accidents are more common in the young and falls more common in the elderly. Men are injured more frequently than women, with a 2:1 ratio.[23] Approximately one-half of all patients who have mild head injury are between the ages of 15 and 34. Approximately 20% to 40% of people who have mild head injuries in the United States do not seek treatment.

US Military

Approximately 20% of veterans of Operations Enduring Freedom (Afghanistan) and Iraqi Freedom sustained a TBI, the signature wound of the conflicts.[24] According to the Congressional Research Service,[25] "Of the total 253,330 TBI cases between January 1, 2000, and August 20, 2012, 194,561 have been mild, 42,083 have been moderate, 6476 have been severe or penetrating, and 10,210 have not been classifiable." Blast exposure is the most common mechanism of injury, contributing to 75% of mild TBI.[26]

Sports

In the United States, 1.6 to 3.8 million persons per year sustain sport-related mild TBI, with many not obtaining immediate medical attention.[27] The incidences of concussion among high school and college football players per 1000 games were 1.55 and 3.02, respectively.[28] Female players have more concussions in high school and college basketball and soccer (highest rates) compared with male players. The rates per 1000 games for soccer are as follows: high school male players, 0.59; high school female players, 0.97; college male players, 1.38; college female players, 1.80.

Postcraniotomy

Iatrogenic trauma may also cause headaches. In the only prospective study of patients for the risk of headaches after treatment of intracranial aneurysms followed for 4 months after the procedure, the incidence of headache was 28 of 51 cases (54.9%) after surgery compared with 12 of 47 cases (25.5%) after embolization.[29] Less than a third had persistent headaches for more than 3 months. In another study of postcraniotomy headaches during the 6 months after craniotomy for the treatment of supratentorial intracranial aneurysms, there was an incidence of postcraniotomy headache of 40%, with 30% having migrainous headaches at 6 months.[30]

In a study of patients undergoing supratentorial craniotomy for epilepsy, 11.9% had ongoing headaches 1 year after surgery with 4% medically uncontrolled.[31] In another study of 107 patients who underwent craniotomies for brain tumors or epilepsy, no patients had debilitating headaches.[32] In a meta-analysis of 1653 patients who underwent resection of acoustic neuromas, long-term significant headaches were reported by 36% of those who underwent a retrosigmoid approach compared with 16% and 1% of those who underwent translabyrinthine and middle fossa approaches, respectively.[33] Some patients with chronic headaches after acoustic nerve resection have occipital nerve injuries improving after excision of the greater and lesser occipital nerves.[34] There is a single case report of a patient with new-onset hemicrania continua 2 days after resection of a large left-sided acoustic neuroma with complete resolution of headache on indomethacin (50 mg twice daily).[35]

HEADACHES

Headaches are estimated as occurring variably in 30% to 90% of persons who are symptomatic after mild head injury.[36] Head and neck injury account for approximately 15% of chronic daily headaches.[37] Paradoxically, headache prevalence and lifetime duration is greater in those who have mild head injury compared with those who have more severe trauma.[38,39] Posttraumatic headaches are more common in those who have a history of headache.[40]

Time of Onset

According to International Headache Society criteria, the onset of the headache should be less than 7 days after the injury.[41] The less than 7-day onset is arbitrary, particularly because the cause of posttraumatic migraine is not understood. For example, posttraumatic epilepsy may have a latency of months or years. Similarly, it would not be surprising if there were a latency of weeks or months for posttraumatic migraine to develop. Conversely, because migraine is a common disorder, the longer the latency between the trauma and onset, the more likely the trauma may not have been causative. Consider the hypothetical case of a 27-year-old man who develops new-onset migraine 2 months after a mild head injury in a motor vehicle accident. The incidence of migraine in men under the age of 30 is 0.25% per year or, in this case, 0.042% per 2 months.[42] Was the new-onset migraine the result of the mild head injury or coincidence?

Consider the increased incidence of new or worse headaches found with onset after 7 days at 3-month assessment in 3 studies. In a prospective study of 212 subjects hospitalized with mild TBI for observation or other injuries, an additional 59% of subjects reported new or worse headache (compared with preinjury) at 3 months who had not previously reported headache within the first 7 days after injury (baseline assessment).[43] Two other studies found a high percentage of new-onset headache with onset after 7 days: 23% additional headaches at the 3-month assessment in consecutive patients with moderate to severe TBI[44] and 19% in a retrospective cohort of US Army soldiers.[45] Three months seems a more reasonable latency for onset than 7 days[43,46] although a small percentage of patients with new-onset primary headaches are misdiagnosed as having posttraumatic headaches.

Epidemiology of Phenotypes

Civilians

In a meta-analysis[47] of 5 studies of posttraumatic headaches,[7,48–51] most headaches were of the tension type (ranging from 6.9% to 85.7%, mean 33.6%) and the second-most type had migraine characteristics (ranging from 1.9% to 40.7%, mean 28.6%). The following features were present: mild to moderate intensity pain, approximately 60%; bilateral, 72.5%; nonthrobbing, 83%; light sensitivity, 35.8%; noise sensitivity, 29.1%; and aggravation by routine physical activities, 71.1%. Analgesic overuse was reported as present in 18.8% to 45.8%. The percentage of mixed or unclassifiable headaches ranged from 4.2% to 36.5%.

In a prospective 1-year study of 212 subjects that included headaches with onset at any time, up to 49% of headaches met criteria for migraine and probable migraine, up to 40% met tension-type criteria, 4% were cervicogenic, and up to 16% were unclassified.[43] Of the up to 27% of subjects who reported having headaches several times per week to daily, 62% of the headache types were migraine in this highest frequency group at 1 year. Individuals over age 60 were significantly more likely to report no headaches over time and at all time points.

In another prospective 1-year study (that included headaches with onset at any time) of 378 subjects who sustained moderate to severe TBIs, migraine occurred in up to 38%, probable migraine in up to 25%, tension-type headache in up to 21%, cervicogenic headache in up to 10%, and unclassifiable headache in up to 30%.[52] Women were more likely to have preinjury migraine than men and to have migraine or probable migraine at all time points after injury.

US military

Migraine is the most common type of posttraumatic headache, occurring in 60% to 97% of cases.[53] Blast trauma had been sustained by 77% of soldiers with chronic posttraumatic headaches.[54] The onset of posttraumatic headaches after injury was within 1 week for nearly 40%, within 1 month for 20%, and beyond 1 month for 40%.[55]

There was a high prevalence of migraine in US soldiers deployed to combat in Iraq without physical trauma, with 17.4% of men and 34.9% of women reporting a headache consistent with migraine during the prior year, much greater than a civilian population.[56]

Athletes

There are few studies describing the types of headaches among athletes. In a study of 296 student athletes ages 12 to 25 years who sustained sport-related concussions, migraines occurred in 52, headache in 176, and no headache in 68.[57] Female athletes were 2.13 times more likely than male athletes to report posttraumatic migraine characteristics. Those with migraine characteristics had prolonged symptom recovery, including cognitive, neurobehavioral, and somatic symptoms. Only 1 patient reported migraine at 90 days. Another study of high school and college athletes found that those with posttraumatic migraines had significantly greater neurocognitive deficits compared with those who had concussions with nonmigraine headaches and controls.[58]

Possible overdiagnosis of migraine

Tension-type, cervicogenic headaches, and occipital neuralgia have the potential for being misdiagnosed as migraine because light and noise sensitivity are commonly associated with PCS[5] and nausea may also be present in early PCS and in those with associated dizziness.

Neck injuries commonly accompany head trauma and can produce headaches, such as those associated with whiplash injuries,[59] discussion of which is beyond the scope of this review. Although not part of PCS, headaches associated with subdural and epidural hematomas also are described.

CASES

Case 1. Migraine from Blast Trauma

A 39-year-old US male army soldier was standing outside of his truck in Afghanistan when 3 rocket-propelled grenades hit the truck. The blast threw him 25 to 30 feet, resulting in loss of consciousness for 3 to 4 minutes and confusion following. He had a mild headache immediately following and developed severe headaches 2 days later, which were initially 2 to 3 times per week and then became daily 10 months after the trauma. He was started on amitriptyline (50 mg) at bedtime and the headaches decreased to 1 to 2 times per week. He described a right-sided, especially frontoparietal, throbbing with an intensity ranging from 3 of 10 to 10 of 10 associated with nausea, vomiting at times, and light and noise sensitivity but no aura. The headache would resolve in approximately 40 minutes with an oral triptan but without medication could last 24 hours. Weightlifting and stomach crunches were triggers. There was no prior history of headaches. An MRI of the brain was normal. He also had posttraumatic stress disorder.

Comment

This is a typical case of posttraumatic migraine with onset within 1 week after blast trauma in a soldier associated with comorbid posttraumatic stress disorder.

Case 2. Footballer's Migraine

Late in the first quarter of Super Bowl XXXII on January 25, 1998, Terrell Davis, a 25-year-old running back for the Denver Broncos with a history of migraine with and without aura since age 7, was unintentionally kicked in the helmet by a Green Bay Packers defender.[60] A few minutes later, he went to the sidelines with a migraine visual aura. Coach Shanahan sent him back in for one more play that was a fake where Elway kept the ball and ran into the end zone. Davis was given his usual migraine medication, dihydroergotamine nasal spray, on the sideline by the trainer. He went into the locker room and his severe headache was gone by the start of the third quarter, with the benefit of the extra Super Bowl halftime minutes. When he returned for the second half, he had 20 carries for 90 yards, including the winning touchdown, and won the game's most valuable player (MVP) award.[61] He had a Super Bowl–record 3 rushing touchdowns.

Comment

This is the most famous example of footballer's migraine, witnessed by 800 million viewers and occurring in American football rather than in soccer, as originally described. Early treatment of migraine can get patients back to school or work and even enable them to be a Super Bowl MVP.

TYPES AND FEATURES OF HEADACHES
Tension-Type Headache

Tension-type headaches occur in a variety of distributions, including generalized, nuchal-occipital, bifrontal, bitemporal, caplike, or headband. The headache, which may be constant or intermittent with variable duration, usually is described as pressure, tight, or dull aching. Temporomandibular joint injury can be caused by either direct trauma or jarring associated with the head injury. Patients may complain of temporomandibular joint area pain with chewing and hemicranial or ipsilateral frontotemporal aching or pressure headaches, although the pain may be referred anywhere in the trigeminal and cervical complex.[62]

Occipital Neuralgia

The term, occipital neuralgia, is in some ways a misnomer because the pain is not necessarily from the occipital nerve and usually does not have a neuralgic quality. Greater occipital neuralgia is a common posttraumatic headache[63] and also is seen frequently without injury. The aching, pressure, stabbing, or throbbing pain may be in a nuchal-occipital or parietal, temporal, frontal, periorbital, or retroorbital distribution. Occasionally, a true neuralgia may be present with paroxysmal shooting-type pain. The headache may last for minutes, hours, or days and be unilateral or bilateral.

Occasionally, referred ipsilateral facial paresthesias or subjective numbness, especially in the cheek, which is a diagnosis of exclusion, may be present due to convergence of the C2 afferents, which supply the greater occipital nerve and trigeminal afferents on second-order neurons within the trigeminocervical complex.[64] Lesser occipital neuralgia similarly can occur with pain generally referred more laterally over the head with reproduction of symptoms by digital pressure over the nerve.

The headache may be the result of an entrapment of the greater occipital nerve in the aponeurosis of the superior trapezius or semispinalis capitis muscle or instead be referred pain without nerve compression from trigger points in these or other suboccipital muscles. Digital pressure over the greater occipital nerve reproduces the headache. Pain referred from the C2-3 facet joint[65] or other upper cervical spine pathology and posterior fossa pathology, however, may produce a similar headache.

Migraine

Recurring attacks of migraine with or without aura can result from mild head injury or preexisting migraine may be exacerbated. Medication overuse for treatment of other types of posttraumatic pain can also increase the frequency of migraine, whether de novo or preexisting.

Impact also can cause acute migraine episodes in adolescents who have a family history of migraine. This originally was termed, footballer's migraine, to describe headaches in young men who play soccer who had multiple migraines with aura attacks triggered only by impact.[66] Similar attacks can be triggered by mild head injury in any sport (see Case 2).

After minor head trauma, children, adolescents, and young adults can develop a variety of transient neurologic sequelae that are not always associated with migraine and are perhaps the result of vasospasm. Five clinical types can cause the following: hemiparesis; somnolence, irritability, and vomiting; a confusional state[67]; transient blindness, often precipitated by occipital impacts; and brainstem signs.[68]

Trigeminal Autonomic Cephalalgias and Hemicrania Continua

Cluster headaches rarely result from mild head injuries, with 19 reports in the literature.[69] There are case reports of posttraumatic chronic paroxysmal hemicranias with aura[70]; short-lasting unilateral neuralgiform headache attacks with conjunctival injection, tearing, sweating, and rhinorrhea[71]; short-lasting unilateral headache with cranial autonomic symptoms[72]; and hemicrania continua.[73]

Supraorbital and Infraorbital Neuralgia

Injury of the supraorbital branch of the first trigeminal division as it passes through the supraorbital foramen just inferior to the medial eyebrow can cause supraorbital neuralgia.[74] Similarly, infraorbital neuralgia can result from trauma to the inferior orbit. Shooting, tingling, aching, or burning pain along with decreased or altered sensation and sometimes decreased sweating in the appropriate nerve distribution may be present. The pain can be paroxysmal or fairly constant. A dull aching or throbbing pain also may occur around the area of injury.

Scalp Lacerations and Local Trauma

Dysesthesias over scalp lacerations occur frequently. In the presence or absence of a laceration, an aching, soreness, tingling, or shooting pain over the site of the original trauma can develop. Symptoms may persist for weeks or months but rarely for more than 1 year.

Subdural Hematomas

Tearing of the parasagittal bridging veins (which drain blood from the surface of the hemisphere into the dural venous sinuses) leads to hematoma formation within the subdural space. Even minor injuries without loss of consciousness, such as bumps on the head or riding a roller coaster,[75] can result in this tearing. Falls and assaults are more likely to cause subdural hematomas than motor vehicle accidents.

Subdural hematomas usually are located over the hemispheres, although other locations, such as between the occipital lobe and tentorium cerebelli or between the temporal lobe and base of the skull, can occur. A subdural hematoma becomes subacute between 2 and 14 days after the injury when there is a mixture of clotted and fluid blood and becomes chronic when the hematoma is filled with fluid more than 14 days after the injury. Rebleeding can occur in the chronic phase. Most patients who have chronic subdural hematomas are late middle aged or elderly. Subdural hematomas can be present with a normal neurologic examination.

Headaches associated with subdural hematomas are nonspecific, ranging from mild to severe and paroxysmal to constant.[76] Unilateral headaches usually are the result of ipsilateral subdural hematomas. Headaches associated with chronic subdural hematomas have at least one of the following features in 75% of cases: sudden onset; severe pain; exacerbation with coughing, straining, or exercise; and vomiting and or nausea.

Epidural Hematomas

Bleeding into the epidural space from a direct blow to the head produces an epidural hematoma. The source of the bleeding is variable and can be arterial or venous or both. In the supratentorial compartment, bleeding is of the following origins: middle meningeal artery, 50%; middle meningeal veins, 33%; dural venous sinus, 10%; and other sources, including hemorrhage from a fracture line, 7%. Most epidural hematomas in the posterior fossa are the result of dural venous sinus bleeding. The locations of epidurals are as follows: temporal region (usually under a fractured squamous temporal bone), 70%; frontal convexity, 15%; parieto-occipital, 10%; and parasagittal or posterior fossa, 5%; 95% of epidurals are unilateral.

Epidural hematomas usually occur between the ages of 10 and 40 and much less frequently in those under 2 or over 60. Motor vehicle accidents and falls are the most common causes. Trivial trauma without loss of consciousness can be a cause.

Forty percent of patients who have an epidural hematoma present with a Glasgow Coma Scale score of 14 or 15. Less than one-third of patients have the classic lucid interval (initially unconscious, then recovery, and then unconscious again).

Up to 30% of epidural hematomas are of the chronic type.[77] The patient often is a child or young adult who sustains what seems to be a trivial injury often without loss of consciousness.[78] A persistent headache then develops, often associated with nausea, vomiting, and memory impairment, which might seem consistent with PCS. After the passage of days to weeks, focal findings develop. The headaches of acute and chronic epidural may be unilateral or bilateral and can be nonspecific.

Other Causes

Trauma can cause a cerbrospinal fluid (CSF) leak through a dural root sleeve tear or a cribiform plate fracture and result in a low CSF pressure headache with the same features as a post–lumbar puncture headache.[79] Hemorrhagic cortical contusions can cause a headache resulting from subarachnoid hemorrhage. Headaches can be the only symptom of posttraumatic carotid and vertebral artery dissections. Cerebral venous thrombosis[80] and carotid-cavernous fistulas[81] are other rare causes.

PATHOGENESIS
Neurobiologic Factors

Mild TBI may result in cortical contusions after coup and contrecoup injuries or diffuse axonal injury resulting from sheer and tensile strain damage.[82] Release of excitatory neurotransmitters, including acetylcholine, glutamate, and aspartate, may be a neurochemical substrate for mild TBI. Impairment in cerebral vascular autoregulation can occur. TBI can also lead to neuroinflammation with activation of glial cells, disruption of the blood-brain barrier leading to extravasation of cytoxic peripheral blood components, and activation of cytokines.[83] Neuroimaging studies, including MRI, single-photon emission CT, positron emission tomography, magnetic source imaging, magnetic resonance diffusion tension imaging, functional MRI, and MRI spectroscopy can demonstrate structural and functional deficits.[84–86] Although these findings may help explain cognitive deficits, the causes of posttraumatic headaches are poorly understood.

Nonorganic Explanations

There are several nonorganic explanations for PCS that suggest an origin for subjective symptoms other than TBI for some people, including psychogenic, sociocultural, and psychosocial factors; base rate misattribution, expectation as etiology, chronic pain, compensation and litigation, and malingering.[87]

Psychogenic factors
A psychogenic contribution to PCS is suggested by several empiric and clinical observations. The symptom complex of PCS (headache, dizziness, and sleep impairment) is similar to the somatization seen in psychiatric disorders, including depression, anxiety, and posttraumatic stress disorder. In addition, anxiety and depression can produce subjective and objective cognitive deficits that are similar to those seen in PCS and that improve with antidepressant treatment.[88]

Several studies suggest that both psychiatric predispositions (poor coping skills, limited social support, and negative perceptions) and psychiatric comorbidity (depression, anxiety and panic, and acute and posttraumatic stress disorder) are more prevalent in patients with PCS compared with general population controls and/or with head-injured patients who do not develop persistent PCS.[26,89–92]

Studies of the interaction of depression, anxiety, and cognitive performance in TBI are limited, however. Some studies have not found a substantial correlation between the level of depressive symptoms and cognitive deficits in patients with mild TBI,[93] whereas others have found a correlation in the response to antidepressant treatment in a subset of patients.[94]

The association of psychiatric disease and PCS is not established. Limitations in methodology, including cross-sectional design and patient and control group selection bias, preclude firm conclusions. Also, such an association could have several explanations. Patients with premorbid psychiatric disease may be more likely to suffer head injury as a result of more prevalent alcoholism, motor or physical impairments resulting from their disease or medications, and other reasons. Alternatively, patients with psychiatric disease may be more prone to develop PCS after head injury. Finally, head injury may cause or precipitate psychiatric disease in susceptible individuals.

Sociocultural and psychosocial factors
The very low, even absent, rates of postconcussion symptomatology in some countries (Lithuania) and in children sometimes reported might suggest a prominent role for sociocultural factors in the pathogenesis of PCS, perhaps because of misattribution or litigation.[95,96] The Lithuanian studies have been criticized, however, because of the high incidence of chronic daily headache in the control group.[97] Another prospective study of 100 patients with acute mild head injury in Austria found none developed posttraumatic headaches at follow-up at 90 to 100 days.[98] Some studies have found poor social support and increased social adversity among patients who suffered prolonged symptoms than among those whose symptoms had remitted.[99]

Base rate misattribution
A high base rate level of PCS symptoms in the general population can lead to misattribution of symptoms to PCS. In one study of 104 healthy university community adults (61% women) with a mean age of 23 years, the following percentages endorsed the following symptoms from the *International Classification of Diseases, Tenth Revision*

criteria for PCS as present in the prior 2 weeks: fatigue, 76%; irritable, 72%; nervous or tense, 63%; poor sleep, 62%; poor concentration, 61%; sad, 61%; temper problems, 53%; headaches, 52%; memory problems, 51%; dizziness, 42%; extrasensitive to noises, 40%; nausea, 38%; and difficulty reading, 36%.[100] Several studies have compared patients with mild TBI to non–head-injured controls, finding a high prevalence of the same symptoms in both groups, indicating a high prevalence of base rate symptoms in the general population[101] similar to those with persistent PCS.[102]

Expectation as etiology

Volunteers with no history of head trauma can correctly identify the symptoms of persistent PCS present 6 months after the injury. Because patients may expect PCS symptomatology after an injury, they and their physicians may mistakenly attribute their common base rate complaints to the head injury, when they are actually unrelated.

Chronic pain

Patients with chronic pain have symptoms of PCS at a rate similar to a comparison group of patients after head injury.[103,104] Similar patterns of cognitive deficits may be seen in patients with chronic pain and PCS. It is not clear whether this reflects a shared prevalence of psychiatric disorders among sufferers of PCS and chronic pain syndromes, suggests that PCS is a manifestation of a chronic pain syndrome, or reflects the ubiquitous nature of these symptoms.[88]

Effects of compensation and litigation

Patients who have litigation are similar to those who do not in the following respects: symptoms that improve with time,[105] types of headaches, cognitive test results,[105] and response to migraine medications.[106] Symptoms usually do not resolve with the settlement of litigation.[107] Pending litigation may increase the level of stress for some claimants and may result in increased frequency of symptoms after settlement. Skepticism of physicians also may accentuate the level of stress and compel some patients to exaggerate so that the doctors take them seriously.

Malingering

There are, however, some patients who have persistent complaints resulting from secondary gain,[108] malingering, and psychological disorders. Potential indicators of malingering after mild head injury include the following: premorbid factors (antisocial and borderline personality traits, poor work record, and prior claims for injury); behavioral characteristics (uncooperative, evasive, or suspicious); neuropsychologic test performance (missing random items, giving up easily, inconsistent test profile, or stating frequently, "I don't know"); postmorbid complaints (describing events surround the accident in great detail or reporting an unusually large number of symptoms); and miscellaneous items (engaging in general activities not consistent with reported deficits, having significant financial stressors, resistance, and exhibiting a lack of reasonable follow-through on treatments).[109]

In a study of mild head-injured litigants, Andrikopoulos[110] compared 72 patients who had no improvement or worsening headache with 39 patients who had improving headache. Those who had no improvement or worsening performed worse on cognitive tests and had greater psychopathology on the Minnesota Multiphasic Personality Inventory-2 than those who had improving headaches, suggesting the possibility of malingering.

TREATMENT OF HEADACHES

There is a dearth of randomized placebo-controlled trials of medications for posttraumatic headaches. Only 5 studies, all done without controls, have been performed for the prevention of posttraumatic headaches. Three studies in civilians, which involved either monotherapy or combined therapy with propranolol, amitriptyline,[106,111] or valproate,[112] showed efficacy although a small study showed no benefit with amitriptyline.[113]

There are 2 open-label retrospective studies of chronic posttraumatic headaches among US soldiers. One found no significant benefit of treatment with low-dose tricyclic antidepressants but improvement with preventive treatment with topiramate. The second found benefit from onabotulinum toxin A injections, with 56% reporting more than one headache type.[114] Triptans may be effective for posttraumatic migraine.[51,115]

There are anecdotal reports of posttraumatic tension-type and migraine-type headaches treated with the usual symptomatic and preventative medications used for nontraumatic headaches. Physicians should be concerned about the potential for medication rebound headaches with the frequent use of over-the-counter medications, such as acetaminophen, aspirin, combination products containing caffeine, and prescription drugs containing narcotics, butalbital, and benzodiazepines. In one survey, more than 70% of those with headache during the first year after mild TBI used acetaminophen or a nonsteroidal antiinflammatory drug (NSAID), which was usually not effective.[116] Habituation also is a concern with narcotics, butalbital, and benzodiazepines. Although chronic posttraumatic migraine may respond to onabotulinum toxin A, this treatment is not effective for cervicogenic headaches.[117] Posttraumatic chronic daily headache may respond to an intravenous DHE regimen.

No strong evidence from clinical trials supports the use of biofeedback, cognitive behavioral therapy, physical therapy and manual therapy, immobilization devices, and ice.[118] A small study suggests benefit from cognitive behavioral training.[119]

Occipital neuralgia may improve with local anesthetic nerve blocks, which are effective alone or combined with an injectable corticosteroid if patients do not respond adequately to local anesthetics alone (eg, 3 mL of 1% xylocaine or 2.5 mL of 1% xylocaine and 3 mg of betamethasone).[63,120] Natsis and colleagues,[121] based on a cadaver study, recommend injecting approximately 20 mm to 25 mm below the external occipital protuberance and approximately 15 mm lateral from the midline, starting infiltration shortly after the injection needle has overcome the resistance of the trapezius muscle aponeurosis. Other investigators recommend injecting one-third of the way laterally along an imaginary line connecting the occipital protuberance to the mastoid process.[120] Before injection, physicians should aspirate to avoid inadvertent vascular injection.

Anecdotally, NSAIDs and muscle relaxants may also be beneficial. If there is a true occipital neuralgia with paroxysmal lancinating pain, baclofen, tizanidine, carbamazepine, gabapentin, or pregabalin may help. Physical therapy and transcutaneous nerve stimulators may help some headaches. A variety of other treatments have been proposed for refractory cases, including pulsed radiofrequency therapy[122,123] and occipital nerve stimulation.[124]

There are studies suggesting benefit from occipital nerve decompression, including one of 76 patients with complete benefit in 89.5% with patient selection based on complete but temporary improvement after an occipital nerve block.[125] There remain questions about the efficacy of decompression because of differences in definitions and diagnosis of occipital neuralgia and suggestions for a sham surgery comparison group.

Treatment of posttraumatic headaches arising from the neck and temporomandibular joint are discussed in other articles in this issue.[62,65]

EDUCATION

One of the most important roles of physicians is education of patients and family members, other physicians, and, when appropriate, employers, attorneys, and representatives of insurance companies. There is widespread ignorance about the potential effects of mild head injury because of what Evans has termed, "the Hollywood head injury myth" [43]. Patient complaints of chronic daily headaches of any type, especially posttraumatic, often are met with skepticism by much of the public, who cannot imagine that headaches occur with such frequency.

Most people's knowledge of the sequelae of mild head injuries largely is the result of movie magic. Some of the funniest scenes in slapstick comedies and cartoons depict a character sustaining single or multiple head injuries, looking dazed, and then recovering immediately. In cowboy movies, action and detective stories, and boxing and martial arts films, seemingly serious head trauma often is inflicted by blows from guns and heavy objects, motor vehicle accidents, falls, fists, and kicks, all without lasting consequences. Our experience is minimal compared with the thousands of simulated head injuries seen in the movies and on television.

Physicians can provide education by summarizing the literature and using vivid examples from sports. The public is familiar with dementia pugilistica, or punch-drunk syndrome, of cumulative head injury in boxers. The examples of Joe Louis and Floyd Patterson are well known. Many have witnessed powerful punches resulting in dazed, disoriented boxers or knockouts. There also is growing awareness of the effects of cumulative concussions in professional football (eg, quarterbacks Steve Young, Troy Aikman, and Stan Humphries) and hockey (eg, Pat Lafontaine) and the fear of chronic traumatic encephalopathy. Reports of headaches preventing athletes from returning to play make the sports pages on a regular basis.

PROGNOSIS

The percentage of patients who have headaches at 1 month varies from 31.3%[33] to 90%,[126] at 3 months from 47%[127] to 78%,[128] and at 1 year from 8.4%[129] to 35%[126]; 24% of patients have persisting headaches at 4 years.[130]

In a prospective cohort study of children with mild TBI (n = 402) or arm injury (n = 122), 43% of those with mild TBI and 26% of those with an arm injury had headache 3 months after injury.[131] Headache at both the 3-month and 12-month follow-up or persistent headache was present in 28% of mild TBI versus 19% with arm injuries, which did not have statistical significance. Persistent headache was associated with female gender, family history of headache, chronic pain prior to injury, lower quality of life, prior NSAID use, and low income but was not associated with injury characteristics.

In a 36-month follow-up study of adolescents after TBI (83% mild), persistent pain (an intensity of 3/10 at each assessment in months 3, 12, 24, and 36) of any site was present in 35 of 144 subjects, with headache reported by 86%, and infrequent pain in 109 of 144 subjects, with headache reported by 45.9%.[132] Female gender and increased symptoms of depression at 3 months after injury were risk factors for persistent pain.

REFERENCES

1. Evans RW. Postconcussion syndrome. In: Basow DS, editor. UpToDate. Waltham (MA): UpToDate; 2014.

2. Giza CC, Kutcher JS, Ashwal S, et al. Summary of evidence-based guideline update: evaluation and management of concussion in sports: report of the Guideline Development Subcommittee of the American Academy of Neurology. Neurology 2013;80:2250–7.
3. Bazarian JJ, Wong T, Harris M. Epidemiology and predictors of post-concussive syndrome after minor head injury in an emergency population. Brain Inj 1999;13: 173–89.
4. Edna TH, Cappelen J. Late postconcussional symptoms in traumatic head injury. An analysis of frequency and risk factors. Acta Neurochir (Wien) 1987;86:12–7.
5. Paniak C, Reynolds S, Phillips K, et al. Patient complaints within 1 month of mild traumatic brain injury: a controlled study. Arch Clin Neuropsychol 2002;17(4): 319–34.
6. Alexander MP. Mild traumatic brain injury: pathophysiology, natural history, and clinical management. Neurology 1995;45:1253–60.
7. Baandrup L, Jensen R. Chronic post-traumatic headache–a clinical analysis in relation to the international headache classification 2nd edition. Cephalalgia 2005;25(2):132–8.
8. Trimble M. Post-traumatic neurosis: from railway spine to the whiplash. Chichester (England): Wiley; 1981.
9. Evans RW. The post-concussion syndrome: 130 years of controversy. Semin Neurol 1994;14:32–9.
10. Erichsen JE. On railway and other injuries of the nervous system. Philadelphia: Henry C. Lea; 1867.
11. Rigler I. Ueber die Verletzungen auf Eisenbahnen Insbesondere der Verletzungen des Rueckenmarks. Berlin: Reimer; 1879.
12. Miller H. Accident neurosis. Br Med J 1961;1:919–25.
13. Symonds C. Concussion and its sequelae. Lancet 1962;1:1–5.
14. Evans RW, Evans RI, Sharp M. The physician survey on the post-concussion and whiplash syndromes. Headache 1994;34:268–74.
15. Feigin VL, Theadom A, Barker-Collo S, et al, BIONIC Study Group. Incidence of traumatic brain injury in New Zealand: a population-based study. Lancet Neurol 2013;12(1):53–64.
16. Faul M, Xu L, WaldM, et al. Traumatic brain injury in the United States: emergency department visits, hospitalizations and deaths 2002–2006. US Department of Health and Human Services Centers for Disease Control and Prevention; 2010. Available at: http://www.cdc.gov/traumaticbraininjury/pdf/blue_book.pdf. Accessed August 11, 2013.
17. Mannix R, O'Brien MJ, Meehan WP 3rd. The epidemiology of outpatient visits for minor head injury: 2005 to 2009. Neurosurgery 2013;73(1):129–34.
18. Cassidy JD, Carroll LJ, Peloso PM, et al. Incidence, risk factors and prevention of mild traumatic brain injury: results of the WHO Collaborating Centre Task Force on Mild Traumatic Brain Injury. J Rehabil Med 2004;43(Suppl):28–60.
19. Bernstein DM. Recovery from mild head injury. Brain Inj 1999;13:151–72.
20. Gordon WA, Brown M, Sliwinksi M. The enigma of "hidden" traumatic brain injury. J Head Trauma Rehabil 1998;13:39–56.
21. Jennett B, Frankowski RF. The epidemiology of head injury. In: Brinkman R, editor. Handbook of clinical neurology, vol. 13. New York: Elsevier; 1990. p. 1–16.
22. Thurman DJ, Alverson C, Dunn KA, et al. Traumatic brain injury in the United States: a public health perspective. J Head Trauma Rehabil 1999;14(6): 602–15.

23. Langlois JA, Kegler SR, Butler JA, et al. Traumatic brain injury related hospital discharges: results from a 14-state surveillance system, 1997. MMWR Surveill Summ 2003;52(4):1–20.

24. Tanielian TL, Jaycox LH, editors. Invisible wounds of war: psychological and cognitive injuries, their consequences, and services to assist recovery. Santa Monica (CA): RAND Corporation; 2008.

25. Fischer HU. Military casualty statistics: operation new dawn, operation iraqi freedom, and operation enduring freedom. Report ID # – RS22452. Congressional Research Service. 2013. Available at: http://www.fas.org/sgp/crs/natsec/RS22452.pdf. Accessed August 11, 2013.

26. Hoge CW, McGurk D, Thomas JL, et al. Mild traumatic brain injury in U.S. Soldiers returning from Iraq. N Engl J Med 2008;358(5):453–63.

27. Langlois JA, Rutland-Brown W, Wald MM. The epidemiology and impact of traumatic brain injury: a brief overview. J Head Trauma Rehabil 2006;21:375–8.

28. Gessell LM, Fields SK, Collins CL, et al. Concussions among United States high school and collegiate athletes. J Athl Train 2007;42:495–503.

29. Magalhães JE, Azevedo-Filho HR, Rocha-Filho PA. The risk of headache attributed to surgical treatment of intracranial aneurysms: a cohort study. Headache 2013;53:1613–23.

30. Rocha-Filho PA, Gherpelli JL, de Siqueira JT, et al. Post-craniotomy headache: characteristics, behaviour and effect on quality of life in patients operated for treatment of supratentorial intracranial aneurysms. Cephalalgia 2008;28(1):41–8.

31. Kaur A, Selwa L, Fromes G, et al. Persistent headache after supratentorial craniotomy. Neurosurgery 2000;47(3):633–6.

32. Gee JR, Ishaq Y, Vijayan N. Postcraniotomy headache. Headache 2003;43(3):276–8.

33. Schaller B, Baumann A. Headache after removal of vestibular schwannoma via the retrosigmoid approach: a long-term follow-up study. Otolaryngol Head Neck Surg 2003;128(3):387–95.

34. Ducic I, Felder JM 3rd, Endara M. Postoperative headache following acoustic neuroma resection: occipital nerve injuries are associated with a treatable occipital neuralgia. Headache 2012;52(7):1136–45.

35. Kalidas K, Levy W. New onset hemicrania continua after acoustic neuroma resection. Cephalalgia 2013;33(Suppl 8):205–6.

36. Minderhoud JM, Boelens ME, Huizenga J, et al. Treatment of minor head injuries. Clin Neurol Neurosurg 1980;82:127–40.

37. Couch JR, Lipton RB, Stewart WF, et al. Head or neck injury increases the risk of chronic daily headache: a population-based study. Neurology 2007;69(11):1169–77.

38. Yamaguchi M. Incidence of headache and severity of head injury. Headache 1992;32:427–31.

39. Couch JR, Bearss C. Chronic daily headache in the posttrauma syndrome: relation to extent of head injury. Headache 2001;41:559–64.

40. Russell MB, Olesen J. Migraine associated with head trauma. Eur J Neurol 1996;3:424–8.

41. Headache Classification Committee of the International Headache Society (IHS). The international classification of headache disorders, 3rd edition (beta version). Cephalalgia 2013;33(9):629–808.

42. Limmroth V, Cutrer FM, Moskowitz MA, et al. Age- and sex-specific incidence rates of migraine with and without visual aura. Am J Epidemiol 1991;134:1111–20.

43. Lucas S, Hoffman JM, Bell KR, et al. A prospective study of prevalence and characterization of headache following mild traumatic brain injury. Cephalalgia 2013. [Epub ahead of print].

44. Hoffman JM, Lucas S, Dikmen S, et al. Natural history of headache after traumatic brain injury. J Neurotrauma 2011;28(9):1719–25.

45. Theeler BJ, Erickson JC. Mild head trauma and chronic headaches in returning US soldiers. Headache 2009;49(4):529–34.

46. Solomon S. Posttraumatic migraine. Headache 1998;38:772–8.

47. Lew HL, Lin PH, Fuh JL, et al. Characteristics and treatment of headache after traumatic brain injury: a focused review. Am J Phys Med Rehabil 2006;85: 619–27.

48. Haas DC. Chronic post-traumatic headaches classified and compared with natural headaches. Cephalalgia 1996;16:486–93.

49. Bettucci D, Aguggia M, Bolamperti L, et al. Chronic post-traumatic headache associated with minor cranial trauma: a description of cephalalgic patterns. Ital J Neurol Sci 1998;19:20–4.

50. Radanov BP, Di Stefano G, Augustiny KF. Symptomatic approach to posttraumatic headache and its possible implications for treatment. Eur Spine J 2001; 10:403–7.

51. Bekkelund SI, Salvesen R. Prevalence of head trauma in patients with difficult headache: the North Norway Headache Study. Headache 2003;43:59–62.

52. Lucas S, Hoffman JM, Bell KR, et al. Characterization of headache after traumatic brain injury. Cephalalgia 2012;32(8):600–6.

53. Theeler B, Lucas S, Riechers RG 2nd, et al. Post-traumatic headaches in civilians and military personnel: a comparative, clinical review. Headache 2013; 53(6):881–900.

54. Erickson JC. Treatment outcomes of chronic post-traumatic headaches after mild head trauma in US soldiers: an observational study. Headache 2011; 51(6):932–44.

55. Theeler BJ, Flynn FG, Erickson JC. Headaches after concussion in US soldiers returning from Iraq or Afghanistan. Headache 2010;50(8):1262–72.

56. Theeler BJ, Mercer R, Erickson JC. Prevalence and impact of migraine among US Army soldiers deployed in support of Operation Iraqi Freedom. Headache 2008;48(6):876–82.

57. Mihalik JP, Register-Mihalik J, Kerr ZY, et al. Recovery of posttraumatic migraine characteristics in patients after mild traumatic brain injury. Am J Sports Med 2013;41(7):1490–6.

58. Mihalik JP, Stump JE, Collins MW, et al. Posttraumatic migraine characteristics in athletes following sports-related concussion. J Neurosurg 2005;102(5):850–5.

59. Evans RW. Whiplash injuries. In: Greenamyre JT, editor. Medlink neurology. San Diego (CA): MedLink Corp; 2014. Available at: www.medlink.com.

60. Domowitch P. Migraine couldn't slow down Super Bowl Mvp, then or now. Philly.com The Inquirer. 1998. Available at: http://articles.philly.com/1998-05-20/sports/25742035_1_migranal-migraine-dihydroergotamine-mesylate. Accessed September 15, 2013.

61. Pennington B. SUPER BOWL XXXII; even a migraine doesn't slow down davis on his way to the M.V.P. New York Times 1998.

62. Graff-Radford SB, Bassiur JP. Temporomandibular disorders and headaches. Neurol Clin 2013;32(2).

63. Hecht JS. Occipital nerve blocks in postconcussive headaches: a retrospective review and report of ten patients. J Head Trauma Rehabil 2004;19(1):58–71.

64. Evans RW. Greater occipital neuralgia can cause facial paresthesias. Cephalalgia 2009;29:801.
65. Bogduk N. The neck and headaches. Neurol Clin 2013;32(2).
66. Matthews WB. Footballer's migraine. BMJ 1972;2:326–7.
67. Soriani S, Cavaliere B, Faggioli R, et al. Confusional migraine precipitated by mild head trauma. Arch Pediatr Adolesc Med 2000;154:90–1.
68. Weinstock A, Rothner AD. Trauma-triggered migraine: a cause of transient neurologic deficit following minor head injury in children. Neurology 1995; 45(Suppl 4):A347–8.
69. Lambru G, Matharu M. Traumatic head injury in cluster headache: cause or effect? Curr Pain Headache Rep 2012;16(2):162–9.
70. Matharu MS, Goadsby PJ. Posttraumatic chronic paroxysmal hemicranias (CPH) with aura. Neurology 2001;56:273–5.
71. Putzki N, Nirkko A, Diener HC. Trigeminal autonomic cephalalgias: a case of post-traumatic SUNCT syndrome? Cephalalgia 2005;25(5):395–7.
72. Jacob S, Saha A, Rajabally Y. Post-traumatic short-lasting unilateral headache with cranial autonomic symptoms (SUNA). Cephalalgia 2008;28(9):991–3.
73. Evans RW, Lay CL. Posttraumatic hemicrania continua? Headache 2000;40: 761–2.
74. Stewart M, Boyce S, McGlone R. Post-traumatic headache: don't forget to test the supraorbital nerve! BMJ Case Rep 2012;21:2012.
75. Fukutake T, Mine S, Yamakami I, et al. Roller coaster headache and subdural hematoma. Neurology 2000;54:264.
76. Jensen TS, Gorelick PB. Headache associated with ischemic stroke and intracranial hematoma. In: Olesen J, Tfelt-Hansen P, Welch KM, editors. The headaches. 2nd edition. Philadelphia: Lippincott Williams & Wilkins; 2000. p. 781–7.
77. Milo R, Razon N, Schiffer J. Delayed epidural hematoma. A review. Acta Neurochir (Wien) 1987;84:13–23.
78. Benoit BG, Russell NA, Richard MT, et al. Epidural hematoma: report of seven cases with delayed evolution of symptoms. Can J Neurol Sci 1982;9:321–4.
79. Vilming ST, Campbell JK. Low cerebrospinal fluid pressure. In: Olesen J, Tfelt-Hansen P, Welch KM, editors. The headaches. 2nd edition. Philadelphia: Lippincott Williams & Wilkins; 2000. p. 831–9.
80. D'Alise MD, Fichtel F, Horowitz M. Sagittal sinus thrombosis following minor head injury treated with continuous urokinase infusion. Surg Neurol 1998; 49(4):430–5.
81. Kaplan JB, Bodhit AN, Falgiani ML. Communicating carotid-cavernous sinus fistula following minor head trauma. Int J Emerg Med 2012;5(1):10.
82. Graham DI, Saatman KE, Marklund N, et al. Neuropathology of brain injury. In: Evans RW, editor. Neurology and trauma. 2nd edition. New York: Oxford; 2006. p. 45–94.
83. Mayer CL, Huber BR, Peskind E. Traumatic brain injury, neuroinflammation, and posttraumatic headaches. Headache 2013;53(9):1523–30.
84. Vagnozzi R, Signoretti S, Cristofori L, et al. Assessment of metabolic brain damage and recovery following mild traumatic brain injury: a multicentre, proton magnetic resonance spectroscopic study in concussed patients. Brain 2010; 133(11):3232–42.
85. Shenton ME, Hamoda HM, Schneiderman JS, et al. A review of magnetic resonance imaging and diffusion tensor imaging findings in mild traumatic brain injury. Brain Imaging Behav 2012;6(2):137–92.

86. Mendez MF, Owens EM, Reza Berenji G, et al. Mild traumatic brain injury from primary blast vs. blunt forces: post-concussion consequences and functional neuroimaging. NeuroRehabilitation 2013;32(2):397–407.

87. Evans RW. Persistent post-traumatic headache, postconcussion syndrome, and whiplash injuries: the evidence for a non-traumatic basis with an historical review. Headache 2010;50:716–24.

88. Nicholson K, Martelli MF, Zasler ND. Does pain confound interpretation of neuropsychological test results? NeuroRehabilitation 2001;16(4):225–30.

89. McCauley SR, Boake C, Levin HS, et al. Postconcussional disorder following mild to moderate traumatic brain injury: anxiety, depression, and social support as risk factors and comorbidities. J Clin Exp Neuropsychol 2001;23:792–808.

90. McCauley SR, Boake C, Pedroza C, et al. Postconcussional disorder: are the DSM-IV criteria an improvement over the ICD-10? J Nerv Ment Dis 2005;193: 540–50.

91. Tatrow K, Blanchard EB, Hickling EJ, et al. Posttraumatic headache: biopsychosocial comparisons with multiple control groups. Headache 2003;43: 755–66.

92. van Veldhoven LM, Sander AM, Struchen MA, et al. Predictive ability of preinjury stressful life events and post-traumatic stress symptoms for outcomes following mild traumatic brain injury: analysis in a prospective emergency room sample. J Neurol Neurosurg Psychiatry 2011;82:782–7.

93. Sherman EM, Strauss E, Slick DJ, et al. Effect of depression on neuropsychological functioning in head injury: measurable but minimal. Brain Inj 2000;14:621–32.

94. Fann JR, Uomoto JM, Katon WJ. Cognitive improvement with treatment of depression following mild traumatic brain injury. Psychosomatics 2001;42:48–54.

95. Mickeviciene D, Schrader H, Obelieniene D, et al. A controlled prospective inception cohort study on the post-concussion syndrome outside the medicolegal context. Eur J Neurol 2004;11:411–9.

96. Stovner LJ, Schrader H, Mickeviciene D, et al. Headache after concussion. Eur J Neurol 2009;16:112–20.

97. Couch JR, Lipton R, Stewart WF. Is post-traumatic headache classifiable and does it exist? Eur J Neurol 2009;16:12–3.

98. Lieba-Samal D, Platzer P, Seidel S, et al. Characteristics of acute posttraumatic headache following mild head injury. Cephalalgia 2011;31(16):1618–26.

99. Fenton G, McClelland R, Montgomery A, et al. The postconcussional syndrome: Social antecedents and psychological sequelae. Br J Psychiatry 1993;162:493–7.

100. Iverson GL, Lange RT. Examination of "postconcussion-like" symptoms in a healthy sample. Appl Neuropsychol 2003;10(3):137–44.

101. Gouvier WD, Uddo-Crane M, Brown LM. Base rates of post-concussional symptoms. Arch Clin Neuropsychol 1988;3(3):273–8.

102. Dean PJ, O'Neill D, Sterr A. Post-concussion syndrome: prevalence after mild traumatic brain injury in comparison with a sample without head injury. Brain Inj 2012;26:14–26.

103. Iverson GL, McCracken LM. Postconcussive symptoms in persons with chronic pain. Brain Inj 1997;11(11):783–90.

104. Smith-Seemiller L, Fow NR, Kant R, et al. Presence of post-concussion syndrome symptoms in patients with chronic pain vs mild traumatic brain injury. Brain Inj 2003;17(3):199–206.

105. Leininger BE, Gramling SE, Farrell AD, et al. Neuropsychological deficits in symptomatic minor head injury patients after concussion and mild concussion. J Neurol Neurosurg Psychiatry 1990;53:293–6.

106. Weiss HD, Stern BJ, Goldberg J. Posttraumatic migraine: chronic migraine precipitated by minor head or neck trauma. Headache 1991;31:451–6.
107. Packard RC. Posttraumatic headache: permanence and relationship to legal settlement. Headache 1992;32:496–500.
108. Binder LM, Rohling ML. Money matters: a meta-analytic review of the effects of financial incentives on recovery after closed-head injury. Am J Psychiatry 1996; 153:7–10.
109. Ruff RM, Wylie T, Tennant W. Malingering and malingering-like aspects of mild closed head injury. J Head Trauma Rehabil 1993;8:60–73.
110. Andrikopoulos J. Post-traumatic headache in mild head injured litigants. Headache 2003;43:553.
111. Tyler GS, McNeely HE, Dick ML. Treatment of posttraumatic headache with amitriptyline. Headache 1980;20:213–6.
112. Packard RC. Treatment of chronic daily posttraumatic headache with divalproex sodium. Headache 2000;40:736–9.
113. Saran A. Antidepressants not effective in headache associated with minor closed head injury. Int J Psychiatry Med 1988;18:75–83.
114. Yerry JA, Finkel AG, Lewis SC, et al. Onabotulinum toxin A for the treatment of chronic post-traumatic headache in service members with a history of mild traumatic brain injury. Cephalalgia 2013;33(11):984–5.
115. Gawel MJ, Rothbart P, Lacobs H. Subcutaneous sumatriptan in the acute treatment of acute episodes of PTH headache. Headache 1993;33:96–7.
116. DiTommaso C, Hoffman JM, Lucas S, et al. Medication usage patterns for headache treatment after mild traumatic brain injury. Headache, in press.
117. Linde M, Hagen K, Salvesen O, et al. Onabotulinum toxin A treatment of cervicogenic headache: a randomized, double-blind, placebo-controlled crossover study. Cephalalgia 2011;31:797–807.
118. Watanabe TK, Bell KR, Walker WC, et al. Systematic review of interventions for post-traumatic headache. PM R 2012;4(2):129–40.
119. Gurr B, Coetzer B. The effectiveness of cognitive-behavioural therapy for post-traumatic headaches. Brain Inj 2005;19:481–91.
120. Blumenfeld A, Ashkenazi A, Napchan U, et al. Expert consensus recommendations for the performance of peripheral nerve blocks for headaches–a narrative review. Headache 2013;53(3):437–46.
121. Natsis K, Baraliakos X, Appell HJ, et al. The course of the greater occipital nerve in the suboccipital region: a proposal for setting landmarks for local anesthesia in patients with occipital neuralgia. Clin Anat 2006; 19(4):332–6.
122. Gabrhelík T, Michálek P, Adamus M. Pulsed radiofrequency therapy versus greater occipital nerve block in the management of refractory cervicogenic headache - a pilot study. Prague Med Rep 2011;112(4):279–87.
123. Huang JH, Galvagno SM Jr, Hameed M, et al. Occipital nerve pulsed radiofrequency treatment: a multi-center study evaluating predictors of outcome. Pain Med 2012;13(4):489–97.
124. Palmisani S, Al-Kaisy A, Arcioni R, et al. A six year retrospective review of occipital nerve stimulation practice - controversies and challenges of an emerging technique for treating refractory headache syndromes. J Headache Pain 2013;14(1):67.
125. Li F, Ma Y, Zou J, et al. Micro-surgical decompression for greater occipital neuralgia. Turk Neurosurg 2012;22(4):427–9.
126. Denker PG. The postconcussion syndrome: prognosis and evaluation of the organic factors. N Y State J Med 1944;44:379–84.

127. Levin HS, Matti S, Ruff RM, et al. Neurobehavioral outcome following minor head injury: a three-center study. 1. Neurosurgery 1987;66:234–43.
128. Rimel RW, Giordani B, Barth JT, et al. Disability caused by minor head injury. Neurosurgery 1981;9:221–8.
129. Rutherford WH, Merrett JD, McDonald JR. Symptoms at 1 year following concussion from minor head injuries. Injury 1978;10:225–30.
130. Edna TH. Disability 3–5 years after minor head injury. J Oslo City Hosp 1987;37:41–8.
131. Blume HK, Temkin N, Wang J, et al. Headache following mild TBI in children: what are the risks? Cephalalgia 2013;33(Suppl 8):244–5.
132. Tham SW, Palermo TM, Wang J, et al. Persistent pain in adolescents following traumatic brain injury. J Pain 2013;14(10):1242–9.

Headaches Caused by Vascular Disorders

John F. Rothrock, MD

KEYWORDS

- Stroke • Headache • Migraine • Intracerebral hemorrhage

KEY POINTS

- The clinical association between stroke and headache is complex, ranging from the largely irrelevant to the highly specific.
- Headache may acutely accompany or chronically complicate all the subtypes of stroke, and especially in the case of ischemic stroke the likelihood of concomitant acute headache often is highly dependent on the specific stroke etiology.
- Because they are potentially lethal and may respond to therapeutic intervention, there are five major stroke syndromes that the clinician must recognize and respond to with alacrity: aneurysmal SAH, cerebellar stroke or hemorrhage, cerebral sinus thrombosis, basilar thrombosis, and hypertensive encephalopathy.
- The symptoms and signs of hypertensive encephalopathy occur not only in the classic setting of a patient who has chronic hypertension and has stopped his or her medications but also in the typically normotensive individual who has developed acute hypertension as a result of sympathomimetic drug use, acute migraine, eclampsia, pheochromocytoma, or a variety of other predisposing conditions.

OVERVIEW OF STROKE AND HEADACHE

Although the brain itself seems to be largely insensate, the dural sinuses, the dura itself, large cerebral arteries located at the skull base, meningeal arteries, and some fibers of the 5th, 9th, and 10th cranial nerves are pain-sensitive. Regional inflammation and traction or compression involving these structures produces headache.

The clinical association between stroke and headache is complex, ranging from the largely irrelevant to the highly specific. In a certain few instances, the primary disorder producing headache (eg, migraine) may even be causal, serving to initiate the stroke process. As for its diagnostic significance in the setting of acute stroke, headache may be little more than an historical afterthought, overshadowed by the focal neurologic deficits resulting from neuronal dysfunction, or it may represent a key, even sole, manifestation of the stroke process. In any event, the incidence and clinical relevance of

Department of Neurosciences, University of Nevada (Reno) School of Medicine, Renown Neurosciences Institute, 75 Pringle Way, Suite 401, Reno, NV 89502, USA
E-mail address: JRothrock@renown.org

Neurol Clin 32 (2014) 305–319
http://dx.doi.org/10.1016/j.ncl.2013.11.003
0733-8619/14/$ – see front matter © 2014 Elsevier Inc. All rights reserved.

neurologic.theclinics.com

acute headache is highly dependent on stroke subtype and etiology. In this article the issue of headache accompanying acute stroke is addressed in some detail.

Mechanistically, there are two major types of stroke (hemorrhagic and ischemic) and four subtypes (subarachnoid hemorrhage [SAH], intracerebral hemorrhage [ICH], embolic stroke, and thrombotic stroke). Thrombotic stroke may be subdivided further based on the size of the vessel involved (ie, small vs large vessel) and whether or not the thrombosis involves an artery or a cerebral sinus. Myriad specific etiologies produce each subtype of stroke. Headache may acutely accompany or chronically complicate all the subtypes, and especially in the case of ischemic stroke, the likelihood of concomitant acute headache often is highly dependent on the specific stroke etiology. For example, headache, facial pain, or both occur much more frequently with internal carotid thrombosis from arterial wall dissection than from atherothrombosis.

Because they are potentially lethal and may respond to therapeutic intervention, there are five major stroke syndromes that the clinician must recognize and respond to with alacrity: (1) aneurysmal SAH, (2) cerebellar stroke or hemorrhage, (3) cerebral sinus thrombosis (CST), (4) basilar thrombosis, and (5) hypertensive encephalopathy. The last is not discussed in detail in this article, but it is important to recall that the symptoms and signs of hypertensive encephalopathy occur not only in the classic setting of a patient who has chronic hypertension and has stopped his or her medications but also in the typically normotensive individual who has developed acute hypertension as a result of sympathomimetic drug use, acute migraine, eclampsia, pheochromocytoma, or a variety of other predisposing conditions.

HEADACHE AS A SYMPTOM ACCOMPANYING ACUTE STROKE
Hemorrhagic Stroke and SAH

SAH is the stroke subtype most commonly accompanied by acute headache, and rupture of a congenital "berry" aneurysm is the most common cause of spontaneous SAH. Intracranial aneurysms are not rare. Autopsy studies suggest that approximately 5% of the population dies with, if not from, an intracranial aneurysm.[1] Nearly 30,000 cases of aneurysmal SAH occur annually in the United States, yielding an incidence rate of 0.012%.

With high-volume aneurysmal SAH, the intracranial pressure (ICP) rises suddenly and dramatically in parallel with excruciating headache, and in nearly half of cases severe headache is the presenting complaint.[2] Rarely does an awake and communicative patient who has suffered aneurysmal SAH fail to report intense head pain.

Warning leaks associated with aneurysmal expansion may precede major, clinically devastating SAH in half of cases.[3,4] These premonitory leaks typically occur hours, several days, or even weeks before high-volume hemorrhage occurs and are manifested symptomatically by so-called "sentinel" headache, typically involving sudden "thunderclap" headache pain that may be precipitated by physical exertion, may persist for hours to days, may be frontal or occipital in location, and may or may not be accompanied by neck stiffness. Nausea, vomiting, and interscapular pain also are common; the neck and interscapular pain may be delayed for 24 hours or more, and the spinal area pain may confuse the diagnostic process if the headache itself has improved or resolved. Migraineurs who experienced sentinel headache report that the characteristics of the headache are distinctly different from those of their typical migraines, and even in patients who have long-standing migraine, a suddenly developing, severe and "different from usual" headache should alert the clinician to the possibility of a bleeding aneurysm.

The importance of early diagnosis and management after initial aneurysmal SAH cannot be overemphasized. Whether low or high volume, an initial aneurysmal bleed imposes a risk of rebleed that peaks within the first 24 hours, occurring in as many as 17% of patients, and persists at an incidence of approximately 1.5% per day for the ensuing 2 weeks. Aneurysmal rebleeding is associated with high mortality (up to 80%) and significant morbidity in survivors.

Although lumbar puncture (LP) is the gold standard for detecting acute SAH, noncontrasted brain computed tomography (CT) is quite sensitive in detecting SAH within the first 12 hours after symptom onset.[5] In one recent study involving patients who presented less than 6 hours after symptom onset, brain CT was 100% sensitive in diagnosing SAH.[6] By 24 hours, however, the sensitivity of CT begins to decline, and at 1 week CT fails to detect SAH in approximately 50% of cases.[7] Even in the acute setting, signs of SAH on CT can be subtle, and the near 100% sensitivity accorded to CT presumes the scan is read by an experienced clinician.

Brain magnetic resonance imaging (MRI) is not considered to be a first-line diagnostic test for evaluating potential SAH, but such imaging may be useful if the findings from brain CT are negative but the results from LP are abnormal. In one study, investigators found that T2-weighted MRI was highly sensitive for detecting SAH in the acute and subacute phases, and other investigators have reported that fluid-attenuated inversion recovery MRI can identify SAH more effectively than CT in the subacute to chronic phase.[8–10]

If the clinical suspicion of SAH is high and brain imaging fails to demonstrate subarachnoid blood, LP is indicated. This clearly is a clinical setting wherein one wishes to avoid a traumatic tap. Although immediate spinal puncture at a higher level may help settle the issue of true SAH versus a traumatic tap, comparing the results of the first and last tubes drawn is unreliable, as is assessing the presence versus absence of crenated red cells. A search for xanthochromia is marginally more useful. Xanthochromia appears within 12 hours of SAH and persists for weeks; testing for xanthochromia by spectrophotometry is more sensitive than visual inspection after immediate centrifugation of the cerebrospinal fluid (CSF). In the end, however, cerebral angiography (eg, magnetic resonance angiography) typically is required to assist in excluding aneurysm as the cause of the bloody CSF.

More than 50% of patients presenting to an emergency department (ED) who have sentinel headache and SAH are misdiagnosed, and the most common reasons for misdiagnosis of SAH are failure to obtain an appropriate brain imaging study, failure to perform an LP, or misinterpretation of the results from brain imaging or CSF analysis. All patients who have thunderclap headache should be evaluated thoroughly to exclude SAH. If SAH is suspected by history and documented by noncontrasted brain CT, LP, or both, cerebral angiography and neurosurgical consultation should follow promptly. The following case exemplifies the hazards of failing to diagnosis a sentinel headache.

A 41-year-old woman with a long-standing history of migraine without aura abruptly developed a severe headache during orgasm. Two hours later in the ED her examination was normal; she complained of neck stiffness, but her neck was described as "supple." She was diagnosed as having benign sexual headaches/explosive type and given a prescription for indomethacin. Three nights later she again developed a severe headache during orgasm, and over the next 30 minutes her level of consciousness progressively declined. In the ED 1 hour after headache onset she was densely stuporous and exhibited intermittent spontaneous decerebrate posturing. Noncontrasted brain CT and subsequent cerebral arteriography were performed. The CT demonstrated extensive SAH, and the arteriogram demonstrated a large basilar tip aneurysm. Progressive transtentorial herniation continued despite aggressive medical management of her increased ICP and ventriculostomy placement with CSF drainage. The patient died on the second hospital day.

It seems that few patients who have chronic or recurrent headache are able to escape undergoing at least one brain imaging procedure. Given the prevalence of cerebral aneurysms in the general population, it is not surprising that a percentage of patients who have primary headache disorders are found to have an incidental, asymptomatic aneurysm. Because many of these individuals are young and likely to live for many more decades, the issue of prophylactic aneurysm surgery or catheter-based intervention takes on major significance. How is a clinician to determine which aneurysms require such invasive treatment? The most recent published data suggest that "size does matter." In the patient who has no history of SAH, aneurysms less than 7 mm in size are associated with a low risk of future hemorrhage, whereas those greater than 25 mm convey approximately a 27% risk of SAH over the ensuing 5 years. Location also plays a role; small (<7 mm) aneurysms within the anterior circulation have a low risk of rupture, whereas aneurysms within the posterior circulation generally are more likely to bleed.[11]

Hemorrhagic Stroke and ICH

Headache accompanies acute ICH in roughly one-third of cases. Although multiple studies consistently have demonstrated that headache is more strongly associated with ICH than with ischemic stroke, that association is not sufficient to provide reliable diagnostic use.[12]

Regardless of the underlying cause, ICH tends to occur during wakeful activity and most often produces smoothly progressive neurologic deterioration over the hours after stroke onset. Acute headache may accompany ICH but is far from invariable. Only a third or less of patients is sufficiently alert to report acute headache, and a similar proportion exhibit vomiting.[13] Although far lower than the incidence rate of headache in aneurysmal SAH, the combination of headache and vomiting is at least three times greater in ICH than in ischemic stroke. Although the absence of these symptoms does not exclude ICH, their presence, especially when combined with acute hypertension, focal neurologic deficits, a depressed level of consciousness, and an early clinical course characterized by progressive deterioration, should lead to strong consideration of the diagnosis.

Headache is more common with lobar hemorrhage than with deep ICH, and in the latter headache occurs more often with putaminal hemorrhage than with hemorrhage involving the caudate nucleus or thalamus.[14–16] The location of the headache accompanying ICH often is of no value in lesion localization, but lobar occipital bleeds do tend to produce ipsilateral orbital/periorbital pain, with more anteriorly situated hemorrhages causing headache that may be periauricular, temporal, or frontal.[17]

Whatever the cause of supratentorial ICH (chronic hypertensive arteriopathy, amyloid angiopathy, use of cocaine or other sympathomimetic drugs, or a host of other, rare causes) there is little in the way of direct therapeutic intervention that is likely to produce a favorable clinical outcome. Specifically, surgical intervention does not seem to provide any clear benefit over medical management alone, and the best treatment of ICH therefore remains a priori prevention of the hemorrhage (most commonly through adequate control of chronic hypertension).[15,16,18]

Cerebellar Hemorrhage

Because of its location within the tightly confined posterior fossa, cerebellar hemorrhage may produce rapid neurologic deterioration, tonsillar (foramen magnum) herniation, and death. With large (>3 cm) cerebellar hematomas or hematomas accompanied by progressive neurologic worsening (as evidenced by declining level of consciousness or evolving brainstem signs and symptoms), emergent craniotomy and surgical decompression of the affected hemisphere should be considered strongly.[19,20] This intervention assumes particular importance not only because it may be lifesaving but also because patients may adapt extremely well over time to loss of the surgically excised cerebellar tissue. The same holds true for cerebellar infarction and associated edematous swelling, but the prospects of a favorable outcome recede if there is coexisting ischemic injury within the brainstem.

Headache, vomiting, and dizziness are common symptoms accompanying cerebellar hemorrhage. If present, headache most often is occipital but at times may radiate frontally.[20] Affected patients typically are unable to walk, stand, or even sit without listing or falling toward the affected side.[21,22] Patients with even anatomically large cerebellar hematomas may exhibit little or no neurologic deficit if simply examined while supine. If one suspects cerebellar stroke, the patient must be examined for evidence of truncal ataxia while sitting, standing, and attempting to walk.

Noncontrasted brain CT is sensitive in detecting acute cerebellar hemorrhage. However, the ability of CT to demonstrate acute ischemic stroke involving the cerebellum is notoriously poor, and if cerebellar stroke is suspected on clinical grounds and brain CT is unremarkable, immediate brain MRI is indicated.

The following case illustrates the classic features of cerebellar hemorrhage. A 54-year-old man with a history of insulin-dependent diabetes presented to the ED complaining of bioccipital headache, "dizziness," and difficulty walking. His symptoms had begun acutely when he arose from bed that morning and had persisted without change throughout the day. His examination was notable for truncal ataxia; he exhibited a pronounced tenderness to fall consistently toward the right when attempting to sit or stand. He was diagnosed as having acute vestibular neuritis and treated with intravenous diazepam. His dizziness improved, but he continued to exhibit truncal ataxia. He was hospitalized, and later that evening his nurses noted that he had vomited in bed and was difficult to arouse. Noncontrasted brain CT performed shortly thereafter demonstrated a large hemorrhage within the right cerebellar hemisphere, compression/distortion of the fourth ventricle, and findings consistent with obstructive hydrocephalus. Emergency craniotomy, ventriculostomy, and evacuation of the right cerebellar hematoma were performed. The patient survived, and his examination 1 month after surgery was notable only for mild gait instability.

Clinical Pearls: Diagnosis of Hemorrhagic Stroke
- In cases of ICH, focal deficits typically trump headache
- The presence (or absence) of headache is not sufficient to distinguish hemorrhagic stroke from ischemic
- In cases of SAH, headache typically trumps focal deficits
- If acute cerebellar stroke is strongly suspected and noncontrasted CT is negative or equivocal, obtain brain MRI immediately
- If acute or recent aneurysmal SAH is suspected and noncontrasted CT is negative or critical, perform an LP immediately

Ischemic Stroke and Transient Ischemic Attack

Headache accompanies acute ischemic stroke in slightly more than 25% of cases.[23] Except in a subset of clear-cut cases (eg, atrial fibrillation or mechanical cardiac valve with clinically significant ischemic stroke involving the middle cerebral artery distribution and no evidence of anatomic disease within the cervical carotid), it often is difficult to determine whether cerebral infarction results from primary intravascular thrombosis or embolism. For example, when stroke occurs in the carotid distribution and a vascular imaging study demonstrates occlusion of the internal carotid at its origin, was the mechanism involved distal hypoperfusion or embolism originating from a fresh intraluminal clot?

This issue becomes yet more problematic when one considers transient ischemic attack (TIA). The incidence of headache accompanying TIA varies widely in published case series, but headache or no, it is even more difficult to establish a specific cause for TIA than it is for ischemic stroke.[24,25] The presence or absence of associated headache is probably of little importance; in cases of TIA, the clinical significance and diagnostic usefulness of associated headache seem low. In one retrospective series involving patients with TIA, investigators found that the presence versus absence of headache had no prognostic value and that headache, when present, was often of no localizing value and did not predict angiographic findings.[25]

Several studies have suggested that with cerebral infarction acute headache tends to be more common with stroke involving areas supplied by the posterior circulation, with strokes of larger size and greater associated deficit and, perhaps, with strokes occurring in patients with an established history of migraine.[25–27] A more recent study found that a previous history of migraine, younger age, female gender, and cerebellar or right hemispheric location each was independently associated with a greater likelihood of headache at stroke onset.[23] The higher frequency of headache occurrence with infarcts involving the posterior circulation has been hypothesized to reflect the comparatively higher density of cervical and trigeminal nociceptive afferents within the region supplied or to ischemia involving the trigeminal or serotonergic nuclei.[28]

When present, the headache accompanying acute ischemic stroke tends to be nonpulsatile and ipsilateral to the involved hemisphere.[29–31] Headache is more common with large infarcts related to thromboembolism but still occurs with surprising frequency in the setting of small vessel (lacunar) stroke.[32,33] In the author's experience, acute headache is reported most commonly when the ischemic stroke is large in size, conveys major neurologic deficit, involves the cortex, and seems to be either cardioembolic in origin or accompanied by imaging evidence of symptomatic carotid, vertebral, or basilar artery occlusion; it should be noted, however, that other investigators dispute some of these associations.[26,27]

How do TIA and stroke cause headache? Explanations advanced in the past have included dilatation of collaterals supplying the ischemic region, distention of the occluded parent vessel itself, ischemia of arterial muscle, acute hypertension, or stroke-associated edema. More recently, evidence has pointed to a role for aggregating platelets, with associated release of serotonin and other vasoactive peptides, or to stroke-induced alteration in the concentrations of neurotransmitters linked to setting the pain threshold or regulating cranial blood flow.[31,34,35]

SPECIFIC CLINICAL SETTINGS
Giant Cell (Temporal) Arteritis

The list of arteritides that may produce headache and, at times, stroke is long (**Box 1**), but giant cell arteritis (GCA) is deserving of special mention.

GCA produces acute blindness (anterior ischemic optic neuropathy) much more commonly than stroke, but carotid and vertebrobasilar distribution strokes do occur. They generally do so within the first few weeks of active disease and may occur (rarely) even in patients who have a normal erythrocyte sedimentation rate (ESR), a normal temporal artery biopsy, and despite concomitant treatment with a corticosteroid.[36,37] Although stroke generated by GCA typically involves the extracranial portions of the carotid and vertebrobasilar systems, intracranial arteritis has been reported.[38]

Box 1
Types of vasculitis causing headache and stroke

Primary angiitis of the central nervous system

Polyarteritis nodosa

Churg-Strauss syndrome

Takayasu arteritis

Wegener granulomatosis

Giant cell arteritis

Drug-induced vasculitis

Lupus[a]

Reversible cerebral vasoconstriction syndrome[b]

[a] True vasculitis is present in only about 10% of patients with systemic lupus, and stroke from lupus-associated vasculitis is uncommon.
[b] Cerebral arteriography in cases of reversible cerebral vasoconstriction syndrome may demonstrate "beating" suggestive of vasculitis, but this multifactorial disorder is a vasculopathy rather than a vasculitis; there are no associated inflammatory changes.

Afflicted patients usually are older than 65 years of age but may be as young as 50. There is a 3:1 female-to-male preponderance. Associated headache is little short of invariable and either is an unprecedented symptom for the patient or is described as "different from usual" by patients who have antecedent or coexisting headache disorders. The pain typically is constant, most often temporal (with radiation to the scalp, face, jaw, or occiput), and may be pulsatile. The pain often is especially prominent at night, interfering with sleep. There may be associated scalp tenderness, jaw claudication, or systemic symptoms (fever, weight loss, fatigue, malaise, or arthralgias). More than one-half of patients with GCA have accompanying polymyalgia rheumatica, and slightly less than half of patients who have polymyalgia rheumatica develop GCA.

If involved by the arteritic process, the superficial temporal arteries may be swollen, nodular, pulseless, and tender to palpation. The ESR is increased in approximately 90% of cases and usually is more than 40 mm/h in afflicted patients older than age 60. The C-reactive protein may be a more specific marker of acute inflammation.[38] A mild to moderate normocytic or slightly hypochromic anemia may be present. Arterial biopsy of the involved area is often diagnostic, but the tendency of GCA to be patchy, producing "skip lesions," or acute steroid therapy may reduce the diagnostic yield.

The symptoms of GCA typically respond to high-dose steroid therapy, but blindness from anterior ischemic optic neuropathy, posterior ischemic optic neuropathy, or central retinal artery occlusion may occur even in patients on treatment. The visual loss rarely is reversible, and blindness of the second eye or ophthalmoplegia may occur. Most patients require treatment for 1 to 2 years, and alternate-day steroid therapy does not seem to suffice. This consequently is one of those unhappy situations wherein the treatment (ie, daily and high-dose steroid therapy and an older population) may be worse than the disease. Following the ESR and C-reactive protein may enable a clinician to judge better when steroid dose reduction or treatment cessation is appropriate.

In the author's experience, GCA is a diagnosis often considered and much sought after...but seldom encountered.

Clinical Pearls: Giant Cell Arteritis
- Rare before age 50
- Head pain may be the sole manifestation
- ESR normal at approximately 10%
- Most common clinical complication: ischemic optic neuropathy causing irreversible blindness
- Stroke (rarely) may complicate GCA
- Establish the diagnosis/arterial biopsy typically indicated; the treatment required is potentially hazardous

Cervical Arterial Dissection

Cervical arterial dissection results from a tear in the intimal lining of the involved vessel, occurring spontaneously or in response to trivial or major trauma. "Trivial" is an appropriate adjective in many cases; such mundane activities as coughing, swimming, head turning while driving, or neck hyperextension during dental procedures or hairwashing all have been reported to cause cervical arterial dissection, and the association between chiropractic neck manipulation and vertebral artery dissection (VAD) long has been recognized.[39,40]

Only in a minority of cases is there evidence of pre-existing arteriopathy, and the arteriopathy most commonly identified is fibromuscular dysplasia. Given the high frequency of fibromuscular dysplasia in the general population, however, uncertainty persists as to whether or not there exists a true causal relationship between the two conditions.[39,41,42]

Although intracranial arterial dissection is rare, dissection of the extracranial internal carotid or vertebral artery, typically occurring at the C1-2 vertebral level, is an important cause of ischemic stroke in young and middle-aged patients. Carotid artery dissection (CAD) has an annual incidence rate of approximately 3 per 100,000, and in patients younger than 45 years of age VAD is the most common cause of Wallenberg syndrome (ie, stroke involving the distribution of the posterior inferior cerebellar artery). In CAD or VAD, blood within the involved vessel's true lumen may escape through the intimal tear and form an intramural hematoma; aneurysmal dilatation (pseudoaneurysm) of the artery may occur at the dissection site. The intramural hematoma may compress the true lumen of the parent vessel, producing hypoperfusion or distal embolism.

The clinical manifestations of CAD range from none to fatal stroke. In a significant minority of patients who have CAD, an ipsilateral oculosympathetic palsy (Horner syndrome) may be present, and pulsatile tinnitus (or other subjective bruits), dysgeusia, or visual scintillations also are common.[43]

Acute headache accompanies CAD in at least 60% of cases and occurs at a somewhat lower rate with VAD.[41,44] Isolated head or neck pain is the only symptom of cervical artery dissection in 8%.[45] With CAD the pain almost always is ipsilateral to the dissection, often is felt most intensely in the eye or face, is commonly accompanied by ipsilateral neck pain, and may precede the occurrence of TIA or stroke by several days.[46] The onset of pain typically is gradual, but thunderclap headache may occur.[46] With VAD, headache usually is occipital in location.

For years acute anticoagulation was considered to be the treatment of choice for CAD, but more recent evidence suggests that such treatment conveys little or no benefit over antiplatelet therapy alone. Cases reported in the medical literature suggest that progression of acute dissection-related stroke, early recurrent stroke, or even late recurrent stroke is rare, regardless of what, if any, treatment is administered. Anatomic resolution of CAD and associated stenosis or occlusion is common, usually occurring within the first 3 months after anatomic dissection. This may be documented noninvasively by serial brain MRI, magnetic resonance angiography, CT angiography, or carotid duplex testing.[47,48]

Cerebral Sinus Thrombosis

CST may occur in individuals who are prothrombotic as a result of any of a host of causes, including acute or chronic infection, dehydration, oral contraceptive use, non-iatrogenic or surgical trauma, malignancy, puerperium, inflammatory disease (eg, Behçet syndrome), nephrotic syndrome, and hereditary factors.[49] The superior sagittal and transverse sinuses are most frequently involved sites, and the spectrum of clinical presentations is broad.

Headache is present in up to 90% of cases and may be the sole manifestation of CST in as many as 10%.[50,51] The headache may be of the thunderclap type in approximately 15% of cases, but in the remainder the headache of CST has little in the way of distinguishing characteristics.[52] Afflicted patients may exhibit symptoms, signs, and LP findings characteristic of intracranial hypertension, and the associated headache may evolve and persist over days to years.[53] Other patients experience a more fulminant, clinically devastating, and potentially fatal course, with progressive focal neurologic deficits and multiple seizures; unfortunately they seem to comprise most cases.[49] The following case is typical of the more fulminant variety.

An 18-year-old woman with no prior history of significant headache was 3 days postpartum when she developed a sudden, severe headache that was of maximal intensity at onset ("the worst headache of my life"). Her general and neurologic examinations revealed no abnormal findings, and brain CT performed with and without contrast and obtained 1 hour after symptom onset was normal. LP was performed and revealed an opening pressure elevated to 320 mm H_2O and rusty-colored CSF with more than 16,000 red blood cells per cubic millimeter, glucose 75 mg/dL, and protein 220 mg/dL. Brain MRI demonstrated increased signal intensity within much of the superior sagittal sinus (consistent with acute thrombosis), and MR venography demonstrated absence of the anterior two-thirds of that sinus.

Anticoagulation with full-dose intravenous heparin was initiated, but within the first minutes of heparin infusion she developed a partial motor seizure that began in the left leg and spread to involve the left arm. After the seizure her examination was notable for marked left leg weakness. Intravenous heparin was continued, and treatment with intravenous phenytoin was begun.

She exhibited no further neurologic deterioration and experienced no further seizure activity. Her examination 1 month after hospital discharge was notable for moderately severe left hemiparesis, with her leg markedly weaker than her arm.

Puerperial and prothrombotic, this patient suffered thrombotic occlusion involving most of her superior sagittal sinus. The consequent obstruction of venous return from the head led to a rapid increase in ICP and thunderclap headache. Brain CT, a relatively insensitive test for detecting CST, was performed largely to exclude aneurysmal SAH; although this was not an unreasonable diagnostic consideration, such bleeds are more common during the last trimester of pregnancy, and postpartum thunderclap headache results more often from eclampsia, CSF oligemia from "wet" epidural anesthesia, CST, or "crash" migraine. The elevated opening pressure and CSF findings from the LP were characteristic of CST, and LP may represent the most sensitive, specific, and clinically effective initial screening test for detection of that condition. Although brain MRI may demonstrate clot within the involved cerebral sinus, that test is somewhat insensitive and nonspecific. As for MR or catheter venography, the venous anatomy is highly variable, and detection of an abnormality (eg, absence of the transverse sinus or nonvisualization of a portion of the superior sagittal sinus) may leave the clinician uncertain as to whether the finding simply represents a congenital anomaly or indicates acute thrombosis. Finally, this patient's clinical course after the LP suggests propagation of the thrombus and obstruction of a tributary vein, consequent venous infarction, secondary hemorrhage involving the leg cortex, and the typical seizure activity and motor deficit associated with hemorrhagic infarction in that region.

The role of antithrombotic therapy for CST remains somewhat controversial. Although anticoagulation long was shunned for its presumed potential to aggravate the bleeding already induced by venous infarction, the more recent published case series and results from a single randomized trial suggest that acute treatment with intravenous heparin may be safe and effective even when CT or MRI demonstrates evidence of hemorrhagic infarction.[54–56] Use of thrombolytic therapy, either intravenous or catheter-delivered, is advocated by some and used by a few, but such treatment currently lacks a credible scientific basis. Even less enthusiasm exists for surgical thrombectomy.

MIGRAINE AND STROKE
Migraine as a Risk Factor for Stroke

Results from several case-control studies, cohort studies, and meta-analyses indicate that migraine is associated with an increased risk of stroke in individuals of both genders.[57–64] The magnitude of this risk and its variance according to age and gender remain issues of some uncertainty, but investigators in the field generally concur that migraine imposes roughly a two-fold increased risk of ischemic stroke, that the risk is higher in females (especially those of ages 45–55), probably higher in those who smoke or in females using an oral contraceptive pill, and lower (if increased at all) in migraineurs of either gender lacking any history of aura. Women who are experiencing active migraine with aura are reported to have more than twice the risk of hemorrhagic stroke than women with no history of migraine, whereas female migraineurs with no history of aura apparently possess a risk of hemorrhagic stroke roughly equal to that of females free of migraine.[64]

Case-control studies have indicated that MRI evidence of brain white matter hyperintensities is four times more likely to be found in the migraine population than in age- and gender-matched individuals who are migraine-free; the association is strongest in women with migraine with aura and a higher frequency of migraine attacks.[65] The Netherlands-based CAMERA-1 study demonstrated migraine with aura in midlife to be associated with a seven-fold increase in the late-life prevalence of cerebellar infarction as demonstrated by MRI.[66] A more recent study confirmed a significant association between migraine with aura and MRI evidence of brain infarcts; contrasting with the findings from CAMERA-1 and other published reports, in that study the infarcts typically were located in areas other than the cerebellum or brainstem.[67] Regardless, the clinical significance of these MRI finding remains unclear. In particular, data from a 9-year longitudinal follow-up to CAMERA-1 suggested that although the MRI-measured deep white matter hyperintensities initially identified seemed to progress in the female subpopulation, that association did not convey any adverse effect on cognition.[68]

Migraine-associated Stroke

Most strokes occurring in migraineurs do not take place during an acute migraine attack. From this observation naturally follows the proposal that migraine may serve as a marker for another, associated disorder that itself is directly operative in producing stroke. Mitral valve prolapse seems to be more prevalent in migraineurs than in control populations, and this has led some investigators to postulate that migraine-associated strokes result from valvular emboli. A hospital-based study of patients with migrainous infarction, however, demonstrated a relatively low prevalence of mitral valve prolapse.[69]

Anzola and colleagues[70] found an increased prevalence of patent foramen ovale in individuals with migraine and proposed patent foramen ovale–related paradoxic emboli as a source of cerebral infarction in this group. The patent foramen ovale/migraine association subsequently was confirmed by several other investigative groups, and evidence emerged that seemed to link migraine with aura, anatomically prominent patent foramen ovale, atrial septal aneurysm, and stroke.[71–73] Studies evaluating patent foramen ovale closure for either stroke prevention or migraine prophylaxis, however, have failed to demonstrate evidence of benefit.

Others have proposed that migraine may be associated with endothelial dysfunction, which may impair vascular reactivity and induce a prothrombotic, proinflammatory, and proliferative state.[74] Individuals with migraine also seem to be at increased risk for cervical artery dissection, and investigators have postulated that endothelial dysfunction and increased activity of elastase and metalloprotease may predispose to disruption of the arterial wall.[65]

Migrainous Infarction

How can acute migraine directly cause stroke? Cerebral arteriography performed at the time of acute migrainous infarction or shortly thereafter has demonstrated findings consistent with arterial spasm, but such abnormalities have been reported only in a handful of cases.[75,76] Oligemia related to the migraine process itself has been proposed as a potential source of migrainous infarction. The association of migraine with MELAS (mitochondrial encephalopathy, lactic acidosis and stroke-like episodes) and CADASIL (cerebral autosomal dominant arteriopathy with subcortical infarcts and leukoencephalopathy) and the occurrence of nonatherosclerotic angiopathies in both

---

Box 2
Thunderclap headache: common causes

- Aneurysmal SAH
- Nonaneurysmal subarachnoid hemorrhage SAH
- Unruptured cerebral aneurysm
- Cervical artery dissection
- Cerebral sinus thrombosis
- Pituitary apoplexy
- Intracerebral hemorrhage
- Dural tear/intracranial hypotension
- Benign sexual headache/explosive type
- Benign exertional headache
- Cough headache
- "Crash" migraine
- Idiopathic recurrent thunderclap headache

disorders may offer clues as to the molecular underpinnings of more typical migraine-induced stroke.

Regardless of its underlying causes, migrainous infarction is rare. Even so, current criteria from the International Classification of Headache Disorders for the diagnosis of migrainous infarction require that the afflicted individual possess an antecedent history of migraine with aura and experience acute stroke symptoms "typical of previous attacks." If migrainous infarction does occur in individuals who lack any history of aura or at times produces deficits that do not match up with previous aura symptoms, these criteria may be overly restrictive and thus diagnostically insensitive.

THUNDERCLAP HEADACHE

In closing, the alarming symptom of thunderclap headache deserves yet more attention. The most common causes of thunderclap headache are listed in **Box 2**. Of these causes, some are benign and others potentially lethal; seven are vascular in origin. It is of critical importance that the clinician recognizes thunderclap headache for what it is and immediately take pains to exclude the more serious etiologies. Of these, sentinel aneurysmal SAH arguably is the most important to identify. Put simply, the sun should not set on an undiagnosed thunderclap headache.

REFERENCES

1. Stornelli SA, French JD. Subarachnoid hemorrhage—factors in prognosis and management. J Neurosurg 1964;21:769–80.
2. Findlay JM, Weir BK, Kanamaru K, et al. Arterial wall changes in cerebral vasospasm. Neurosurgery 1989;25:736.
3. Leblanc R. The minor leak preceding subarachnoid hemorrhage. J Neurosurg 1987;66:35–9.
4. Auer LM. Unfavorable outcome following early surgical repair of ruptured cerebral aneurysms—a critical review of 238 patients. Surg Neurol 1991;35:152–8.
5. Boesiger B, Shiber J. Subarachnoid hemorrhage diagnosed by computed tomography and lumbar puncture: are fifth generation CT scanners better at identifying SAH? J Emerg Med 2005;29:23–7.
6. Backes D, Rinkel G, Kemperman H, et al. Time-dependent test characteristics of head computed tomography in patients suspected of nontraumatic subarachnoid hemorrhage. Stroke 2012;43:2115–9.
7. Sames T, Storrow A, Finklestein J, et al. Sensitivity of degeneration computed tomography in subarachnoid hemorrhage. Acad Emerg Med 1996;3:16–20.
8. Mitchell P, Wilkinson I, Hoggard N, et al. Detection of subarachnoid haemorrhage with magnetic resonance imaging. J Neurol Neurosurg Psychiatry 2001; 70:205–11.
9. Noguchi K, Ogawa T, Inugami A, et al. Acute subarachnoid hemorrhage: MR imaging with fluid-attenuated inversion recovery pulse sequences. Radiology 1995;196:773–7.
10. Noguchi K, Ogawa T, Seto H, et al. Subacute and chronic subarachnoid hemorrhage: diagnosis with fluid-attenuated inversion recovery MR imaging. Radiology 1997;203:257–62.
11. Weibers DO, Whisnant JP, Huston J III, et al, International Study of Unruptured Intracranial Aneurysms Investigators. Unruptured intracranial aneurysms: natural history, clinical outcome, and risks of surgical and endovascular treatment. Lancet 2003;362:103–10.

12. Runchey S, McGee S. Does this patient have a hemorrhagic stroke? Clinical findings distinguishing hemorrhagic stroke from ischemic stroke. JAMA 2010; 30:2280–6.
13. Mohr JP, Caplan LR, Melski JW, et al. The Harvard Cooperative Stroke Registry: a prospective registry. Neurology 1978;28:754–62.
14. Walshe TM, Davis KR, Fisher CM. Thalamic hemorrhage: a computed tomographic clinical correlation. Neurology 1977;27:217–22.
15. Barraquer-Bordas L, Illa I, Escartin A, et al. Thalamic hemorrhage: a study of 23 patients with a diagnosis by computed tomography. Stroke 1981;12:524–7.
16. Stein RW, Kase CS, Hier DB, et al. Caudate hemorrhage. Neurology 1984;34: 1549–54.
17. Ropper AH, Davis KR. Lobar cerebral hemorrhages: acute clinical syndromes in 24 cases. Ann Neurol 1980;8:141–7.
18. McKissock W, Richardson A, Taylor J. Primary intracerebral hemorrhage: a controlled trial of surgical and conservative treatment in 180 unselected cases. Lancet 1961;2:221–6.
19. Little JR, Tubman DE, Ethier R. Cerebellar hemorrhage in adults: diagnosis by computerized tomography. J Neurosurg 1978;48:575–9.
20. Ott KH, Kase CS, Ojemann RG, et al. Cerebellar hemorrhage: diagnosis and treatment. Arch Neurol 1974;31:160–7.
21. Fisher CM, Picard EH, Polak A, et al. Acute hypertensive cerebellar hemorrhage: diagnosis and surgical treatment. J Nerv Ment Dis 1965;140:38.
22. Dinsdale HB. Spontaneous hemorrhage in the posterior fossa: a study of primary cerebellar and pontine hemorrhage with observations on the pathogenesis. Arch Neurol 1964;10:200.
23. Tentschert S, Wimmer R, Greisenegger S, et al. Headache at stroke onset in 2196 patients with ischemic stroke or transient ischemic attack. Stroke 2005;3:e1–3.
24. Gorelick PB, Hier DB, Caplan LR, et al. Headache in acute cerebrovascular disease. Neurology 1986;36:1445–50.
25. Grindal A, Toole JF. Headache and transient ischemic attacks. Stroke 1974;5: 603–6.
26. Jorgensen HS, Jespersen HF, Nakayama H, et al. Headache in stroke: the Copenhagen stroke study. Neurology 1994;44:1793–7.
27. Kumral E, Bogousslavsky J, Melle GV, et al. Headache at stroke onset: the Lausanne Stroke Registry. J Neurol Neurosurg Psychiatry 1995;58:490–2.
28. Evans R, Mitsias P. Headache at the onset of acute cerebral ischemia. Headache 2009;49:902–8.
29. Fisher CM. Headache in cerebrovascular disease. In: Vinken PJ, Bruyn GW, editors. Handbook of clinical neurology, vol. 5. Amsterdam: North Holland Publishing; 1968. p. 124.
30. Medina J, Diamond S, Rubino S. Headaches in patients with transient ischemic attacks. Headache 1975;15:194.
31. Edmeads J. The headaches of ischemic cerebrovascular disease. Headache 1979;19:345–9.
32. Arboix A, Massons J, Oliveres M, et al. Headache in acute cerebrovascular disease: a prospective clinical study in 240 patients. Cephalalgia 1994;14:37.
33. Ferro JM, Melo TP, Oliveiro AV, et al. A multivariate study of headache associated with ischemic stroke. Headache 1995;35:315–9.
34. Pickard JD, Mackenzie ET, Harper AM. Serotonin and prostaglandins: intracranial and extracranial effects with reference to migraine. In: Greene R, editor. Current concepts in migraine research. New York: Raven Press; 1978. p. 101.

35. Sicuteri F. Migraine, a central biochemical dysnociception. Headache 1976; 16:145.

36. Howard GF, Ho SU, Kim KS, et al. Bilateral carotid occlusion resulting from giant cell arteritis. Ann Neurol 1984;15:204.

37. Säve-Söderbergh J, Malmvall BO, Andersson R, et al. Giant cell arteritis as a cause of death: report of nine cases. JAMA 1986;255:493.

38. Hayreh SS, Podhajsky PA, Raman RI, et al. Giant cell arteritis: validity and reliability of various diagnostic criteria. Am J Ophthalmol 1997;123:285–96.

39. Hart RG, Easton JD. Dissections of cervical and cerebral arteries. Neurol Clin 1983;1:155–82.

40. Hufnagel A, Hammers A, Schonle PW, et al. Stroke following chiropractic manipulation of the cervical spine. J Neurol 1999;246:683–8.

41. Fisher CM, Ojemann RG, Roberson GH. Spontaneous dissection of cervico-cerebral arteries. Can J Neurol Sci 1978;5:9–19.

42. Schievink WI, Mokri B, O'Fallon WM. Recurrent spontaneous cervical-artery dissection. N Engl J Med 1994;330:393–7.

43. Mokri B, Sundt TM Jr, Houser OW. Spontaneous internal carotid dissection, hemicrania, and Horner's syndrome. Arch Neurol 1979;36:677–80.

44. Biousse V, D'Anglejan-Chatillon J, Massiou H, et al. Head pain in non-traumatic carotid artery dissection: a series of 65 patients. Cephalalgia 1994;14:33–6.

45. Arnold M, Cumurciuc R, Stapf C, et al. Pain as the only symptom of cervical artery dissection. J Neurol Neurosurg Psychiatry 2006;77:1021–4.

46. Silbert PL, Mokri B, Schievink WI. Headache and neck pain in spontaneous internal carotid and vertebral artery dissections. Neurology 1995;45:1517–22.

47. Rothrock JF, Lim V, Press G, et al. Serial magnetic resonance and carotid duplex studies in the management of carotid dissection. Neurology 1989;39:686–92.

48. Kasner SE, Hankins LL, Bratina P, et al. Magnetic resonance angiography demonstrates vascular healing of carotid and vertebral artery dissections. Stroke 1997;28:1993–7.

49. Bousser M, Barnett H. Cerebral venous thrombosis. In: Barnett H, Mohr J, Stein B, et al, editors. Stroke: pathology, diagnosis and management. 2nd edition. New York: Churchill and Livingstone; 1992. p. 522.

50. Stam J. Thrombosis of the cerebral veins and sinuses. N Engl J Med 2005;352: 1791–8.

51. Uzar E, Ekici F, Acar A, et al. Cerebral venous sinus thrombosis: an analysis of 47 patients. Eur Rev Med Pharmacol Sci 2012;1:1499–505.

52. de Bruijn SF, Stam J, Kappell LJ. Thunderclap headache as first symptom of cerebral venous sinus thrombosis. CVST Study Group. Lancet 1996;348:1623–5.

53. Barnes BD, Winestock DP. Dynamic radionuclide scanning in the diagnosis of thrombosis of the superior sagittal sinus thrombosis. Neurology 1977;27: 656–61.

54. Einhäupl KM, Villringer A, Meister W. Heparin treatment in sinus venous thrombosis. Lancet 1971;358:597–600.

55. Bousser MG, Chiras J, Sauron B, et al. Cerebral venous thrombosis: a review of 38 cases. Stroke 1985;16:199–213.

56. Levine SR, Twyman RE, Gilman S. The role of anticoagulation in cavernous sinus thrombosis. Neurology 1988;38:517–22.

57. Henrich J, Horwitz R. A controlled study of ischemic stroke risk in migraine patients. J Clin Epidemiol 1989;42:773–80.

58. Tzourio C, Tehindrazanarivelo A, Iglesias S, et al. Case-control study of migraine and risk of ischemic stroke in young women. BMJ 1995;310:830–3.

59. Buring J, Hebert P, Romero J, et al. Migraine and subsequent risk of stroke in the Physician's Health Study. Arch Neurol 1995;52:129–34.
60. Carolei A, Marini C, Cematteis G, et al. History of migraine and risk of cerebral ischemia in young adults. Lancet 1996;347:1503–6.
61. Merikangas K, Fenton B, Cheng S, et al. Association between migraine and stroke in a large-scale epidemiological study of the United States. Arch Neurol 1997;54:362–8.
62. Chang C, Donaghy M, Puolter N. Migraine and stroke in young women: case-control study. BMJ 1999;318:13–8.
63. Tzourio C, Iglesias S, Hubert J, et al. Migraine and risk factors of ischemic stroke: a case control study. BMJ 1993;307:289–92.
64. Kurth T, Slomke M, Kase C, et al. Migraine, headache and the risk of stroke in women: a prospective study. Neurology 2005;64:1020–6.
65. Alhazzani A, Goddeau R. Migraine and stroke: a continuum of association in adults. Headache 2013;53:1023–7.
66. Kruit M, Launer L, Ferrari M, et al. Infarcts in the posterior circulation territory in migraine. The population-based MRI CAMERA study. Brain 2005;128:2068–77.
67. Kurth T, Mohamed S, Maillard P, et al. Headache, migraine and structural brain lesions and function: population-based epidemiology of vascular ageing-MRI study. BMJ 2011;342:c7357.
68. Palm-Menders I, Koppen H, Kruit M, et al. Structural changes in migraine. JAMA 2012;308(18):1889–97.
69. Rothrock JF, Dittrich HC, Meyerhoff B, et al. Migraine, stroke and mitral valve prolapse. Neurology 1988;38(Suppl 1):296.
70. Anzola G, Magoni M, Guindani M, et al. Potential source of cerebral embolism in migraine with aura: a transcranial Doppler study. Neurology 1999;52:1622–5.
71. Milhaud D, Bogousslavsky J, Van Melle G, et al. Ischemic stroke and active migraine. Neurology 2001;57:1805–11.
72. Rothrock J, Walicke P, Swenson M, et al. Migrainous stroke. Arch Neurol 1988;45:63–7.
73. Schwedt T, Denaerschalk B, Dodick D. Patent foramen ovale and migraine: a quantitative systemic systematic review. Cephalalgia 2008;28:531–40.
74. Tietjen G, Herial N, White L, et al. Migraine and biomarkers of endothelial activation in young women. Stroke 2009;40:2977–82.
75. Rothrock J, Walicke P, Swenson M, et al. Migrainous stroke. Arch Neurol 1988;45:63–7.
76. Bogousslavsky J, Regli F, Van Melle G, et al. Migraine stroke. Neurology 1988;38:223.

Headaches and Vasculitis

David S. Younger, MD[a,b],*

KEYWORDS

- Headaches • Vasculitis • Central nervous system • Intracranial vessels

KEY POINTS

- Vasculitides are potentially treatable life-threatening disorders.
- Emperic treatment with immunosuppressive agents should not be attempted without proof of the diagnosis.
- Diagnostic histopathology and suggestive findings on neuroimaging are the corner stones of accurate diagnosis of CNS vasculitis.

INTRODUCTION

Since my earlier review nearly a decade ago,[1] notable progress has been made in vasculitis of the nervous system, as reflected in a recently published monograph.[2] This review has been adapted and in some portions reproduced from a contemporaneously updated textbook chapter on adult and childhood vasculitis of the nervous system.[3]

CLASSIFICATION AND NOSOLOGY

The 2012 Revised International Chapel Hill Consensus Conference (CHCC) Nomenclature of Vasculitides[4] is now the most widely used classification for the vasculitides. It categorized the clinicopathologic entities based on the involved vessels and updated the nosology of the vasculitic syndromes, using specific descriptive terminology that conveyed pathophysiologic specificity. Recognizing the validity and usefulness of a classification based on vessel caliber[3] and current nosology,[4] **Box 1** shows a current recommended categorization for the vasculitides. The Pediatric Rheumatology European Society and the European League against Rheumatism[5] proposed specific classification criteria for the commonest childhood vasculitis syndrome based on vessel size, similar to the CHCC nomenclature.[4]

[a] Department of Neurology, New York University School of Medicine, 550 First Avenue, New York, NY 10016, USA; [b] Division of Neurology, Department of Medicine, Lenox Hill Hospital, 100 East 77th Street, New York, NY 10021, USA
* 333 East 34th Street, Suite 1J, New York, NY 10016.
E-mail address: david.younger@nyumc.org

Neurol Clin 32 (2014) 321–362
http://dx.doi.org/10.1016/j.ncl.2013.11.004
0733-8619/14/$ – see front matter © 2014 Elsevier Inc. All rights reserved.

Box 1
Classification of CNS vasculitis

Large-vessel vasculitis

  Giant cell arteritis

  Takayasu arteritis

  Idiopathic aortitis (IgG-4)

Medium-vessel vasculitis

  Polyarteritis nodosa

  Kawasaki disease

Small-vessel vasculitis

  ANCA-associated vasculitis

    Microscopic polyangiitis

    Granulomatosis with polyangiitis (Wegener)

    Eosinophilic granulomatosis with polyangiitis (Churg-Strauss)

  Immune complex vasculitis

    Cryoglobulinemia

    IgA vasculitis (Henoch-Schönlein)

    Hypocomplementemic urticarial vasculitis (anti-C1q)

Variable-vessel vasculitis

  Behçet disease

  Cogan syndrome

Single-organ vasculitis

  Primary CNS vasculitis

Vasculitis associated with systemic collagen vascular disease

  Systemic lupus erythematosus

  Rheumatoid arthritis

Vasculitis associated with illicit substance abuse

  Amphetamines

  Cocaine

  Heroin

Vasculitis associated with infection

  Acute bacterial meningitis

  Mycobacterial tuberculous infection

  Spirochete disease

    Neurosyphilis

    Lyme neuroborreliosis

  Varicella zoster virus–related vasculopathy

  Fungal infection

  Human immunodeficiency virus/AIDS

BLOOD-BRAIN BARRIER

The past decade has witnessed extraordinary progress in the understanding of the blood-brain barrier (BBB) and has in turn shed new insights into current understanding of the etiopathogenesis of headache in cerebral vasculitis. The neurovascular unit comprising local neuronal circuits, glia, pericytes, and vascular endothelium plays a vital role in the dynamic modulation of blood flow, metabolism, and electrophysiologic regulation,[6] which together ensure a well-controlled internal environment, provided by cellular exchange mechanisms in the interface between blood, cerebrospinal fluid (CSF), and the brain.[7] Many of the influx and efflux mechanisms of the BBB are present early in the developing brain, encoded by genes at higher levels than in the adult.[8]

The evolution of migraine attacks, which is understood as a constellation of reversible premonitory symptoms associated with reversible activation of discrete brain regions, neurotransmitter systems, and neurovascular coupling in the brainstem, thalamus, hypothalamus, and cortex,[9] is unassociated with breakdown or leakage of the BBB during an attack.[10] However, loss of BBB integrity has been shown during inflammatory neurologic disease in human and experimental animal models,[11] which includes disruption of tight junctions, increase in transcytosis, change in transport properties, and increased leukocyte infiltration and trafficking. The molecules implicated in the pathologic breakdown of the BBB include the vasoactive protein vascular endothelial growth factor, matrix metalloproteinase, the inflammatory cytokines interleukin 1 (IL-1), IL-6, tumor necrosis factor α (TNF-α), metalloproteinase type 2 and 9, and the leukocyte adhesion molecules P-selectin and E-selectin, and immunoglobulin (Ig) superfamily molecules vascular cell adhesion molecule type 1, and intercellular adhesion molecule type 1. The disruption of tight and adherens junctions, enzymatic degradation of the capillary basement membrane or both, leads to altered expression and function of membrane transporters or enzymes, increased passage of inflammatory cells across the BBB from the blood to the central nervous system (CNS), with dysfunction of astrocytes and other components.[7] Although transient breakdown is associated with varying neuronal dysfunction and damage, extended BBB disruption leads to aberrant angiogenesis, neuroinflammation, concomitant vasogenic edema, accumulation of toxic substances in the brain interstitial fluid, and oxidative stress. Further investigation is necessary in understanding the unique BBB alterations and sequelae that cause or contribute to vascular inflammation and brain tissue injury in primary and secondary CNS vasculitis.

CLINICOPATHOLOGIC CORRELATIONS
Large-Size Vessel Vasculitis

Two disorders, giant cell arteritis (GCA) and Takayasu arteritis (TAK), which fall under the category of large-size vessel vasculitis, and a third disorder, isolated aortitis, which affects large vessels, but is generally considered in the category of a single-organ vasculitis (SOV), can all be associated with headache.

Giant Cell Arteritis

Two-thirds of patients with temporal GCA present with headache, often in association with musculoskeletal complaints, in individuals of both genders and age older than 50 years.[12,13] The headache emanates along tender granulomatous lesions of inflamed extracranial vessels, including branches of the external carotid artery, including the superficial temporal, occipital, facial, and internal maxillary arteries, as well as ophthalmic, posterior ciliary, and central retinal vessels, and in the vertebral and carotid arteries to the point of dural investment. There may be tender red cords along the temple, with scalp tenderness or occipital and nuchal pain. Untreated or inadequately recognized unilateral or bilateral blindness, the result of arteritis of the intraorbital posterior ciliary and central retinal arteries, is the commonest dreaded complication, seen in up to one-half of patients. There may be oculomotor disturbances resulting from vasculitis of the extraocular muscles; vertigo and hearing impairment resulting from acute auditory artery involvement; cervical myelopathy resulting from anterior spinal artery involvement; brainstem strokes and transient ischemic attacks resulting from vasculitic involvement of the proximal intracranial carotid artery and extracranial vertebral artery. The erythrocyte sedimentation rate (ESR) is typically increased to 100 mm/h or more. Temporal artery biopsy is the only sure way of establishing the diagnosis; however, false-negative findings on the contemplated affected side may be caused by inadvertent sampling of a vasculitic-free length of vessel. Noninvasive imaging using ultrasonography, high-resolution contrast-enhanced magnetic resonance imaging (MRI), and [18F]fluorodeoxyglucose (FDG) positron emission tomography (PET) can facilitate recognition of GCA and assist the surgeon in centering on an involved segment of vessel.[14] Ultrasonography may show hypoechoic circumferential wall thickening, which occurs around the arterial lumen, termed the halo sign. Contrast-enhanced high-resolution MRI shows areas of active inflammation. [18F]FDG PET, which can examine all of the involved vessels with a single examination, shows areas of abnormal vascular uptake typically synonymous with vessel wall inflammation. The earliest lesions in GCA consist of vacuolization of vascular smooth muscle of the media, with enlargement of mitochondria, infiltration of lymphocytes, plasma cells, and histiocytes (**Fig. 1**A). Over time, inflammation extends into the intima and adventitia, leading to segmental fragmentation and necrosis of the elastic lamina, granuloma formation, and proliferation of connective tissue along the vessel wall (see **Fig. 1**B). The classic histologic picture of granulomatous vasculitis, which is observed in about one-half of affected patients, eventuates in infiltration of vessel cell by giant cells at the junction between the intima and media, leading to thrombosis, intimal hyperplasia, and fibrosis.[15]

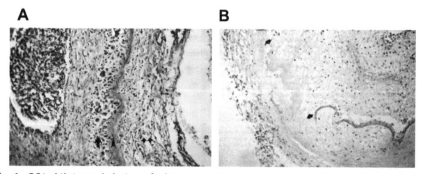

Fig. 1. GCA. (*A*) An early lesion of a large muscular artery, necrosis, inflammation, and giant cell formation (*single arrow*) can be seen immediately adjacent to the internal elastic lamina (*arrowhead*), which is undergoing degenerative changes, and there is some intimal proliferation (*double arrows*) (stain, hematoxylin-eosin, original magnification ×100). (*B*) This more advanced lesion has complete segmental destruction of the internal elastic lamina and virtually the entire media (*arrows*). Marked intimal proliferation has nearly occluded the lumen, and few inflammatory cells remain (stain, hematoxylin-eosin, original magnification ×50). (*From* Younger DS. Adult and childhood vasculitis of the nervous system. In: Younger DS, editor. Motor disorders. New York: Younger DS; 2013. p. 235–80; with permission.)

Takayasu Arteritis

Individuals younger than 50 years, particularly women of Asian descent with granulomatous arteritis affecting the aorta and its branches, are most susceptible to TAK.[4] About two-thirds of patients manifest systemic reactions at onset, including malaise, fever, stiffness of the shoulders, nausea, vomiting, night sweats, anorexia, weight loss, and irregularity of menstrual periods weeks to months before the local signs of vasculitis were recognized.[16] Headache is associated with visual loss, absent pulses in the neck and limbs with symptoms of claudication, and syncope on bending of the head backward, caused by vasculitis-related circulatory insufficiency along the aorta and branches to the brain, face, and limbs.[16,17] Other investigators ascribe headache to associated neck pain and carotid arterial inflammation[18] and increased propensity to migraine.[18,19] There may be ischemic presentations of amaurosis fugax, monocular blindness, subclavian steal and carotid sinus syndrome, audible neck and limb bruits, and asymmetry of pulses, all resulting from granulomatous vasculitis of the ascending and descending aorta and its major branches.[20,21] Although arterial biopsy is impractical given the restriction of lesions to the aorta and its branches, cerebral magnetic resonance angiography (MRA) and conventional angiography show vessel irregularities, stenosis, poststenotic dilatations, aneurysmal formation, occlusions, and increased collateralization. Although the mechanism and distribution of headache differs between patients with GCA and TAK, and pervasiveness of headache is greater in GCA than in TAK, there are strong similarities and subtle differences in the distribution of arterial disease on cerebral arteriography that suggest that the 2 disorders may exist along a spectrum of the same or similar disease.[22]

Isolated aortitis

Isolated noninfectious aortitis comprises disorders characterized by chronic inflammation restricted to the aortic wall[23] and IgG-4 infiltrating plasma cells. Headache was an initial feature among 14% of patients with aortitis who had concomitant GCA or TAK,[24] without which the diagnosis of coexisting aortitis might have been overlooked.[25] Headache may also be a clue to infectious aortitis when headache occurs in association with fever, or as a constitutional symptom in noninfectious aortitis when associated with another systemic inflammatory disorder.[25] The risk factors for aortitis include advanced age, history of connective tissue disease, IgG4-related systemic disease, diabetes mellitus, and heart valve pathology.[26]

Medium-Size Vessel Vasculitis

Two distinct disorders, polyarteritis nodosa (PAN) and Kawasaki disease (KD) belong to the category of medium-vessel vasculitis, each of which can have associated headache symptoms.

Polyarteritis Nodosa

There are only a few well-documented postmortem series of patients with PAN to investigate the clinicopathologic correlation of the vasculitis and headache. Kernohan and colleagues[27] estimated that 8% of patients with PAN had CNS involvement. In a description of the postmortem findings of five pathologically studied patients with PAN, headache was nonetheless a complaint in four of them during the course of their illness, with involvement of epineurial vessels of the PNS, medium vessels of the systemic vasculature, and small meningeal arteries and large named vessels of the CNS, as follows. Patient 1 with weakness and paresthesia of the legs, and lightening pains in the limbs and head, nonetheless showed PAN involvement of epineurial vessel sparing systemic and CNS vasculature. Patient 2, who developed fatal progressive worsening of PAN with associated pain in the legs and suboccipital region, had widespread systemic PAN at postmortem examination; however, the brain was not examined. Patient 4, who complained of right supraorbital, mandibular, and aural pain, which was attributed to infected sinuses and nonerupted wisdom tooth, developed confusion, left-sided weakness and sensory loss, followed by stupor and coma before death. Postmortem examination showed near complete obstruction of the right middle cerebral artery (MCA) caused by chronic PAN involvement. Patient 5, who developed severe headache as though his head was in a vise at the onset of PAN, also died after progressive stupor and coma. Postmortem examination showed diffuse system PAN with involvement of small meningeal arteries. In these patients, headache, which was a pervasive feature at any stage of the illness, did not always correlate with the observed histopathology. The neuropathologic changes included characteristic hyalinelike necrosis of a portion of the media and the internal elastic lamina, followed by extension of the inflammatory process to the adventitia by periarteritis (**Fig. 2**). The perivascular inflammation was secondary thus to the lesion in media of the artery, and although periarteritis developed, there was usually proliferation of the intima, leading to narrowing of the vessel lumen. When present, aneurysms developed during the subacute stage of the disease, leading to the gross nodosa or nodule features. Vasculitic involvement of arterioles, capillaries, and venules, and glomerulonephritis are typically absent, and there is no association with antineutrophilic cytoplasmic antibodies (ANCA), the latter of which proves to be a useful discriminatory feature.[4]

Kawasaki Disease

This disorder was named in the honor of the investigator,[28] who described acute febrile mucocutaneous syndrome with lymphoid involvement and desquamation of the fingers and toes in children. It affects medium and small arteries, particularly the coronary arteries, leading to aneurysm and ectasia formation.[4] Endothelial damage occurs in the acute stages of the illness.[29] Headache is an associated symptom, along with cough, abdominal pain, arthralgia, and seizures, which are noted in up to one-quarter of untreated patients.[30] Those with abdominal pain and headache are older by a decade or more than those without these symptoms.[30] Migraine and Raynaud

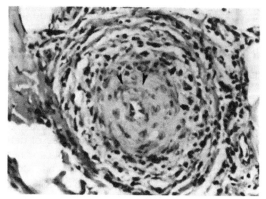

Fig. 2. This small muscular artery from muscle is from a patient with PAN. In the third, or proliferative, phase shown here, chronic inflammatory cells replace the neutrophils of the second phase; there is evidence of necrosis of the media (*arrows*), early intimal proliferation (*arrowheads*), and fibrosis. The lumen is almost completely occluded. In the healing phase, this process is replaced by dense, organized connective tissue (stain, hematoxylin-eosin, original magnification ×250). (*From* Younger DS. Adult and childhood vasculitis of the nervous system. In: Younger DS, editor. Motor disorders. New York: Younger DS; 2013. p. 235–80; with permission.)

phenomenon, which coexist in some patients with KD, may be reflective of similar vascular lesions that indicate the late consequences of extracoronary endothelial cell dysfunction.[31]

Small-Vessel Size Vasculitis

The category of small-size vessel vasculitis (SVV) includes several disorders that fall under the designations of ANCA-associated vasculitis (AAV) and immune complex vasculitis. The category of AAV, which is associated with necrotizing vasculitis with few or no immune deposits, predominantly affects small vessels, including capillaries, venules, arterioles, and small arteries, and is associated with myeloperoxidase (MPO) ANCA or proteinase 3 (PR3) ANCA. It includes three disorders: microscopic polyangiitis (MPA), granulomatosis with polyangiitis (GPA), formerly termed Wegener disease, and eosinophilic GPA (EGPA), formerly termed Churg-Strauss syndrome (CSS). The other major category of SVV are the immune complex vasculitides, characterized by moderate to marked vessel wall deposits of Ig and complement components all along small arteries and veins. Immune complex SVV includes the entities of antiglomerular basement membrane disease, cryoglobulinemic vasculitis (CV), hypocomplementemic urticarial vasculitis (HUV) mediated by anti-C1q antibodies, and IgA vasculitis, formerly termed Henoch-Schönlein purpura (HSP).

Microscopic Polyangiitis

Fever, arthralgia, purpura, hemoptysis, pulmonary hemorrhage, abdominal pain, and gastrointestinal bleeding precede the explosive phase of systemic necrotizing SVV, which affected the kidney and lungs, with rapidly progressive glomerulonephritis and pulmonary capillaritis. Cerebral signs and symptoms, including headache, was noted at presentation in 18% of patients.[32] Abnormal ANCA serology was noted in up to 80% of patients. Two of five deaths were attributed to CNS involvement by vasculitis during periods of disease at 4 and 8 months, respectively; however, that hypothesis could not be confirmed, because postmortem examinations were not performed. Microscopic polyangiitis is associated with MPO-ANCA in 58% of patients and PR3 in 26%, respectively, attributing disease activity to MPO-AAV and PR-AAV.[33]

Granulomatosis with Polyangiitis

Nervous system involvement in GPA was recognized by Drachman,[34] who described a patient with one month of dull bifrontal-vertex headache, which had awakened him from sleep for one month. This headache was followed by early complaints of rhinitis, nasal obstruction, epistaxis, and sensory and motor mononeuropathy multiplex, and later by disorientation, confusion, and hypertension. Many patients with GPA complain of severe constant headache attributed to destructive sinusitis early in the course of the illness; possible causes for headache and cerebral involvement were attributed pathologically to vasculitis of large arterial branch vessels, particularly over the surface of the brain; hypertensive encephalopathy suggested by microscopic infarction in the basal ganglia in close relation to arteries showing fibrinoid impregnation of their walls; and meningeal infiltration by many plasma cells. Autoantibodies against neutrophil granule serine protease 3 are detected in two-thirds of patients, and MPO in 24% of patients, respectively, attributing disease activity to PR3-AAV and MPO-AAV.[33]

Eosinophilic Granulomatosis with Polyangiitis

In 1951, Churg and Strauss[35] described the clinicopathologic findings of EGPA among 13 patients with so-called allergic granulomatosis, allergic angiitis, and periarteritis nodosa. Clinically, severe asthma, fever, and hypereosinophilia was noted, in association with widespread vascular lesions at postmortem examination, comprising fibrinoid collagen changes and granulomatous proliferation of epithelioid cells and giant cells, the so-called allergic granuloma, both within vessel walls and in connective tissue throughout the body. Other manifestations included cutaneous and subcutaneous nodules and granulomatous lymphadenitis. Contrary to the characterization that CNS involvement was rare in CSS yet conferred a poorer prognosis,[36] clinical CNS involvement, presumably headache as well, was noted in 8 (62%) of patients, varying from disorientation to convulsions and coma. Three patients with CNS involvement died of cerebral (2 patients) or subarachnoid hemorrhages (1 patient). Involvement of the peripheral nervous system, which is a principal criterion for the diagnosis according to the American College of Rheumatology (ACR),[37] may provide a clue to the nature of the CNS lesions. Epineurial necrotizing vasculitis, noted in 54% of patients of one cohort,[38] was typified by CD8-positive suppressive/cytotoxic and CD4-positive helper T-lymphocytes, in addition to eosinophils in inflammatory infiltrates, with only occasional CD20-positive B-lymphocytes, and scare deposits of IgG, C3d, and IgE.

Cryoglobulinemia

The presence in the serum of one or more immunoglobulins that precipitate lower than core body temperatures and redissolve on rewarming is termed cryoglobulinemia.[39] Wintrobue and Buell[40] described the first patient with cryoglobulinemia, a 56-year-old woman who presented with progressive frontal headache, left face and eye pain; and right shoulder, neck, and lumbar discomfort after a bout of shingles. These symptoms were followed by Raynaud symptoms, recurrent nosebleeds, exertional dyspnea and palpitation, and changes in the eye ground attributed to central vein thrombosis. Postmortem examination showed infiltrating myeloma of the humerus and lumbar vertebra, and splenic enlargement. A unique plasma protein was detected, which spontaneously precipitated with cold temperature and solubilized at high temperature and which differed from Bence-Jones proteinuria of other patients with myeloma. Gorevic and colleagues[41] provided a complete description of the main clinical features and biological features of mixed CV in 40 patients, the clinical features of which included palpable purpura in all patients, polyarthralgia in three-quarters, renal disease in slightly more than half, and deposits of IgG, IgM, and complement, or renal arteritis in one-third. All cryoglobulins have rheumatoid activity consisting of IgM and polyclonal IgG, and one-third had monoclonal IgM κ components. Brouet and colleagues[42] provided modern classifications of cryoglobulinemia among 86 patients, which included type 1, composed of a single monoclonal immunoglobulin; and types II and III as mixed cryoglobulinemia, composed of different immunoglobulin, with a monoclonal component in type II, and polyclonal immunoglobulin in type III. In the absence of well-defined disease, the presence of mixed cryoglobulinemia was termed essential. Agnello and colleagues[43] reported a strong association with concomitant hepatitis C virus (HCV) infection and a high rate of false-negative serologic tests in type II cryoglobulinemia. The frequency of headache has not been specifically cited in any published cases of cryoglobulinemia. However, headache could be a presenting feature in those with CNS involvement, as noted in two patients with lacunar cerebral strokes and associated subcortical white matter changes on brain MRI,[44,45] two patients with cortical stroke syndromes and associated cortical gray matter infarction on brain MRI,[46] one patient with a temporal arteritislike syndrome with associated ischemic cerebral infarction,[47] three patients with relapsing encephalopathy,[48] two patients with cerebral hemorrhage,[45] two others with ischemic subcortical infarcts,[44] and in five others[41,49] with postmortem evidence of CNS involvement clinically alone or pathologically with widespread vasculitis, including the brain.[41] With an overall mortality of 8.7%,[50] and a 33% fatality rate among those with CNS involvement,[51] the symptom set of CNS involvement including headache seems to be important in prognosis.

Hypocomplementemic Urticarial Vasculitis

This uncommon disorder presents with recurrent attacks of erythematous, urticarial, and hemorrhagic skin lesions lasting up to 24 hours at a time, associated with recurrent attacks of fever, joint swelling, and variable abdominal distress. Serum complement levels are depressed; however, immunodiffusion against purified preparations of human C1q shows strong reactivity. Skin biopsies show varied patterns of polymorphonuclear infiltration involving the vessel wall characteristic of necrotizing vasculitis, infiltration scattered diffusely through the dermis typical of anaphylactoid purpura, or mild nonspecific perivascular infiltration. Renal biopsy may show mild to moderate glomerulonephritis indistinguishable from those seen in other forms of chronic membranoproliferative glomerulonephritis. The differences in HUV from systemic lupus erythematosus (SLE) include more urticarial and purpuric skin lesions, mild or absent renal involvement, or other visceral involvement. Moreover, serum speckled antinuclear and anti-DNA antibodies, and basement membrane Ig deposits, are characteristically absent in HUV. Among 14 patients with HUV reported by Wisnieski and colleagues,[52] 1 patient with orbital pseudotumor complained of headache. It is unlikely that the headache in HUV would favor SLE in an individual patient, because prospective studies suggest that headache occurs in SLE at a frequency equal to normal controls.[53] Buck and colleagues[54] and Grotz and colleagues[55] cited aseptic meningitis and pseudotumor cerebri, both typified by headache, as a possible neurologic manifestation of HUV.

IgA Vasculitis

Osler[56] described cerebral manifestations in association with attacks of purpura in a patient with transient hemiparesis, in 3 others with potentially fatal hemorrhage, including one with a history of childhood attacks culminating in subdural hemorrhage, and in two others who progressed to the comatose state, one of whom had postmortem confirmation of a subdural hemorrhage; however, headache was not mentioned. Green[57] quoted a personal communication from Dr Eli Davis (St Andrew's Hospital, UK) indicating the frequency of blood in CSF in 2 of 1000 patients and reporting a child with headache and xanthochromia that followed onset of fever, malaise, sore throat, arthralgia, rash, and meningeal symptoms after presumed streptococcal illness. The first mention of headache in this disorder was provided by Lewis and Philpott[58] in the description of three patients with neurologic complications of HSP, two of whom manifested severe headache concomitant at onset followed shortly afterward by meningeal signs and xanthochromic CSF, which indicates subarachnoid hemorrhage; a third patient without complaints of headache rapidly lapsed into coma after repeated convulsions. Postmortem examination in the only patient who died was limited to the abdominal cavity, which showed subacute nephritis and arteriolitis. Belman and colleagues[59] estimated the incidence of headache to be 8.9% and noted that it was the presenting symptom in one of their three reported patients, specifically a child with a prodrome of febrile irritability, colic, nausea, and vomiting, who later developed palpable purpuric rash, hematuria, and skin biopsy, which showed leukocytoclastic vasculitis. The other two patients differed in development of other neurologic signs, which included transient postictal hemiparesis or mononeuropathy multiplex. Recognized as a distinct entity for more than 200 years, HSP is the commonest vasculitis in children, with an incidence of 10 patients per 100,000 a year and an association with a variety of pathogens, drugs, and other environmental exposures.[60] Positive throat cultures are noted in up to one-third of cases, with group A β-hemolytic *Streptococcus* and titers to anti-streptolysin O increased in up to one-half of cases. Recognized neurologic complications include headache, obtundation, seizures, paresis, cortical blindness, chorea, ataxia, cranial nerve palsies, peripheral neuropathy, and myositis.[60] IgA seems to play a pivotal role in the pathogenesis of increased serum and polymeric levels of IgA,[61] IgA-containing immune complexes and rheumatoid factor,[62] and selective deposition of IgA1 in glomerular mesangium in renal biopsies in virtually all patients with HSP nephritis and IgA nephropathy.[63]

Variable-Size Vessel Vasculitis

This category of vasculitis can affect vessels of any size, including those that are small, medium, and large, and of any type, including arteries, veins, and capillaries. Behçet disease (BD) and Cogan syndrome are two examples of a primary variable-size vessel vasculitis (VVV) with a propensity for vasculitis, CNS involvement, and headache.

Behçet Disease

This disorder is characterized by relapsing aphthous ulcers of the mouth, eye, and genitalia.[64] Nervous system involvement has been estimated at from 10%[65] to 25%[66] in clinicopathologically confirmed patients, with approximately one-third showing parenchymal involvement and two-thirds vascular involvement.[65] Headache was the commonest neurologic symptom, independent of neurologic involvement in two-thirds of patients in one study cohort,[67] and noted to be primary in 38%, with 24% manifesting tension-type and 15% migraines, and secondary to tandem neurologic involvement in 5%. Frontal and occipital headache and deep-seated pain around the eyes were presenting symptoms in several patients with imminent florid involvement later studied at postmortem examination,[68–71] or a clue to silent neurologic involvement in other cohorts.[72] Siva and Saip[73] classified neurologic involvement into 2 major primary types, one caused by vascular inflammatory mechanisms with focal or multifocal parenchymal involvement, presenting most often as a subacute brainstem syndrome, and another with few symptoms and a more favorable prognosis, caused by isolated cerebral venous sinus thrombosis and intracranial hypertension. A secondary form results instead from cerebral emboli due to cardiac disease, intracranial hypertension from superior vena cava syndrome, and neurotoxicity of specific mediations used in treatment. Mortality among neurologically complicated clinicopathologically-confirmed cases[66] was 41%, with 59% occurring within one year of onset of neurologic involvement. Among nonfatal cases, residual neurologic signs were not uncommon. The neuropathologic findings in BD in brain biopsies and postmortem examination have been remarkably consistent among patients over the past several decades, showing perivascular cuffing of small meningovascular and parenchymal arteries and veins,[66,68,69,71,74] rarely medium-sized arteries showing fibrinoid degeneration and recanalization, and examples of venous thrombosis.[70] The inflammatory cell infiltrates are generally comprised lymphocytes, both T-cells and B-cells, macrophages, rarely plasma cells and eosinophils, with reactive astrocytosis and microscopic gliosis in neighboring cerebral, cerebellar, and brainstem white matter. Neuroimaging in those with neural parenchymal involvement showed a mesodiencephalic junction lesion, with edema extending along certain long tracts of the brainstem and diencephalon in 46% of patients, with the next most common location of involvement along the pontobulbar region in 40% of cases supporting a small-vessel vasculitis.

Cogan Syndrome

Mogan and Baumgartner[75] described a 26-year-old man with recurrent headachelike pain, spasm, and redness of the left eye with photophobia, excessive tearing, and marked conjunctival injection, followed by severe attack of dizziness, tinnitus, vertigo, nausea, vomiting, ringing in the ears, profuse perspiration, and deafness. A diagnosis of recurrent interstitial keratitis (IK) and explosive Menière disease was made. In retrospect, this was probably the first reported patient with Cogan Syndrome of nonsyphilitic IK with vestibuloauditory symptoms.[76] Symptoms of IK develop abruptly and gradually resolve, associated with photophobia, lacrimation, and eye pain (which may be unilateral or bilateral), and tend to recur periodically for years, before becoming quiescent. Vestibuloauditory dysfunction is manifested by sudden onset of Menière-like attacks of nausea, vomiting, tinnitus, vertigo, and frequently, progressive hearing loss, which characteristically occurs before or after the onset of IK. With probably fewer than 100 reported patients with this rare disorder of childhood and young adulthood, most reported patients with typical Cogan Syndrome have appeared as single case reports or patient series, often without pathologic confirmation or evidence of systemic vasculitis in a biopsy or at postmortem examination. Headache was described by Norton and Cogan[77] during the acute illness or at onset in a patient with atypical Cogan Syndrome, who manifested a superior central retinal artery branch occlusion and orbital edema, as well as by Cody[78] and Cody and Williams[79] among three of five patients with typical Cogan Syndrome and one of two patients with atypical Cogan Syndrome. More recently, Gluth and colleagues[80] noted headache in 24 of 60 (40%) patients with Cogan Syndrome of mean age 38 years (range 9–70 years), whereas Pagnini and colleagues[81] noted headache at onset in 17% of children of mean age 11 years (range 4–18 years) and in association with other systemic features, including fever, arthralgia, myalgia, arthritis, and weight loss in up to 48% of children. Haynes and colleagues[82] found headache less common in typical Cogan Syndrome in 17% of patients at onset, compared with 27% with atypical Cogan Syndrome, a finding that correlated with CNS involvement identified in 4% of patients with typical Cogan Syndrome compared with 15% with atypical Cogan Syndrome, respectively.

Pathologically proven necrotizing vasculitis in association with Cogan Syndrome was confirmed at postmortem examination in three patients,[83–85] by examination of subcutaneous nodular tissue and amputated limbs, and postmortem examination in one patient,[86] or examination of biopsy tissue alone in ten living patients.[83,84,87–92]

Crawford[83] observed three patients with systemic necrotizing vasculitis, both of whom had headache at onset of Cogan Syndrome. Postmortem examination in the first patient (case 1) who had frontal headaches and IK before onset of vestibuloauditory symptoms, showed necrotizing arteritis involving small arteries and arterioles of the brain, gastrointestinal tract, and kidneys, in addition to cerebral edema and petechial hemorrhages.

Single-Organ Vasculitis

Single-organ vasculitis affects arteries or veins of any size in a single organ without features to indicate that it is a limited expression of a systemic vasculitis.[4] Involvement of small, medium, and large vessels of a single organ can be multifocal or diffuse as in those leading to an isolated organ-related clinicopathologic syndrome of the CNS, kidneys, peripheral nerves, coronary and pulmonary vessels, and retina, or focally in the breast, genitourinary, gastrointestinal system, or aorta, particularly after incidental biopsy or surgical resection because of a related or unrelated vasculitic process.[93]

Primary CNS vasculitis

Isolated angiitis of the CNS (IACNS), granulomatous angiitis of the brain, and granulomatous angiitis of the nervous system (GANS), primary angiitis of the CNS (PACNS), and primary CNS vasculitis (PCNSV) are terms used to describe vasculitis restricted to the CNS; however, they connote different entities. The identification of angiographic beading in two patients and a sausage appearance in another patient at sites of presumed arteritis, the sine qua non of cerebral vasculitis (**Fig. 3**), was first noted by Hinck and colleagues in GCA,[94] and later by Cupps and Fauci[95] in IACNS. The latter observation, along with preliminary efficacy of a combination immunosuppressive regimen of oral cyclophosphamide and alternate-day prednisone in three patients with IACNS defined angiographically alone, and in one other patient with histologically proven GANS of the filum terminate, led to prospective diagnostic and therapeutic recommendations.[96] At that time, investigators at the National Institutes of Health regarded IACNS and GANS as equivalent entities, with the former term emphasizing the restricted nature of the vasculitis and the latter the granulomatous histology. Giant cells and epithelioid cells, usually found at autopsy in GANS, were an inconsistent finding in a meningeal and brain biopsy and were therefore considered unnecessary for antemortem diagnosis. In 1988, Calabrese and Mallek[97] proposed criteria for the diagnosis of PACNS, which like IACNS, relied on either classic angiographic or histopathologic features of angiitis within the CNS in the absence of systemic vasculitis or another cause for the observed findings. The typical patient presented with headache of gradual onset, often accompanied by the signs and symptoms of dementia, and only later developing focal neurologic symptoms and signs. The clinical course might be rapidly progressive over days to weeks or at times insidiously over many months, with seemingly prolonged periods of stabilization. In the same year, Younger and colleagues[98] described four patients with GANS defined by the presence of granulomatous giant cell and epithelioid cell infiltration in the walls of arteries of various caliber

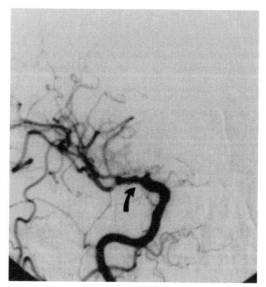

Fig. 3. Radiographic features of cerebral vasculitis. Ectasia and beading in the M1 segment and lack of flow in the A1 segment of the right anterior cerebral artery (*arrow*). (*From* Younger DS. Adult and childhood vasculitis of the nervous system. In: Younger DS, editor. Motor disorders. New York: Younger DS; 2013. p. 235–80; with permission.)

from named cerebral vessels to small arteries and veins at postmortem examination (**Fig. 4**A, B). One each was noted in association with Hodgkin lymphoma, herpes zoster, neurosarcoidosis, and no associated disorder. Headache was noted at onset in all four patients, as well as in 57% of patients with GANS, and during the course of the disease in 78%. Moreover, the combination of headache, mental change, increased protein content with or without pleocytosis followed by hemiparesis, quadriparesis, progressive to lethargy and stupor were predictive of a poor prognosis and mandated the need for combined meningeal and brain biopsy to establish the diagnosis with certainty. Although there has not been a prospective study of the outcome of GANS and PACNS, undiagnosed and therefore untreated, the outcome of either is poor. Enthusiasm for treatment with combination chemotherapy using cyclophosphamide has waned with recognition of the apparent risk of fatal side effects and the apparent efficacy at least of corticosteroids and azathioprine in other immunosuppressant medications in 1 retrospective analysis.[99] Salvarani and colleagues[100] diagnosed PCNSV in 31 patients by histopathology and 70 patients angiographically, in whom 18 had a granulomatous inflammatory pattern, 8 lymphocytic pattern, and 5 acute necrotizing pattern. Headache was the commonest symptom in 63% of patients, followed by abnormal cognition, hemiparesis, and persistent neurologic deficit. Hajj-Ali and Calabrese[101] separated GANS from PACNS and the reversible cerebral vasoconstriction syndrome, suggested by sudden, severe thunderclaplike headache with or without associated neurologic deficits and most reversible angiographic findings not caused by true vasculitis.

Childhood IACNS or childhood PACNS (cPACNS) caused by involvement of distal small vessels have a gradual onset of persistent headache, cognitive decline, mood disorder, and focal seizures, and involvement of proximal medium and large arteries leads to large arterial stroke and propensity to subarachnoid hemorrhage.[102] The incurred deficit is influenced not only by the size and distribution of the involved vessels but also by the degrees and number of stenosis. Overall, the commonest presenting features of cPACNS were acute severe headaches and stroke features.[103]

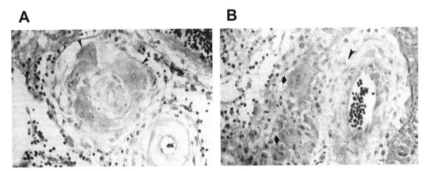

Fig. 4. CNS vasculitis. (*A*) The media and adventitia of this small leptomeningeal artery have been almost completely replaced by multinucleated giant cells (*arrowheads*). There is intimal proliferation with obliteration of the vascular lumen, and a dense, perivascular, mononuclear inflammatory infiltrate can be seen (stain, hematoxylin-eosin, original magnification ×250). (*B*) A larger leptomeningeal vessel shows necrosis of the media and internal elastic lamina with multinucleated giant cell formation (*arrows*), intimal proliferation (*arrowhead*), and lymphocytic infiltration of the adventitia and neighboring meninges (stain, hematoxylin-eosin, original magnification ×250). (*From* Younger DS. Adult and childhood vasculitis of the nervous system. In: Younger DS, editor. Motor disorders; 2013. p. 235–80. New York: Younger DS; with permission.)

Children with angiographically positive progressive cPACNS can present with both focal and diffuse neurologic deficits with multifocal MRI lesions and evidence of both proximal and distal vessel stenosis on angiography. Untreated, they progress beyond three months, acquiring new neurologic deficits and new angiographically confirmed areas of vessel inflammation. Those with angiographically positive nonprogressive cPACNS often present with focal deficits, unilateral MRI lesions, and proximal angiographic vascular stenoses. Such patients instead have monophasic inflammatory large-vessel disease, which usually fails to progress beyond 3 months.[103] Angiographically negative, small-vessel (SV)-cPACNS vasculitis,[104,105] which presents with new onset of severe headaches, seizures, or cognitive decline, warrants prompt consideration of lesional brain biopsy to ascertain the diagnosis before commencement of immunosuppressant treatment, because both corticosteroids and delay in performance of the biopsy can obscure the histopathologic features. In contrast to adult PCNSV, granulomatous inflammation is typically absent. Instead, brain biopsy shows a mixture of lymphocytes and macrophages, with occasional plasma cells, polymorphonuclear cells, and eosinophils in the walls of small arteries, arterioles, capillaries, and venules in the leptomeninges, cortex, and subcortical white matter. The BrainWorks Investigator Group, which prospectively records Canadian children with inflammatory brain diseases, including N-methyl-D-aspartate receptor encephalitis and other neuronal antibody-mediated CNS diseases, progressive and nonprogressive large-vessel and small-vessel vasculitis, and CNS vasculitis associated with infection, recently reported an increase in the diagnoses of primary inflammatory brain disease (IBD) in children.[106]

Vasculitis Associated with Systemic Collagen Vascular Disease

Specific systemic disorders associated with vasculitis, and in turn with headache, include sarcoidosis and the serologically specific collagen vascular disorders such as SLE and rheumatoid arthritis (RA).

Systemic Lupus Erythematosus

The early concepts of the collagen vascular disorders introduced by Klemperer[107,108] stemmed from the appreciation of fibrinoid necrosis using collagen staining in patients with SLE. As collagen swells and fragments, it dissolves to form a homogeneous hyaline and granular periodic acid-Schiff-positive material. The latter fibrinoid material contained immunoglobulins, antigen-antibody complexes, complement, and fibrinogen. The organ-specific responses of the CNS of this fibrinoid material lead to recognizable clinical sequelae caused by vascular and parenchymal damage. Several fluorescent antibody tests provide serologic support of SLE. The antinuclear antibody (ANA) screen produces a homogeneous pattern in most patients, with antibodies to native double-stranded (ds) DNA and reactivity to the Smith (Sm) and ribonucleoprotein (RNP) antigens, the combination of which constitutes the extractable nuclear antigen. Circulating IgG and IgM antibodies with an affinity for charged phospholipids, antiphospholipid antibodies (APA), some of which have procoagulant activity such as the lupus anticoagulant (LAC) and the generic anticardiolipin antibody (ACL) assay using cardiolipin as the antigen probe for APA, are all important determinants of prothrombotic events, especially in the CNS, wherein there is a propensity for occlusive microangiopathy.

Borowoy and colleagues[109] noted a prevalence of neuropsychiatric SLE (NPSLE) of 6.4% in a cohort of 1253 patients with SLE defined by the ACR[110] compared with the reported estimates of NPSLE of 14% to 39% in children and adults. Headache was regarded as a nonspecific minor NPSLE manifestation of chronic disease, along with mild cognitive impairment and depression. According to Tomic-Lucic and colleagues,[111] those with so-called late onset SLE caused by development of disease after age 50 years had a frequency of NPSLE of 6.6% compared with 36.6% in early onset disease along with a higher prevalence of comorbid conditions and higher Systemic Lupus International Collaborating Clinics/ACR damage index, despite less major organ involvement and a more benign course. Once believed to be an important cause of CNS or cerebral lupus, true vasculitis was present in only 12% of postmortem examinations in the series by Johnson and Richardswon.[112] There was no mention of headache or CNS vasculitis among the 150 patients with SLE described by Estes and Christian,[113] nor was there mention of headache among 50 clinicopathologic cases of SLE, one-half of whom had CNS lesions, compiled by Devinsky and colleagues.[114] Feinglass and colleagues[115] noted neuropsychiatric manifestations at onset of SLE among 3% of 140 patients compared with 37% in the course of the illness; however, headache was not specifically tabulated.

Cerebral dysfunction in SLE can be caused by large-vessel or small-vessel involvement or both. In the series by Feinglass and colleagues,[115] vasculitis was noted in 28% of patients, as well as in 46% of those with neuropsychiatric involvement compared with 17% of patients lacking neuropsychiatric involvement. Postmortem examination of the CNS in 10 of the 19 fatalities showed two cases of multiple large and small infarcts, one of which showed inflammatory cell infiltrates in the walls of medium-sized vessels and perivascular infiltrates around small arterioles. Although active CNS vasculitis was absent in the brain and spinal tissue of all 50 cases reported by Devinsky and colleagues,[114] two had evidence of inactive healed CNS vasculitis, suggested by focal disruption of the elastic lamina and mild intimal proliferation of a single medium-sized artery, one of which had active systemic vasculitis of the PAN type, and both of which showed Libman-Sacks endocarditis and embolic brain infarcts. Focal angiitis of the CNS with cystlike formation around affected blood vessels was noted at postmortem in the patient described by Mintz and Fraga,[116] with typical SLE rash, cutaneous vasculitis, and active neuropsychiatric involvement. Trevor and colleagues[117] summarized the literature of large named cerebral vessel occlusions from 1958 to 1965 and noted 1 patient with an MCA stenosis progressing to occlusion and 3 others with angiographic internal carotid artery (ICA) occlusions, adding three new patients and suggesting a relation to the occurrence of cerebral arteritis. Two women, one age 21 years and the other age 42 years, presented with headache followed by focal neurologic symptoms attributed respectively to left MCA, followed by right ICA occlusions, and a right MCA stenosis progressing to occlusion in four months. A third patient had a left ICA occlusion without mention of headache. Johnson and Richardswon[112] attributed the vasculitic nature of this process histopathologically to cerebral vasculitis mediated by acute inflammation and necrosis. Younger and colleagues[118] reported large named cerebral vessel occlusion attributed to circulating anticardiolipin antibodies in a young man in whom a vasculitis mechanism was not evoked.

The pathogenic mechanisms of cerebral SLE are not well understood.[119] Immune complex–mediated vasculitis probably affecting small vessels is believed to account for much of the damage in CNS lupus despite the paucity of cerebral vasculitis evident in the form of inflammatory infiltrates in vessel walls at postmortem examination. In those with discrete vascular infarcts, there is a known association with the presence of circulating pathogenic antibodies, which predisposes some individuals to a high risk of stroke caused by both small-vessel and large-vessel occlusion.[118,120] Lupus cerebritis and meningoencephalitis are two neurologic disturbances that can be associated with preceding headache. These disturbances are noted in up to 75% of patients with SLE depending on criteria,[121] and an etiopathogenesis related to antibody-mediated neuronal dysfunction is likely given the lack of correlation of symptoms of NPSLE and CNS lesions at postmortem examination, together with the transient nature of the disturbance. Patients with SLE are also predisposed to infectious episodes, including those not yet treated because of impaired B-cell function and humoral immunity, in addition to others receiving immunosuppressant medication rendered impaired in T-cell function and cell-mediated immunity.[121]

Rheumatoid Arthritis

The ACR and European League Against Rheumatism Collaborative Initiative[122] published classification criteria for RA. Rheumatoid vasculitis (RV) qualifies as an extra-articular manifestation of RA.[123] There remains only a slight excess mortality in patients with RV compared with RA controls after allowance for general risk factors such as age and sex.[124] Three forms of vasculitis occur in RA, affecting all calibers of blood vessels, from dermal postcapillary venules to the aorta, usually in association with circulating IgM and IgG rheumatoid factor (RF) as measured by the latex fixation test, decreased complement levels, and a positive ANA test. The first form of RV is a proliferative endarteritis of a few organs, notably the heart, skeletal muscle, and nerves characterized by inflammatory infiltration of all layers of small arteries and arterioles, with intimal proliferation, necrosis, and thrombosis. The second form is a fulminant vasculitis indistinguishable from PAN, with less severe leukocytosis, myalgia, renal and gastrointestinal involvement, and bowel perforation. The third type takes the form of palpable purpura, arthritis, cryoglobulinemia, and low complement levels. CNS vasculitis is rare in RV; however, the postmortem findings of nine such patients have been reported,[125–132] and although not mentioned in any of them, headache would not be an unexpected feature. The duration of RA had a range of 1 to 30 years, with most surviving decades. The neurologic presentations included delirium, confusion, seizures, hemiparesis, Gerstmann-like syndrome, blindness, and peripheral neuropathy. Postmortem examination showed widespread systemic vasculitis in 3 patients.[125,127,128]

Vasculitis Associated with Illicit Substance Abuse

Even although headache in an illicit drug abuser should always prompt concern for stroke, hemorrhage, and CNS infection, further separable by neuroimaging and CSF analysis, cerebral vasculitis is rare, with few histologically well-documented patients described in the literature. Three observations cast doubt on the frequent association of substance abuse with true cerebral vasculitis. First, most cases have been diagnosed by beading alone on a cerebral angiogram, without pathologic verification. Second, the vascular insult associated with drug abuse is likely caused by contributory factors, including human immunodeficiency virus type 1 (HIV-1) and acquired immuno defficiency syndrome (AIDS), which frequently accompanies drug abuse. Third, necrotizing arteritis itself is not a feature of an experimental animal model, in which vessel beading develops within 2 weeks of potential administration of amphetamine, postmortem examination of which shows per vascular cuffing, not arteritis.

Amphetamines

Parenteral illicit drug use as a cause of CNS vasculitis was first reported in association with amphetamines in 1970 among 14 drug addicts who suffered strokes and intracranial hemorrhage in association with multiple amphetamine and narcotic drug use.[133] Necrotizing arteritis of the polyarteritis type was found in cerebral arteries and arterioles. Many of the patients had complicating factors, including severe hypertension and hepatitis B antigenemia. Two patients, one abbreviated D.G. and the other E.V., who injected methamphetamine via intravenous injection, had arterial lesions in cerebral, cerebellar, and brainstem pontine vessels; however, detailed histopathologic descriptions were not provided. Cerebral vasculitis was identified in a dubious report[134] of a three-week postpartum woman, who took her first over-the-counter Dexatrim diet pill in many months containing phenylpropanolamine followed 90 minutes later by sudden headache, nausea, and vomiting. Brain computed tomography (CT) showed subarachnoid blood with a frontal lobe hematoma, and bilateral carotid angiography showed diffuse segmental narrowing and dilatation of small, medium, and large vessels and branches of the anterior and posterior circulation. Evacuation and histopathologic analysis of the hematoma showed necrotizing vasculitis of small arteries and veins, with infiltration of polymorphonuclear leukocytes particularly prominent in the intima, with fragmentation of the elastic lamina and areas of vessel occlusion. It was unclear whether the findings were related to primary or drug-related CNS vasculitis.

Cocaine
Nine histologically verified patients with cocaine-related vasculitis have been described.[135–141] In all but one patient who had a long-standing cocaine habit with abuse some time in the six months before admission, onset of neurologic symptoms immediately followed cocaine use, which was intranasally in six, intravenously in two, smoked in one, and acquired via unknown modality in another. Cerebral vasculitis, associated with cerebral hemorrhage in 3 patients and ischemia in seven, typically began with abrupt onset of headache, focal hemiparesis, confusion or agitation, and grand mal seizures, which progressed to stupor, coma, and death. The underlying pathology of cerebral vasculitis established by brain and meningeal biopsy in seven patients and postmortem examination in two was nonnecrotizing, with transmural mononuclear cell inflammation affecting small arteries and veins or veins alone each in three patients, necrosis of small cerebral vessels associated with polymorphonuclear cell inflammation of small arteries and veins or large named vessels in two others, and perivascular cuffing of small arteries and veins in another.

Heroin
No convincing, pathologically confirmed cases of heroin-induced cerebral vasculitis have been described in the literature, nor has cerebral vasculitis been suggested as a likely occurrence in heroin abuse,[142] heroin addiction,[143,144] or acute heroin overdose.[145] Moreover, detailed neuropathologic studies carried out on 134 victims of acute heroin intoxication, including 18 who survived for periods of hours or days,[146] who showed cerebral edema in conjunction with vascular congestion, capillary engorgement, and perivascular bleeding attributed to toxic primary respiratory failure; and ischemic nerve cell damage resembling systemic hypoxia, respectively, showed no evidence of cerebral vasculitis, and only one focus of lymphocytic perivascular inflammation. The brains of 10 intravenous drug abusers who died of heroin overdoses, including one caused by gunshot injury,[147] likewise showed no evidence of cerebral vasculitis at postmortem examination, showing only a few perivascular mononuclear cells associated with pigment deposition.

Vasculitis Caused by CNS Infection

The category of infection-related vasculitides includes acute bacterial and mycobacterial tuberculous (TB) meningitis, spirochete organisms (notably, neurosyphilis and

Lyme neuroborreliosis [LNB]), viral infections (notably, varicella zoster virus [VZV]), mycotic and parasitic infections, and HIV/AIDS. Recognition of an infection is important, because prompt treatment may avert or lessen the severity of both headache and vasculitis.

Acute Bacterial Meningitis

The relationship between vascular and parenchymatous cerebral changes, including vasculitis, and acute and chronic neurologic symptoms and signs, including headache, has not been thoroughly resolved in clinicopathologically studied cases of meningitis. Nor have investigators resolved the origin of vasculitis, whether caused by extension of inflammation from inflamed meninges or the passage of vessels through inflammatory exudation. Twelve of 59 infants younger than two years who suffered from meningitis caused by Haemophilus (H.) influenzae, Meningococcus or Pneumococcus were reported by Dodge and Swartz.[148] Polymorphonuclear infiltration extending to the subintimal region of small arteries and veins was associated with exudative meningitis and anatomic necrosis of the cerebral cortex in all infants studied. However, occlusion of a major venous sinus was found in only two cases, and subarachnoid hemorrhage secondary to necrotizing arteritis was noted in only one case, representing a most unusual pathologic finding, according to Dodge and Swartz.[148] Angiography reflected the localized nature of purulent meningitis in a 6-month-old infant with fatal H influenzae meningitis described by Lyons and Leeds,[149] in whom cerebral angiography showed vasospasm, stenosis, occlusion, and extremely slow arteriovenous circulation and collateral blood supply and a marked decrease in the diameter of bilateral supraclinoid internal carotid arteries. Only one area considered to be a mycotic aneurysm as suggested by irregular dilatations was later shown to be caused by histologically confirmed vasculitis, showing the limited nature of cerebral vasculitis in purulent meningitis. Roach and Drake[150] described five cases of ruptured cerebral aneurysms as suggested by cerebral angiography caused by septic emboli; two of these patients complained of headache; however, none of them had demonstrable vasculitis in histologic examination of the aneurysm specimen after surgery or in postmortem examination of the brain. Focal arteriographic changes in the setting of purulent meningitis may be the result of perivascular inflammation caused by the surrounding exudate.[151]

H. Influenzae Meningitis Headache was a complaint in only 1 patient of 14 clinicopathologically studied children and infants described by Adams and colleagues[152] with H influenzae meningitis; however, all of the other patients were too young (mean age 17 months) to tell of this or other subjective symptoms. Vascular inflammation by neutrophilic cells was noted in 6 (43%) patients, including 3 with associated necrosis in the walls of cortical or meningeal veins associated with ischemic cortical necrosis; or alone without vessel necrosis in three others, including one each in the subintimal region of meningeal or subarachnoid vessels, or in the walls of small to medium subarachnoid arteries associated with ischemic cortical necrosis. Vascular inflammation was absent in 8 (57%) patients, 3 of whom manifested vascular endothelial hyperplasia of meningeal vessels, whereas the remaining five were reported to have no vascular alterations. Based on the clinicopathologic findings, the investigators[152] proposed that from the earliest stages of meningitis, pathologic changes could be found in small and medium-sized subarachnoid arteries and veins, accompanied by endothelial cell swelling, multiplication, and crowding of lumina, a reaction that ensued over 48 to 72 hours. This reaction was followed by infiltration of adventitial connection by neutrophilic cells and in the intima of arteries accompanied by lymphocytes, forming a conspicuous layer. Foci of vascular necrosis occurred in some cases. Vascular inflammation of the adventitia of subarachnoid vessels was believed to be caused by involvement of the arachnoid membrane, which formed the adventitia of the subarachnoid vessels; thus, in a sense, the vessel wall was affected from the beginning by the inflammatory process arising within itself. Subintimal inflammation was believed to have an origin in the foci of necrosis with spread beneath the intima along the line of least resistance. By contrast, spinal and cranial nerves surrounded by purulent exudates from the beginning of the infectious process at the base of the brain were infiltrated by inflammatory cells only after several days and were not pronounced compared with meningeal and cortical vessels, with comparatively more lymphocytes.

Among 34 other patients reported by Smith and Landing[153] with *H. influenzae* meningitis aged 5 months to 8.5 years of age, and duration of 2 to 42 days, in whom headache was also difficult to ascertain, vasculitis involving arterial vessels was noted in six postmortem cases and venous lesions were noted in 10 cases. Cortical necrosis was noted at autopsy in three of the patients with concomitant arteritis and in 5 of those with phlebitis. However, in only one patient (a 10-week-old infant who died the evening of admission) was arteritis believed to be responsible for brain damage. In this infant, postmortem examination disclosed acute inflammation of the walls of several veins and small arteries in the polymorphonuclear meningeal exudate overlying the cortical surface and extending into the superficial cortex, with narrowing of the lumina by endothelial proliferation and fibrin thrombi, associated with extensive early cortical necrosis.

Pneumococcal Meningitis Cairns and Russell[154] described six children and adults with pneumococcal meningitis divided into acute early, intermediate, and late meningitis, depending on whether patients survived a few days, 1 to 2 weeks, or more, respectively, after institution of intravenous penicillin. Five (83%) patients manifested histopathologic features of active or chronic vasculitis, all of whom showed cortical necrosis on postmortem examination of the brain. Headache was noted in 2 of 5 (40%) patients old enough to complain of it and was present in one patient with acute vasculitis and in another with chronic vasculitis. Among three patients who died early, postmortem examination showed acute vasculitis in two patients, including 1 patient aged 3 months with leptomeningeal phlebitis, and another patient aged 21 years with panarteritis of perforating cortical vessels to one frontal lobe. A third patient with early pneumococcal meningitis aged 32 years was noted to have vascular cuffing alone at postmortem examination. In a patient aged 50 years with intermediate survival, postmortem examination showed acute and chronic vasculitis, with subintimal inflammation of arterioles and fibrinoid necrosis of arterioles of the medulla and spinal cord. Among two patients with late meningitis, one patient aged 22 years was noted to have focal intimal hyperplasia of the basilar artery with focal fibrinoid necrosis, and postmortem examination in the other patient aged 15 years showed focal intimal hyperplasia of the basilar artery with endarteritis of fourth ventricle meningeal vessels, which indicates chronic vasculitis. There was a tendency for fibrous deposits to appear in the walls of meningeal arteries with or without purulent panarteritis, with predominance in the brain stem and spinal cord in intermediate and late cases and resemblance to the lesions of PAN with longer survival.

Mycobacterial Tuberculous Infection
Although diagnosis of the different forms of bacterial purulent meningitis was possible only after development of modern bacteriologic methods and the introduction of the lumbar puncture as a diagnostic measure by Quinke in 1891, tuberculous

meningitis was the first type of meningitis to be described clinically as dropsy of the brain in 1768 and subsequently shown to be inflammatory when meningeal tubercles and visceral tubercles were found to be identical in 1830. The tuberculoma, once the commonest intracranial tumor, is now exceptionally rare. The chief neurologic signs and symptoms of tuberculous meningitis reflecting meningeal irritation manifested as neck stiffness and a positive Kernig sign; increased intracranial pressure, notably headache and vomiting; and mental changes, seizures, and focal neurologic signs.

According to Smith and Daniel,[155] arteritis is the rule in the neighborhood of tuberculous lesions, wherein vessel walls are invaded by mononuclear cells, with the adventitia more heavily involved than the media. The subintimal and intimal regions form a layer of homogeneous fibrinoid material that later involves the media, and the vessel lumen is reduced by inflammatory cell exudation beneath the fibrinoid material, the end results of which are reduction or complete obliteration of the lumen, proliferative endarteritis, and cerebral infarction. The vessels most heavily involved were those at the base of the brain and others in the sylvian fissure. Headache was a presenting sign in case 7 reported by Smith and Daniel[155] of an 18-year-old girl with fever, confusion, right hemiplegia, back and neck pain for several days, followed by incontinence, complete flaccid paraplegia, delirium dementia, generalized spasticity, and death. Postmortem examination showed advanced tuberculous meningitis with dense basal adhesions, hydrocephalus, and obliteration of the spinal subarachnoid space by adhesions, hemorrhagic infarction, and widespread arteritis with acute fibrinoid necrosis, without tuberculomas. Case 4 reported by Greitz[156] was a 4-year-old girl with fever, left arm weakness, and increasing disorientation, which rapidly progressed to coma, nuchal rigidity, and spasticity of the legs. Vertebral angiography showed local widening of a branch of the left posterior cerebral artery (PCA) and a posterior fossa mass. The patient died soon afterward, and at postmortem examination, there was tuberculous meningitis with typical tuberculous vasculitis consisting of inflammatory changes in arteries at the base of the brain, notably in small vessels, with intimal swelling, leading to concentric narrowing of vessel lumina.

Leher[157] reported the radiopathologic triad of ventricular dilatation recognized by sweeping of the pericallosal artery; vessel narrowing, typically of the supraclinoid portion of the ICA caused by compression by thickened leptomeninges and exudation, arteritis and spasm; and narrowing or occlusion of smaller and medium-sized arteries with scanty collaterals, local swelling, and early draining veins. Occlusive tuberculous vasculitis is associated with local areas of cerebral infarction of vessels at the base of the brain and arteritis. Headache was a presenting symptom in one of three patients described by Leher,[157] none of whom had a previous history of tuberculosis, and all of whom had diagnostic angiographic abnormalities and histopathologic evidence of tuberculous arteritis. Case 1 was a 33-year-old man with anorexia and insomnia. Carotid angiography showed narrowing of the supraclinoid ICA as well as narrowing of two convexity vessels in the sylvian fissure. At postmortem examination, there was marked eccentric left frontoparietal region arterial narrowing caused by fibroblastic proliferation of the intima, with many inflammatory cells below the elastica. Headache was not mentioned in two other histopathologically confirmed patients with tuberculous vasculitis. Case 2 was a 33-year-old man who presented with fever and stiff neck. Cerebral angiography showed irregularity of the supraclinoid ICA and reduction in the caliber of the convexity MCA vessels. He died shortly thereafter, and postmortem examination disclosed tuberculous leptomeningitis and arteritis of the ICA and MCA with thickened vessel walls and narrowed lumina. Case 4 was a

39-year-old man who presented with confusion and stupor and who was found to have indentation of the lateral aspect of the ICA as it entered the subarachnoid space above the anterior clinoid on cerebral angiography. Ventriculography showed a block at the aqueduct of Sylvius. He died shortly thereafter, and postmortem examination showed widely distributed systemic tuberculosis with binding of vessels at the base of the brain that showed arteritis accompanied by infarction of the basal ganglia and brainstem.

Kopsachilis and colleagues[158] described a 39-year-old man without known tuberculosis who developed sudden visual loss in one eye. Fluorescein angiography showed an inferotemporal branch retinal vein occlusion consisting of blockage with areas of hemorrhage, exudation, and late leakage. This occlusion was followed by optic disk swelling and headache. Biopsy of an enlarged cervical and submandibular lymph node showed caseating epithelioid ant cells confirming tuberculosis. Treatment with antituberculous treatment led to improved visual acuity.

Spirochete Disease
Neurosyphilis Meningovascular syphilis comprises 39% to 61% of all symptomatic cases of neurosyphilis and tends to occur more frequently in patients with concurrently infected HIV/AIDS. It is characterized by obliterative endarteritis, which affects blood vessels of the brain, spinal cord, and leptomeninges, precipitating substantial ischemic injury. Often referred to as Heubner arteritis, it involves medium-sized to large arteries with lymphoplasmacytic intimal inflammation and fibrosis; however, there is a variant form termed Nissl-Alzheimer arteritis, which characteristically affects small vessels and produces both adventitial and intimal thickening. Both types can lead to vascular thrombotic occlusions and cerebral infarction, with preferential involvement of the MCA. The search for the cause of stroke in young adults should include meningovascular syphilis as a potential cause. Sudden acute severe headache heralded onset of occlusion of bilateral vertebral and proximal basilar artery documented by MRA[159] in a 35-year-old African man. He responded to thrombectomy with restoration of blood flow but succumbed to fatal pontine and subarachnoid hemorrhages. Postmortem examination showed reactive plasma reagin and a positive Venereal Disease Research Laboratory (VDRL) test in CSF with CNS vasculitis characterized by mural thrombi along the vertebrobasilar arteries with well-defined lines of Zahn of alternating layers of fibrin, platelet, and red blood cell aggregates, and inflammatory cell infiltration of the arterial walls, particularly in the adventitia. Headache of 2 to 3 weeks in duration was the presenting feature of 2 other patients with stroke syndromes,[160] 1 of whom had narrowing of bilateral M1 segments of the MCA, reactive CSF VDRL-positive *Treponema pallidum* hemagglutin assay and fluorescent treponemal antibody-absorption staining in the CSF, similar to the second patient, who presented with a stroke in the territory of the PCA without focal changes on cerebral angiography; neither of these patients was studied pathologically for true vasculitis. Headache was not mentioned in 1 patient with abrupt onset of confusion, aphasia, and hemiparesis in whom carotid angiography documented a smaller than average caliber with otherwise normal named vessels, abnormal complement fixation test of the blood and CSF, a positive colloidal gold curve test, and leptomeningeal biopsy, which showed lymphocytic infiltration, focal fibrosis, and chronic perivasculitis consistent with meningovascular syphilis.[161] Neither headache nor confirmatory pathologic evidence of CNS vasculitis was mentioned in a patient with basilar artery stenosis and serologically confirmed syphilis in the CSF presumed to be caused by meningovascular syphilis,[162] suggested by a positive string sign of the midbasilar artery at cerebral angiography.

Lyme Neuroborreliosis The term LNB was introduced by Veenendaal-Hilbers and colleagues[163] in 1988 to emphasize CNS involvement caused by *Borrelia (B.) burgdorferi* infection, the causative agent of Lyme disease. Among 20 patients described in the literature with neurovascular clinical syndromes ascribed to CNS vasculitis, for whom detailed information was available, including documentation of positive CSF Lyme serology, two patients[164,165] presented with headache and were noted to have histopathologically confirmed vasculitis on brain biopsy. Patient 3 reported by Oksi and colleagues[164] was an 11-year-old boy with headache and hyperactivity syndrome who developed gait difficulty concomitantly with a stroke visualized on brain MRI. Subsequent craniotomy and biopsy of the area of enhancement disclosed lymphocytic vasculitis of small vessels without fibrinoid necrosis, and CSF *B. burgdorferi* serology was positive. Headache improved with intravenous antimicrobial therapy. Patient 2 reported by Topakian and colleagues[165] presented with headache, fatigue, malaise, nausea, and vomiting, first considered migrainous, then psychosomatic, until subsequent MRI disclosed ischemic brain infarctions, MRA was compatible with diffuse vasculitis, and CSF showed lymphocytic pleocytosis with positive oligoclonal bands, and diagnostic CSF and serum *B. burgdorferi* serology. Brain biopsy showed vasculitis involving leptomeningeal arteries comprising lymphoplasmacytic vessel wall infiltration with focal necrosis. Epithelioid cells were beaded in multiple granulomalike formations in the leptomeninges. There was symptomatic improvement after a course of intravenous antimicrobial therapy. A third patient reported by Miklossy and colleagues,[166] a 50-year-old man with leg spasticity and CSF pleocytosis for 15 months who progressed to hemiparesis and ventilatory support, was later found to have diagnostic *B. burgdorferi* serology in serum and CSF. Postmortem examination showed perivascular lymphocytic inflammation of leptomeningeal vessels, some of which showed infiltration of the vessel walls, duplication of the elastic lamina, narrowing of lumina, and complete obstruction of some leptomeningeal vessels by organized thrombi. Seventeen other patients with presumed CNS vasculitis caused by *B burgdorferi* infection of the CNS were reported, nine of whom presented with headache,[147,163,167–172] whereas headache was unmentioned in the case report of eight others,[173–176] none of whom had histologically-proven CNS vasculitis.

VZV-Related Vasculopathy

The VZV causes chickenpox in childhood and most children manifest only mild neurologic sequelae. After it resolves, the virus becomes latent in neurons of cranial and spinal ganglia of nearly all individuals and reactivates in adult elderly and immunocompromised individuals, to produce shingles. An uncommon but serious complication of virus reactivation is ischemic and hemorrhagic stroke caused by VZV vasculopathy, which affects both immunocompetent and immunocompromised individuals presenting with headache and mental status changes with or without focal neurologic deficits and a spectrum of vascular damage from vasculopathy to vasculitis, with stroke.[177,178] Both large and small vessels can be involved, and MRI shows multifocal ischemic lesions, commonly at gray-white matter junctions. The diagnosis of VZV can be missed when symptoms and signs occur months after zoster, or in the absence of a typical zoster rash. Among 14 patients with VZV-related vasculopathy described in the literature for whom detailed clinicopathologic data were available, only one patient presented with headache, fever, mental status change, and focal neurologic deficits, and focal narrowing of the ICA, anterior cerebral artery (ACA) and MCA, and antibody to VZV in CSF, without a rash,[179] in whom VZV DNA and VZV-specific antigen was found in three of five cerebral arteries examined with histologically confirmed CNS vasculitis involving the circle of Willis. Patient 1 reported by Eidelberg and colleagues,[180] who presented with headache and herpes zoster ophthalmicus (HZO) rash, was deemed to have CNS vasculitis based on complete occlusion of the MCA; however, postmortem examination showed no evidence of vasculitis. Headache was not mentioned in 5 other patients despite histologically proven widespread small-vessel granulomatous angiitis associated with lymphoma in 2 patients[181] and basilar branch vessel involvement of granulomatous angiitis in another.[182] One patient with contralateral hemiplegia one month after HZO was found at postmortem examination to have endarteritis of unilateral ACA, MCA, and PCA[183] with VZV DNA from the involved vessels. One patient with AIDS, unilateral weakness, and garbled speech caused by ischemic infarction in association with lumbosacral zoster rash was found to have CNS vasculitis of vessels of the circle of Willis with VZV DNA without herpetic inclusions at postmortem examination. Neither headache nor supporting histopathology was present in seven other patients with VZV vasculopathy, including five patients with HZO and contralateral hemiparesis,[184] and two patients with HZO and contralateral delayed hemiparesis.[185]

More recently, Nagel and colleagues[186] analyzed virus-infected cerebral and temporal arteries from three patients with VZV vasculopathy. Several characteristic were noted in all VZV-infected arteries studied, including disrupted internal elastic lamina, hyperplastic intima composed of cells expressing smooth muscle actin and smooth muscle myosin heavy chain but not endothelial cells expressing CD31, and decreased medial smooth muscle cells. The location of VZV antigen, degree of neo-intimal thickening, and disruption of the median were related to the duration of disease, wherein the presence of VZV primarily in adventitia early in infection and in the media and intimal later supported the hypothesis that after reactivation from ganglia, VZV spread transaxonally to the arterial adventitia followed by transmural spread of virus. Stroke in VZV vasculopathy appeared to result from changes in arterial caliber and contractility produced in part by abnormal accumulation of smooth muscle cells and myofibroblasts in thickened neointimal and disruption of the media.[186] Nagel and colleagues[187] studied the immune characteristics of virus-infected temporal artery three days after onset of ischemic optic neuropathy, and in the MCA after 10 months of protracted CNS disease. In both early and later VZV vasculopathy, T-cells, activated macrophages, and rare B-cells were found in adventitia and intima, whereas neutrophils and VZV antigen were abundant along with a thickened intima associated with inflammatory cells in vaso vasorum vessels. In the media of late VZV vasculopathy, viral antigen but not leukocytes was found and VZV was not found in inflammatory cells.

Fungal Infection

Four fungal species, *Aspergillus*, *Candida*, *Coccidiodes*, and *Mucormycetes*, can lead to opportunistic infection in immunocompromised and severely disabled hosts and have the capacity to invade arteries of the CNS. Cysticercosis, the most common parasitic infection of the nervous system caused by the tapeworm *Taenia solium*, leads to tissue cysts in the CNS within the subarachnoid space and basal cisterns, producing an arachnoiditis and small-vessel angiitis with resulting tissue infarction. Histopathologically confirmed fungal arteritis of cerebral vasculitis has rarely been reported; however, Shigenaga and colleagues[188] described a 62-year-old farmer with palpitation, shortness of breath, dizziness, malaise, and aplastic anemia treated with corticosteroids. Two months later he developed frontal headache, fever, tetraplegia, and fatal coma. Postmortem examination showed thromboendarteritis of the circle of Willis arteries, leptomeningitis, meningoencephalitis, and softening of the brain. The ACA and MCA showed aspergillotic arteritis involving all layers of the vessel wall by polymorphonuclear leukocytes, lymphocytes, and plasma cells, with complete occlusion of the lumen, distention and thinning of the walls, and extension of the inflammatory reaction to the adventitia. Headache was not mentioned in the description by Davidson and Robertson[189] of a 75-year-old farmer who lapsed into sudden fatal unconsciousness and was found to have a mycotic basilar artery aneurysm. Microscopic examination of the affected vessel showed focal necrosis of all layers and heavy infiltration by neutrophils and occasional mononuclear cells admixed with thrombus of varying ages and *Aspergillus* hyphae situated parallel to the vessel wall. Frontal headache was the presenting symptom of a 74-year-old man described by Wollschlaeger and colleagues,[190] who was later found to have an intrasellar mass on cerebral angiography, biopsy of which showed *Aspergillus* granuloma of the pituitary gland, which infiltrated the ICA within the cavernous sinus, with branching hyphae of septated fungus extending into the lumen of the artery and forming a massive organizing thrombus.

HIV/AIDS

Early in the HIV/AIDS epidemic, it was clear that many infected persons were intravenous drug users. Their associated risk behavior exposed them to infection through sharing of contaminated needles, thereby increasing the risk of spread of HIV and other blood-borne infections. The two postulated periods in the neurobiology of HIV when autoimmune disease manifestations can occur that seem to be significant for the development of cerebral vasculitis are shortly after seroconversion and before the spread of productive infection, and after initiation of highly active antiretroviral therapy (HAART) in association with the immune reconstitution inflammatory syndrome (IRIS).[191] The timing of early HIV invasion has been difficult to ascertain based on the presence of one or more well-recognized clinicopathologic HIV/AIDS syndromes, including HIV encephalitis, HIV-associated dementia, and AIDS dementia complex,[192–194] all of which indicate symptomatic infection.

Headache associated with irritation and confusion was the presenting feature of a 42-year-old homosexual man without evidence of immunodeficiency who developed cerebral granulomatous angiitis in association with human T-lymphotropic virus type III (HTLV-III). At postmortem examination, there was evidence of fibrous intimal scarring and marked luminal narrowing of the ACA, MCA, and PCA and their proximal branches, with mononuclear cell infiltration of the vessel walls and numerous multinucleated giant cells near the internal elastic lamina. However, headache was not mentioned in the description of six presymptomatic HIV-seropositive drug abusers reported by Gray and colleagues[147] with nonnecrotizing cerebral vasculitis studied at postmortem examination, nor in seven other patients reported by Bell and colleagues[195] with lymphocytic infiltration of the walls of leptomeningeal and subarachnoid veins. Headache was also not mentioned in the clinicopathologic description of 23 intravenous drug users from the Edinburgh HIV Autopsy Cohort described by Bell and colleagues[195] who died suddenly after seroconversion but while still in the presymptomatic stage of HIV infection compared with ten HIV-negative intravenous drug users, twelve nonintravenous drug user controls, or in nine patients with full-blown AIDS, who also died suddenly. Seven of the presymptomatic HIV-positive patients showed infiltration of T-cells in the walls of veins in association with low-grade lymphocytic meningitis; seven others showed isolated lymphocytic meningitis, and one patient had focal perivascular lymphocytic cuffing and macrophage collections throughout the central white matter tissue of the brain and in basal ganglia. Headache was not a conspicuous complaint in early HIV-associated hemophilia[196] even among patients who died suddenly of intracranial hemorrhage and liver cirrhosis with comparable neuropathologic changes of gliosis, occasional microglial nodules, perivascular mononuclear infiltrates, and leptomeningeal meningitis, without multinucleated giant cells or evidence of HIV in the brain. The introduction of HAART has changed the incidence, course, and prognosis of the neurologic complications of HIV infection concomitant with almost undetectable viral load in plasma and an increase in circulating T-lymphocytes. Headache was not mentioned in the only pathologically confirmed patient with cerebral vasculitis and IRIS described by van der Ven and colleagues.[197]

LABORATORY EVALUATION

There is general agreement on four principles in the diagnosis of vasculitis. First, vasculitis is a potentially serious disorder, with a propensity for permanent disability, as a result of tissue ischemia and infarction; recognition of the neurologic manifestations is important in developing a differential causative diagnosis. Second, undiagnosed and untreated, the outcome of vasculitis is potentially fatal. Third, a favorable response to an empirical course of immunosuppressive and immunomodulating therapy should never be considered a substitute for the absolute proof of the diagnosis of vasculitis. Fourth, histopathologic confirmation of vasculitis in the nervous system is essential for accurate diagnosis, such as by brain and meninges when there is CNS involvement, and analysis of nerve and muscle biopsy tissue when PNS involvement is postulated.

The laboratory evaluation of vasculitis of the CNS is summarized in **Box 2**. Serologically specific serum studies should be obtained in all patients guided by the clinical presentation and postulated causative diagnosis to avoid excessive cost and spurious results. Electrodiagnostic studies are useful in the initial investigation of systemic vasculitis, because they can identify areas of asymptomatic involvement and sites for muscle and nerve biopsy and distinguish the various neuropathic syndromes associated with peripheral nerve and muscle involvement. A wide sampling of nerves and muscles should be examined, both distal and proximal, using standard recording and needle electrodes for the performance of nerve conduction studies and needle electromyography (EMG), at skin temperatures of 34°C, with comparison to normative data. Most patients with peripheral nerve vasculitis (PNV) show evidence of active axonopathy acutely in an MNM pattern and over time in a distal symmetric or asymmetric pattern. Quantitative motor unit potential analysis can delineate whether proximal wasting and weakness are caused by myopathic or neurogenic disease.

CSF analysis, electroencephalography (EEG), and neuroimaging studies are integral to the diagnostic evaluation of most CNS disorders, including vasculitis. Properly performed, lumbar puncture carries minimal risk and provides potentially useful information regarding possible underlying vasculitis, as suggested by CSF pleocytosis in excess of 5 cells/mm³, increase in protein level greater than 100 mg/dL, and evidence of intrathecal synthesis of immunoglobulin or oligoclonal bands. Molecular genetic, immunoassay, and direct staining techniques to exclude spirochetal, fungal, mycobacterial, and viral infections, as well as cytospin examination of CSF for possible malignant cells, should be performed. Although there are no typical electrographic findings in CNS vasculitis, EEG should be performed to screen for epileptogenic foci. MRI is more sensitive than CT, but both methods lack specificity in histologically-confirmed cases. The most common MRI findings are multiple bilateral cortical and deep white matter signal abnormalities and enhancement of the meninges after gadolinium. MRA and functional imaging of the brain provide complementary findings to conventional MRI. The former is useful in the evaluation of medium-vessel and

---

Box 2
Laboratory evaluation of headache and vasculitis

Blood studies

Screening: CBC, ESR, comprehensive chemistry panel, CK, ANA, T-cell and B-cell subset panel, hepatitis B and C serology, two-tier Lyme (ELISA and confirmatory Western blot), acute and convalescent viral titers, HIV-1.

Disease-specific serology: C1q, CH50, RF, cryoglobulins, SSA, SSB, RNP, Sm IgG, ACL, APL antibodies, LAC, ds DNA antibody, HTLV-III screening antibody, IF ANCA; HLA haplotypes.

Radiologic studies

Screening: 3-T MRI and MRA of the brain and neck vessels; USG of the temporal arteries and great vessels, nuclear medicine perfusion SPECT, EMG and NCS, and EEG.

Second tier: MRI, MRA, and [18F]FDG body PET-CT, systemic and cerebral DSA, and CSF analysis via lumbar puncture (protein, glucose, cell count, IgG level, oligoclonal bands, cytology, VDRL, bacterial Gram stain, India ink; viral encephalitis panel, Lyme total antibody and Western blot, Lyme PCR, viral PCR; bacterial, viral, fungal and TB cultures, Paraneoplastic and antineuronal antibodies).

Histopathologic studies

Punch skin biopsy with immunofluorescence; open biopsy of the sural or superficial fibular sensory nerve and corresponding soleus or peroneus brevis muscle; leptomeningeal and cortical brain biopsy.

Abbreviations: [18F]FDG body PET-CT, [18F]fluorodeoxyglucose body positron emission tomography-computed tomography; ACL, anticardiolipin antibody; ANA, antinuclear antibody; APL, antiphospholipid antibody; CBC, complete blood count; CK, creatine kinase; ds, double stranded; DSA, digital subtraction angiography; EEG, electroencephalography; ELISA, enzyme-linked immunosorbent assay; EMG, electromyography; ESR, erythrocyte sedimentation rate; HIV-I, human immunodeficiency virus type I; HLA; human leukocyte antigen; IF ANCA, immunofluorescence antineutrophil cytoplasmic antibody; LAC, lupus anticoagulant; MRI, magnetic resonance imaging; MRA, magnetic resonance angiography; NCS, nerve conduction studies; PCR, polymerase chain reaction; RNP, ribonucleoprotein; Sm, smith; SPECT, single-photon emission computed tomography; SSA, sjogren SSA/Ro; SSB, sjogren SSB/La; TB, tuberculosis; USG, ultrasonography.

---

large-vessel disease, but miss fine-vessel contours better seen on cut-film or digital subtraction angiography. The abnormal diffuse and focal perfusion patterns seen on single-photon emission CT do not always correlate with neurologic symptoms or distinguish vasculitic from nonvasculitic vasculopathy. Beading of vessels, the sine qua non of cerebral vasculitis, is found in only about a third of patients with histologically-proven CNS vasculitis, as well as in CNS infection, atherosclerosis, cerebral embolism, and vasospasm of diverse cause. Multiple microaneurysms, often seen on visceral angiography in systemic vasculitis, are rare in CNS vessels.

Brain, spinal cord, and meningeal biopsy are the gold standard for the diagnosis of CNS vasculitis, but false-negative results occur because of focal lesions and sampling errors. Radiographic studies that guide the biopsy site toward areas of abnormality probably improve the sensitivity, but this has not been formally studied. The risk of serious morbidity related to biopsy is less than 2.0% at most centers, which is probably less than the cumulative risk of an empirical course of long-term immunosuppressive therapy. There are no certain guidelines as to when to proceed to brain and meningeal biopsy. However, it would certainly be warranted if there were no other explanation for the progressive syndrome of fever, headache, encephalopathy, and focal cerebral signs, in association with CSF pleocytosis, and protein content increase greater than 100 mg/dL, which is suggestive of GANS. Open biopsy of a cutaneous nerve is indispensable in the evaluation of all forms of PNV. First recommended by Harry Lee Parker in a discussion of the article by Woltman and Kernohan in 1938,[27] biopsy of the superficial peroneal musculocutaneous nerve and peroneus brevis muscle was later implemented in the histopathologic diagnosis of PAN in several patients with mononeuritis multiplex.[198,199] A quarter of a century later, a series of investigations established the importance of cutaneous nerve biopsy in the definition of PNV.[200–202] The Peripheral Nerve Society has published guidelines for the histopathologic diagnosis of PNV.[203]

TREATMENT

Neurologists treating vasculitis must choose the sequence and combination of available immunosuppressant and immunomodulating therapies to induce and sustain remission and treat relapses, recognizing the possible beneficial and adverse effects. The management of systemic vasculitis has recently been reviewed.[204] When headache is a result of cerebral vasculitis, it remits along with other features of CNS involvement, such that it is a useful feature to follow with presumptively effective vasculitis therapy. In other circumstances, headache may be a side effect of the vasculitic therapy. The specific treatment and prevention of headache in children and adults apart from vasculitis is beyond the scope of this article and is reviewed elsewhere.[205–207] A systematic approach to the treatment of CNS vasculitis in the setting of headache is shown in **Box 3**.

The usefulness of corticosteroids in the treatment of systemic vasculitis has been appreciated for more than 50 years; however, there has never been a randomized controlled trial conducted to support their use. The beneficial effects of corticosteroids are attributed to a multiplicity of effects on the cell and humoral immune system, including inhibition of activated T-and B-cells, antigen-presenting cells, and leukocytes at sites of inflammation, interferon γ, induced major histocompatibility complex class II expression, macrophage differentiation, pathogenic cytokine expression, complement interactions, and immunomodulating cell adhesion molecules (CAM). Patients receiving long-term corticosteroid therapy for vasculitis should be monitored closely for hypertension, fluid retention, glucose intolerance, cataracts, myopathy, avascular necrosis, osteoporosis, infection, gastric and duodenal ulcers, and psychosis, and followed empirically for the need of short-acting insulin coverage as needed, physiotherapy, calcium supplementation, and bone densitometry. The effectiveness of a daily oral regimen of 2 mg/kg/d or oral cyclophosphamide with prednisone in GPA served as a template for the treatment of virtually all types of systemic vasculitis for decades,[208] and together, they remain the standard treatment of inducing remission in virtually all forms of potentially fatal systemic vasculitis. Although 75% to 90% of patients with GPA and other AAV achieve remission with oral or intravenous cyclophosphamide, few data are available on therapeutic strategies for patients with disease refractory to this first-line therapy. Its favorable effect on vasculitis derives from the preferential T-cell lysis resulting from the inhibition of hematopoietic precursors in the bone marrow, leaving stem cells unharmed. At high doses, this inhibition favors repopulation of the marrow and thus the cellular immune system. After an intravenous dose of cyclophosphamide, the nadir of peripheral leukopenia, which corresponded with peak marrow suppression, occurred in 7 to 18 days. Less

---

Box 3
Recommendations for the treatment of vasculitides

Large-vessel vasculitis: GCA, TAK

    CS[221,222]

    AZA,[223] rituximab,[224] infliximab,[225] anti-TNF-α, anti-IL-6R[226,227] and tocilizumab[228]

    Adjunctive therapy: ASA[229] and AC[230]

Medium-vessel vasculitis: PAN, KD

    CS and CYC[231–233]

Small-vessel vasculitis: AAV, immune complex vasculitis

    ANCA-associated vasculitis

        GPA, EGPA, MPA: induction with CS + CYC[208,234,235] or CS + rituximab[211,212,236–239] and maintenance with rituximab[240–245] or AZA[212,246,247]

    Immune complex vasculitis

        CV: INF-α[248–250] and PegINF-α plus ribovarin[248,251] or rituximab[252] in HCV-associated mixed cryoglobulinemia

        IgA vasculitis: CS[253]

        Supportive

    Hypocomplementic-C1q: antihistamines, IVIg, plasmapheresis

Variable-vessel vasculitis: BD, CS

    CS,[80,254] colchicine or anti-TNF-α[255]

Single-organ vasculitis

    Isolated aortitis

        CS[224,256]

        AZA, MM, MTX[256]

    Primary CNS vasculitis: induction with CS[100,101,257] or CS + CYC,[100,104,257,258] followed by maintenance with AZA,[257] MTX, or MM[259]

Vasculitis associated with systemic disease

    Systemic lupus erythematosus

        Corticosteroids[111] and anticoagulation[118]

    Rheumatoid vasculitis

        CS,[128] rituximab,[260,261] infliximab,[217,262] and AZA or MTX[263]

Vasculitic associated with illicit substance abuse

    Avoid illicit substance

Vasculitis associated with infection

    Antimicrobial agents chosen specifically to treat a given causative organism

Abbreviations: AC, anticoagulation; ASA, aspirin; AZA, azathioprine; CS, corticosteroids; CS, Cogan syndrome; CYC, cyclophosphamide; INF, interferon; IVIg, intravenous immunoglobulin; MM, mycophenolate mofetil; MTX, methotrexate; PegINF, pegylated interferon.

than 20% of labeled cyclophosphamide is excreted unchanged in the urine. The toxic side effects include hemorrhagic cystitis, bladder cancer, bone marrow suppression, and the risk of fatal infection and gonadal toxicity. Bladder toxicity may be reduced by administration of the drug in a single daily oral morning dose followed by hydration, and administration of the drug intravenously as pulse therapy, adjusting the dose to renal function. Intravenous cyclophosphamide, which can be administered as pulse therapy based on body surface area, is as effective as and less toxic than oral cyclophosphamide in achieving remission of AAV.[209,210]

Rituximab is a chimeric monoclonal anti-CD20 antibody that selectively depletes B-cells but not plasma cells. The RITUXVAS (Rituximab Versus Cyclophosphamide in ANCA-Associated Vasculitis) study[211] reported nonsuperiority of rituximab to standard intravenous cyclophosphamide for severe AAV, with high sustained remission rates in both groups. Rituximab-based therapy was not associated with reductions in early adverse events. The RAVE (Rituximab in ANCA-Associated Vasculitis) study[212] found that rituximab was not inferior to daily cyclophosphamide treatment of induction of remission in severe AAV and possibly superior in relapsing disease.

Treatment with activity against TNF-α seems to be important in AAV and other systemic vasculitides. In animal models, inhibition of TNF-α markedly decreased the development of bactericidal granulomas during bacille Calmette-Guérin infection.[213] CD4+ T-cells from patients with GPA are associated with HLA-DR+ CD4+ T-cells showing an unbalanced Th1-type cytokine pattern and increased levels of TNF-α.[214] Moreover, serum levels of TNF-α receptor correlate with disease activity and TNF-α-positive cells infiltrate renal lesions.[215] Treatment with the dimeric soluble TNF receptor etanercept was not effective for the maintenance of remission in patients with GPA, and durable remissions were achieved in only a few patients, with a high rate of treatment-related complications, including the development of solid cancers in 6 patients in the etanercept group compared with none in the control group.[216] In a pilot study, the anti-TNF-α antibody infliximab[217] was well tolerated during short-term follow-up and successfully induced prompt symptomatic responses in those with systemic vasculitis not responding to conventional treatments, including 7 patients with GPA, two with RV, and one with CV of mean duration of 9, 21.5, and 17 years, respectively, with no major side effects.

Oral methotrexate at the dose of 20 to 25 mg/wk with prednisolone was as effective as oral cyclophosphamide 2 mg/kg/d with prednisolone, which was tapered and withdrawn over 12 months in the initial treatment of early nonsevere AAV[218]; however, the methotrexate regimen was less effective for induction of remission in those with extensive disease and pulmonary involvement and associated with more relapses than cyclophosphamide after termination of treatment. The high relapse rates in both treatment groups supported the practice of continuing immunosuppressive treatment beyond 12 months. The reported adverse effects of methotrexate in that study[218] included infection, leukopenia, hypertension, liver dysfunction, nausea, and vomiting.

The purine analogue azathioprine, which metabolizes to the cytotoxic derivative 6-mercaptopurine, exerts favorable action in vasculitis by the inhibition of T-cell activation and T-cell-dependent antibody-mediated responses. Azathioprine is generally considered a safe, although less effective, alternative agent to prednisone and cyclophosphamide in virtually all forms of vasculitis. However, there are 3 drawbacks to its use. First, idiosyncratic side effects, most often gastrointestinal and flulike, occur in approximately 10% of patients and rarely necessitate permanent withdrawal of the medication. However, pancreatitis and gastritis severe enough to warrant hospitalization can occur. Second, bone marrow suppression occurs in nearly all patients, usually manifested by mild pancytopenia. Third, there is typically a long delay in the onset of the therapeutic effect of three months or more. Taking all of these factors into account, most clinicians concur with the slow advancement of the dose over weeks, commencing with 50 mg/d and achieving maintenance levels of 2 to 3 mg/kg/d with careful monitoring of liver and marrow function.

High-dose intravenous immune globulin (IVIg) therapy is the most widely used immunomodulating agent for autoimmune neurologic disorders.[219] It is alternative therapy for CNS and PNS vasculitis, and diverse connective tissue disorders. Among 22 patients with relapsing AAV, including nineteen with GPA and three MPA, IVIg was administered at the dose of 0.5 g/kg/d for four days as additional therapy monthly for 6 months in conjunction with corticosteroids and immunosuppressants (21 patients).[220] IVIg induced complete remissions of relapsed AAV in 13 of 22 patients at nine months. The immunomodulating and anti-inflammatory actions of IVIg are provided by monthly doses of 2000 mg/kg/body weight given 400 to 500 mg/kg per day, respectively, over 4 to 5 days each month at a slow drip with acetaminophen and diphenhydramine pretreatment to prevent the commonest side effects, including headache, fever, chills, rash, erythema, flushing, nausea, myalgia, arthralgia, abdominal cramps, and chest and back pain. True anaphylactic reactions to IVIg can occur in recipients with documented previous allergies to immune globulins or antibodies, especially IgA type. Transient reversible renal insufficiency occurs in individuals with preexisting renal disease. Susceptible individuals can be identified by less than normal expected 24-hour creatinine clearance rates for age and abnormal vascular perfusion on radionuclide scans. Aseptic meningitis rarely occurs several hours after treatment and resolves over several days with discontinuation of therapy.

REFERENCES

1. Younger DS. Headaches and vasculitis. Neurol Clin 2004;22:207–28.
2. Younger DS, Younger AP. CNS vasculitis. In: Coyle P, Rivzi S, editors. Clinical neuroimmunology: multiple sclerosis and related disorders. Springer; 2011. p. 307–29.
3. Younger DS. Adult and childhood vasculitis of the nervous system. In: Younger DS, editor. Motor disorders. New York: Younger DS; 2013. p. 235–80.
4. Jennette JC, Falk RJ, Bacon PA, et al. 2012 revised International Chapel Hill Consensus Conference Nomenclature of Vasculitides. Arthritis Rheum 2013; 65:1–11.
5. Ozen S, Ruperto N, Dillon MJ, et al. EULAR/PRES endorsed consensus criteria for the classification of childhood vasculitides. Ann Rheum Dis 2006;65: 936–41.
6. Neuwelt EA, Bauer B, Fahlke C, et al. Engaging neuroscience to advance translational research in brain barrier biology. Nat Rev Neurosci 2011;12:169–82.
7. Benarroch EE. Blood-brain barrier. Recent developments and clinical correlations. Neurology 2012;78:1268–74.
8. Ek CJ, Dziegielewska KM, Habgood MD, et al. Barriers in the developing brain and neurotoxicology. Neurotoxicology 2012;33:586–604.
9. Charles A. The evolution of a migraine attack–a review of recent evidence. Headache 2013;53:413–9.
10. Edvinsson L, Tfelt-Hansen P. The blood-brain barrier in migraine treatment. Cephalalgia 2008;28:1245–58.
11. Daneman R. The blood brain barrier in health and disease. Ann Neurol 2012;72: 648–72.
12. Blair RJ, Ross JJ, Morris A, et al. A sleeping giant. N Engl J Med 2011;365:72–7.

13. Hunder GG, Bloch DA, Michel BA, et al. The American College of Rheumatology 1990 criteria for the classification of giant cell arteritis. Arthritis Rheum 1990;33: 1122–8.
14. Blockmans D, Bley T, Schmidt W. Imaging for large-vessel vasculitis. Curr Opin Rheumatol 2009;21:19–28.
15. Salvarani C, Cantini F, Boiardi L, et al. Polymyalgia rheumatica and giant-cell arteritis. N Engl J Med 2002;347:261–71.
16. Nakao K, Ikeda M, Kimata SI, et al. Takayasu's arteritis: clinical report of eighty-four cases and immunologic studies of seven cases. Circulation 1967;35:1141–55.
17. Riehl JL, Brown J. Takayasu's disease. Arch Neurol 1965;12:92–7.
18. Kerr GS, Hallahan CW, Giordano J, et al. Takayasu arteritis. Ann Intern Med 1994;120:919–29.
19. Graham JR. Migraine (clinical aspects). Handb Clin Neurol 1968;5:45–58.
20. Manno RL, Levine SM, Gelber AC. More than meets the eye. Semin Arthritis Rheum 2011;40:324–9.
21. Arend WP, Michel BA, Bloch DA, et al. The American College of Rheumatology 1990 criteria for the classification of Takayasu arteritis. Arthritis Rheum 1990;33: 1129–34.
22. Grayson PC, Maksimowicz-McKinnon K, Clark TM, et al. Distribution of arterial lesions in Takayasu's arteritis and giant cell arteritis. Ann Rheum Dis 2012;71: 1329–34.
23. Stone JR. Aortitis, periaortitis, and retroperitoneal fibrosis, as manifestations of IgG4-related systemic disease. Curr Opin Rheumatol 2011;23:88–94.
24. Pipitone N, Salvarani C. Idiopathic aortitis: an underrecognized vasculitis. Arthritis Res Ther 2011;13:119.
25. Gornik HL, Creager MA. Aortitis. Circulation 2008;117:3039–51.
26. Stone JH, Khosroshahi A, Deshpande V, et al. IgG4-related systemic disease accounts for a significant proportion of thoracic lymphoplasmacytic aortitis cases. Arthritis Care Res 2010;62:316–22.
27. Kernohan JW, Woltman HW. Periarteritis nodosa: a clinicopathologic study with special reference to the nervous system. Arch Neurol 1938;39:655–86.
28. Kawasaki T. Acute febrile mucocutaneous syndrome with lymphoid involvement with specific desquamation of the fingers and toes in children. Arerugi 1967;16: 178–222 [in Japanese].
29. Hirose S, Hamashima Y. Morphological observations on the vasculitis in the mucocutaneous lymph node syndrome. A skin biopsy study of 27 patients. Eur J Pediatr 1978;129:17–27.
30. Yun SH, Yang NR, Park SA. Associated symptoms of Kawasaki disease. Korean Circ J 2011;41:394–8.
31. Constantinescu CS. Migraine and Raynaud phenomenon: possible late complications of Kawasaki disease. Headache 2002;42:227–9.
32. Savage CO, Winearls CG, Evans DJ, et al. Microscopic polyarteritis: presentation, pathology and prognosis. QJM 1985;220:467–83.
33. Hagen EC, Daha MR, Hermans J, et al. Diagnostic value of standardized assays for anti-neutrophil cytoplasmic antibodies in idiopathic systemic vasculitis: EC/BCR Project for ANCA Assay Standardization. Kidney Int 1998;53:743–53.
34. Drachman DA. Neurological complications of Wegener's granulomatosis. Arch Neurol 1963;8:45–55.
35. Churg J, Strauss L. Allergic granulomatosis, allergic angiitis, and periarteritis nodosa. Am J Pathol 1951;27:277–301.

36. North I, Strek ME, Leff AR. Churg-Strauss syndrome. Lancet 2003;361:587–94.
37. Masi AT, Hunder GG, Lie JT, et al. The American College of Rheumatology 1990 criteria for the classification of Churg-Strauss syndrome (allergic granulomatosis and angiitis). Arthritis Rheum 1990;33:1094–100.
38. Hattori N, Ichimura M, Nagamatsu M, et al. Clinicopathological features of Churg-Strauss syndrome-associated neuropathy. Brain 1999;122:427–39.
39. Ferri C, Sebastiani M, Giuggioli D, et al. Mixed cryoglobulinemia: demographic, clinical, and serologic features and survival in 231 patients. Semin Arthritis Rheum 2004;33:355–74.
40. Wintrobe MM, Buell MV. Hyperproteinemia associated with multiple myeloma. With report of a case in which an extraordinary hyperproteinemia was associated with thrombosis of the retinal veins and symptoms suggesting Raynauds disease. Bull Johns Hopkins Hosp 1933;52:156–65.
41. Gorevic PD, Kassab HJ, Levo Y, et al. Mixed cryoglobulinemia: clinical aspects and long-term follow-up of 40 patients. Am J Med 1980;69:287–308.
42. Brouet JC, Clauvel JP, Danon F, et al. Biologic and clinical significance of cryoglobulins: a report of 86 cases. Am J Med 1974;57:775–88.
43. Agnello V, Chung RT, Kaplan LM. A role for hepatitis C virus infection in type II cryoglobulinemia. N Engl J Med 1992;327:1490–5.
44. Origgi L, Vanoli M, Carbone A, et al. Central nervous system involvement in patients with HCV-related cryoglobulin. Am J Med Sci 1998;315:208–10.
45. Cacoub P, Sbai A, Hausfater P, et al. Atteinte neurologique central et infection par le virus de l'hèpatite. Gastroenterol Clin Biol 1998;22:631–3 [in French].
46. Petty GW, Duffy J, Huston J. Cerebral ischemic in patients with hepatitis C virus infection and mixed cryoglobulinemia. Mayo Clin Proc 1996;71:671–8.
47. Díaz de Entre-Sotos FZ, Pérez-Aloe MT, Pérez-Tovar JF. Stroke and limb ischaemia in hepatitis C virus-related cryoglobulinaemia. Ir J Med Sci 2004; 173:57.
48. Ince PG, Duffey P, Cochrane HR, et al. Relapsing ischemic encephalopathy and cryoglobulinemia. Neurology 2000;55:1579–81.
49. Abramsky O, Slavin S. Neurological manifestations in patients with mixed cryoglobulinemia. Neurology 1974;24:245–9.
50. Landau DA, Scerra S, Sene D, et al. Causes and predictive factors of mortality in a cohort of patients with hepatitis C virus-related cryoglobulinemic vasculitis treated with antiviral therapy. J Rheumatol 2010;37:615–21.
51. Ramos-Cassals M, Robles A, Brito-Zeron P, et al. Life-threatening cryoglobulinemia: clinical and immunological characterization of 29 cases. Semin Arthritis Rheum 2006;36:189–96.
52. Wisnieski JJ, Baer AN, Christensen J, et al. Hypocomplementemic urticarial vasculitis syndrome. Clinical and serological findings in 18 patients. Medicine 1995;74:24–41.
53. Katsiari CG, Vikelis M, Paraskevopoulou ES, et al. Headache in systemic lupus erythematosus vs multiple sclerosis: a prospective comparative study. Headache 2011;51:1398–407.
54. Buck A, Christensen J, McCarty M. Hypocomplementemic urticarial vasculitis syndrome. A case report and literature review. J Clin Aesthet Dermatol 2012; 5:36–46.
55. Grotz W, Baba HA, Becker JU, et al. Hypocomplementemic urticarial vasculitis syndrome. Dtsch Arztebl Int 2009;106:756–63.
56. Osler W. The visceral lesions of purpura and allied conditions. BMJ 1914;1: 517–25.

57. Green B. Schöenlein-Henoch purpura with blood in the cerebrospinal fluid. Br Med J 1946;1:836.
58. Lewis IC, Philpott MG. Neurologic complications in the Schöenlein-Henoch purpura syndrome. Arch Dis Child 1956;31:369–71.
59. Belman AL, Leicher CR, Moshe SL, et al. Neurologic manifestations of Schoenlein-Henoch purpura: report of three cases and review of the literature. Pediatrics 1985;75:687–92.
60. Saulsbury FT. Clinical update: Henoch-Schönlein purpura. Lancet 2007;369: 976–8.
61. Trygstad CW, Stiehm ER. Elevated serum IgA globulin in anaphylactoid purpura. Pediatrics 1971;47:1023–8.
62. Levinsky RJ, Barratt TM. IgA immune complexes in Henoch-Schönlein purpura. Lancet 1979;2:1100–3.
63. Conley ME, Cooper MD, Michael AF. Selective deposition of immunoglobulin A_1 in immunoglobulin A nephropathy, anaphylactoid purpura nephritis, and systemic lupus erythematosus. J Clin Invest 1980;66:1432–6.
64. Behcet H, Matteson EL. On relapsing, aphthous ulcers of the mouth, eye and genitalia caused by a virus. 1937. Clin Exp Rheumatol 2010;28(Suppl 60): S2–5.
65. Gökçay F, Celebisoy N, Gökçay A, et al. Neurological symptoms and signs in Behcet disease: a Western Turkey experience. Neurologist 2011;17:147–50.
66. Wolf SM, Schotland DL, Phillips LL. Involvement of nervous system in Behçet's syndrome. Arch Neurol 1965;12:315–25.
67. Saip S, Siva A, Altintas A, et al. Headache in Behçet's syndrome. Headache 2005;45:911–9.
68. McMenemey WH, Lawrence TJ. Encephalomyelopathy in Behçet's disease. Report of necropsy findings in two cases. Lancet 1957;273:353–8.
69. Rubinstein LJ, Urich H. Meningo-encephalitis of Behçet's disease. Case report with pathological findings. Brain 1963;86:151–60.
70. Kawakita H, Nishimura M, Satoh Y, et al. Neurological aspects of Behçet's disease. A case report and clinico-pathological review of the literature in Japan. J Neurol Sci 1967;5:417–39.
71. Arai Y, Kohno S, Takahashi Y, et al. Autopsy case of neuro-Behçet's disease with multifocal neutrophilic perivascular inflammation. Neuropathology 2006;26: 579–85.
72. Koseoglu E, Yildirim A, Borlu M. Is headache in Behçet's disease related to silent neurologic involvement? Clin Exp Rheumatol 2011;29(Supp 67):S32–7.
73. Siva A, Saip S. The spectrum of nervous system involvement in Behcet's syndrome and its differential diagnosis. J Neurol 2009;256:513–29.
74. Hadfield MG, Aydin F, Lippman HR, et al. Neuro-Behçet's disease. Clin Neuropathol 1997;16:55–60.
75. Mogan RF, Baumgarten CJ. Meniere's disease complicated by recurrent interstitial keratitis: excellent results following cervical ganglionectomy. West J Surg 1934;42:628.
76. Cogan DG. Syndrome of nonsyphilitic interstitial keratitis and vestibuloauditory symptoms. Arch Ophthal 1945;33:144–9.
77. Norton EW, Cogan DG. Syndrome of nonsyphilitic interstitial keratitis and vestibuloauditory symptoms. A long-term follow-up. Arch Ophthalmol 1959;61:695–7.
78. Cody DT, Williams HL. Cogan's syndrome. Laryngoscope 1960;70:447–78.
79. Cody DT, Williams HL. Cogan's syndrome. Proc Staff Meet Mayo Clin 1962;37: 372–5.

80. Gluth MB, Baratz KH, Matteson EL, et al. Cogan syndrome: a retrospective review of 60 patients throughout a half century. Mayo Clin Proc 2006;81: 483–8.
81. Pagnini I, Zannin ME, Vittadello F, et al. Clinical features and outcome of Cogan syndrome. J Pediatr 2012;160:303–7.
82. Haynes BF, Kaiser-Kupfer MI, Mason P, et al. Cogan's syndrome: studies in thirteen patients, long-term follow-up, and a review of the literature. Medicine 1980; 59:426–41.
83. Crawford WJ. Cogan's syndrome associated with polyarteritis nodosa. A report of three cases. Pa Med J 1957;60:835–8.
84. Eisenstein B, Taubenhaus M. Nonsyphilitic interstitial keratitis and bilateral deafness (Cogan's syndrome) associated with cardiovascular disease. N Engl J Med 1958;258:1074–9.
85. Cogan DG, Dickersin GR. Nonsyphilitic interstitial keratitis with vestibuloauditory symptoms. A case with fatal aortitis. Arch Ophthalmol 1964;71:172–5.
86. Fisher ER, Hellstrom HR. Cogan's syndrome and systemic vascular disease. Analysis of pathological features with reference to its relationship to thromboangiitis obliterans (Buerger). Arch Pathol 1961;72:572–92.
87. Oliner L, Taubenhaus M, Shapira TM, et al. Nonsyphilitic interstitial keratitis and bilateral deafness (Cogan's syndrome) associated with essential polyangiitis (periarteritis nodosa). A review of the syndrome with consideration of a possible pathogenic mechanism. N Engl J Med 1953;248:1001–8.
88. Leff TL. Cogan's syndrome: ocular pathology. N Y State J Med 1967;67: 2249–57.
89. Gelfand ML, Kantor T, Gorstein F. Cogan's syndrome with cardiovascular involvement: aortic insufficiency. Bull N Y Acad Med 1972;48:647–60.
90. Cheson BD, Bluming AZ, Alroy J. Cogan's syndrome: a systemic vasculitis. Am J Med 1976;60:549–55.
91. Del Caprio J, Espinozea LR, Osterland SK. Cogan's syndrome in HLA Bw 17 [letter]. N Engl J Med 1976;295:1262–3.
92. Pinals RS. Cogan's syndrome with arthritis and aortic insufficiency. J Rheumatol 1978;5:294–8.
93. Hernandez-Rodriguez J, Hoffman GS. Updating single-organ vasculitis. Curr Opin Rheumatol 2012;24:38–45.
94. Hinck V, Carter C, Rippey C. Giant cell (cranial) arteritis. A case with angiographic abnormalities. Am J Roentgenol Radium Ther Nucl Med 1964;92: 769–75.
95. Cupps T, Fauci A. Central nervous system vasculitis. Major Probl Intern Med 1981;21:123–32.
96. Cupps TR, Moore PM, Fauci AS. Isolated angiitis of the central nervous system. Prospective diagnostic and therapeutic experience. Am J Med 1983;74: 97–105.
97. Calabrese HL, Mallek JA. Primary angiitis of the central nervous system: report of 8 new cases, review of the literature, and proposal for diagnostic criteria. Medicine 1988;67:20–39.
98. Younger DS, Hays AP, Brust JC, et al. Granulomatous angiitis of the brain. An inflammatory reaction of diverse etiology. Arch Neurol 1988;45:514–8.
99. Younger DS, Calabrese LH, Hays AP. Granulomatous angiitis of the nervous system. Neurol Clin 1997;15:821–34.
100. Salvarani C, Brown RD Jr, Calamia KT, et al. Primary central nervous system vasculitis: analysis of 101 patients. Ann Neurol 2007;62:442–51.

101. Hajj-Ali RA, Calabrese LH. Central nervous system vasculitis. Curr Opin Rheumatol 2009;21:10–8.
102. Lanthier S, Lortie A, Michaud J, et al. Isolated angiitis of the CNS in children. Neurology 2001;56:837–42.
103. Benseler SM. Central nervous system vasculitis in children. Curr Rheumatol Rep 2006;8:442–9.
104. Benseler SM, deVerber G, Hawkins C, et al. Angiographically-negative primary central nervous system vasculitis in children: a newly recognized inflammatory central nervous system disease. Arthritis Rheum 2005;52:2159–67.
105. Elbers J, Halliday W, Hawkins C, et al. Brain biopsy in children with primary small-vessel central nervous system vasculitis. Ann Neurol 2010;68:602–10.
106. Twilt M, Sheikh S, Cellucci T, et al. Recognizing childhood inflammatory brain diseases in Canada. Presse Med 2013;42:670.
107. Klemperer P. Diseases of the collagen system. Bull N Y Acad Med 1947;23:581–8.
108. Klemperer P. The pathogenesis of lupus erythematosus and allied conditions. Ann Intern Med 1948;28:1–11.
109. Borowoy AM, Pope JE, Silverman E, et al. Neuropsychiatric lupus: the prevalence and autoantibody associations depend on the definition: results from the 100 Faces of Lupus Cohort. Semin Arthritis Rheum 2012;42:179–85.
110. The American College of Rheumatology nomenclature and case definitions for neuropsychiatric lupus syndrome. Arthritis Rheum 1999;42:599–608.
111. Tomic-Lucic A, Petrovic R, Radak-Perovic M, et al. Late-onset systemic lupus erythematosus: clinical features, course, and prognosis. Clin Rheumatol 2013;32(7):1053–8.
112. Johnson RT, Richardson EP. The neurological manifestations of systemic lupus erythematosus. Medicine 1968;47:337–69.
113. Estes D, Christian CL. The natural history of systemic lupus erythematosus by prospective analysis. Medicine 1971;50:85–95.
114. Devinsky O, Petito CK, Alonso DR. Clinical and neuropathological findings in systemic lupus erythematosus: the role of vasculitis, heart emboli, and thrombotic thrombocytopenic purpura. Ann Neurol 1988;23:380–4.
115. Feinglass EJ, Arnett FC, Dorsch CA, et al. Neuropsychiatric manifestations of systemic lupus erythematosus: diagnosis, clinical spectrum, and relationship to other features of the disease. Medicine 1976;55:323–39.
116. Mintz G, Fraga A. Arteritis in systemic lupus erythematosus. Arch Intern Med 1965;116:55–66.
117. Trevor RP, Sondheimer FK, Fessel WJ, et al. Angiographic demonstration of major cerebral vessel occlusion in systemic lupus erythematosus. Neuroradiology 1972;4:202–7.
118. Younger DS, Sacco R, Levine SR, et al. Major cerebral vessel occlusion in SLE due to circulating anticardiolipin antibodies. Stroke 1994;25:912–4.
119. Khamashta MA, Cervera R, Hughes GR. The central nervous system in systemic lupus erythematosus. Rheumatol Int 1991;11:117–9.
120. Levine SR, Welch KM. The spectrum of neurologic disease associated with antiphospholipid antibodies. Arch Neurol 1987;44:876–83.
121. McCaffrey LM, Petelin A, Cunha BA. Systemic lupus erythematosus (SLE) cerebritis versus *Listeria monocytogenes* meningoencephalitis in a patient with systemic lupus erythematosus on chronic corticosteroid therapy: the diagnostic importance of cerebrospinal fluid (CSF) of lactic acid levels. Heart Lung 2012;41:394–7.

122. Aletaha D, Neogi T, Silman AJ. 2010 rheumatoid arthritis classification criteria. An American College of Rheumatology/European League Against Rheumatism Collaborative Initiative. Arthritis Rheum 2010;62:2569–81.

123. Turesson C. Extra-articular rheumatoid arthritis. Curr Opin Rheumatol 2013;25: 360–6.

124. Voskuyl AE, Zwinderman AH, Westedt ML, et al. The mortality of rheumatoid vasculitis compared with rheumatoid arthritis. Arthritis Rheum 1996;39: 266–71.

125. Pirani CL, Bennett GA. Rheumatoid arthritis; a report of three cases progressing from childhood and emphasizing certain systemic manifestations. Bull Hosp Joint Dis 1951;12:335–67.

126. Kemper JW, Baggenstoss AH, Slocumb CH. The relationship of therapy with cortisone to the incidence of vascular lesions in rheumatoid arthritis. Ann Intern Med 1957;46:831–51.

127. Sokoloff L, Bunim JJ. Vascular lesions in rheumatoid arthritis. J Chronic Dis 1957;5:668–87.

128. Johnson RL, Smyth CJ, Holt GW, et al. Steroid therapy and vascular lesions in rheumatoid arthritis. Arthritis Rheum 1959;2:224–49.

129. Steiner JW, Gelbloom AJ. Intracranial manifestations in two cases of systemic rheumatoid disease. Arthritis Rheum 1959;2:537–45.

130. Ouyang R, Mitchell DM, Rozdilsky B. Central nervous system involvement in rheumatoid disease. Neurology 1967;17:1099–105.

131. Ramos M, Mandybur TI. Cerebral vasculitis in rheumatoid arthritis. Arch Neurol 1975;32:271–5.

132. Watson P, Fekete J, Deck J. Central nervous system vasculitis in rheumatoid arthritis. Can J Neurol Sci 1977;4:269–72.

133. Citron BP, Halpern M, Mccarron M, et al. Necrotizing angiitis associated with drug abuse. N Engl J Med 1970;283:1003–11.

134. Glick R, Hoying J, Cerullo L, et al. Phenylpropanolamine: an over-the-counter drug causing central nervous system vasculitis and intracerebral hemorrhage. Case report and review. Neurosurgery 1987;20:969–74.

135. Krendel DA, Ditter SM, Frankel MR, et al. Biopsy-proven cerebral vasculitis associated with cocaine abuse. Neurology 1990;40:1092–4.

136. Fredericks RK, Lefkowitz DS, Challa VE, et al. Cerebral vasculitis associated with cocaine abuse. Stroke 1991;22:1437–9.

137. Murrow PL, McQuillen JB. Cerebral vasculitis associated with cocaine abuse. J Forensic Sci 1993;38:732–8.

138. Tapia JF, Schumacher JM. Case records of the Massachusetts General Hospital. Weekly clinicopathological exercises. Case 27-1993. A 32-year-old man with the sudden onset of a right-sided headache and left hemiplegia and hemianesthesia. N Engl J Med 1993;329:117–24.

139. Merkel PA, Koroschetz WJ, Irizarry MC, et al. Cocaine-associated cerebral vasculitis. Semin Arthritis Rheum 1995;25:172–83.

140. Martinez N, Diez-Tejedor E, Frank A. Vasospasm/thrombus in cerebral ischemia related to cocaine abuse [letter]. Stroke 1996;27:147–8.

141. Diez-Tejedor E, Frank A, Gutierrez M, et al. Encephalopathy and biopsy-proven cerebrovascular inflammatory changes in a cocaine abuser. Eur J Neurol 1998;5:103–7.

142. Caplan LR, Hier DB, Banks G. Current concepts of cerebrovascular disease-stroke: stroke and drug abuse. Stroke 1982;13:869–72.

143. Richter RW, Pearson J, Bruun B, et al. Neurological complications of addictions to heroin. Bull N Y Acad Med 1973;49:4–21.

144. Louria DB, Hensle T, Rose J. The major medical complications of heroin addiction. Ann Intern Med 1967;67:1–22.
145. Sporer KA. Acute heroin overdose. Ann Intern Med 1999;130:584–90.
146. Oehmichen M, Meibner C, Reiter A, et al. Neuropathology in non-human immunodeficiency virus-infected drug addicts: hypoxic brain damage after chronic intravenous drug abuse. Acta Neuropathol 1996;91:642–6.
147. Gray F, Marie-Claude L, Keohane C, et al. Early brain changes in HIV infection: neuropathological study of 11 HIV seropositive, non-AIDS cases. J Neuropathol Exp Neurol 1992;51:177–85.
148. Dodge PR, Swartz MN. Bacterial meningitis–a review of selected aspects. II. Special neurologic problems, postmeningitic complications and clinicopathological correlations (concluded). N Engl J Med 1965;272:1003–10.
149. Lyons EL, Leeds NE. The angiographic demonstration of arterial vascular disease in purulent meningitis. Radiology 1967;88:935–8.
150. Roach MR, Drake CG. Ruptured cerebral aneurysms caused by micro-organisms. N Engl J Med 1965;273:240–4.
151. Ferris EJ, Rudikoff JC, Shapiro JH. Cerebral angiography of bacterial infection. Radiology 1968;90:727–34.
152. Adams R, Kubik C, Bonner F. The clinical and pathological aspects of influenza meningitis. Arch Pediatr 1948;65:354–76, 408–41.
153. Smith JF, Landing BH. Mechanisms of brain damage in *H. influenza* meningitis. J Neurosurg 1960;19:248–65.
154. Cairns H, Russell DS. Cerebral arteritis and phlebitis in pneumococcal meningitis. J Pathol Bacteriol 1946;58:649–65.
155. Smith HV, Daniel P. Some clinical and pathological aspects of tuberculosis of the central nervous system. Tuberculosis 1947;28:64–80.
156. Greitz T. Angiography in tuberculous meningitis. Acta Radiol 1964;2:369–77.
157. Lehrer H. The angiographic triad in tuberculous meningitis. A radiographic and clinicopathologic correlation. Radiology 1966;87:829–35.
158. Kopsachilis N, Brar M, Marinescu A, et al. Central nervous system tuberculosis presenting as branch retinal vein occlusion. Clin Exp Optom 2013;96:121–3.
159. Feng W, Caplan M, Matheus M, et al. Meningovascular syphilis with fatal vertebrobasilar occlusion. Am J Med Sci 2009;338:169–71.
160. Adagio N, Muayqil T, Scozzafava J, et al. The re-emergence in Canada of meningovascular syphilis: 2 patients with headache and stroke. CMAJ 2007;176:1699–700.
161. Rabinov KR. Angiographic findings in a case of brain syphilis. Radiology 1963;80:622–4.
162. Flint AC, Liberato BB, Anziska Y, et al. Meningovascular syphilis as a cause of basilar artery stenosis. Neurology 2005;64:391–2.
163. Veenendaal-Hilbers JA, Perquin WV, Hoogland PH, et al. Basal meningovasculitis and occlusion of the basilar artery in two cases of *Borrelia burgdorferi* infection. Neurology 1988;38:1317–9.
164. Oksi J, Kalimo H, Marttila RJ, et al. Inflammatory brain changes in Lyme borreliosis: a report on three patients and review of literature. Brain 1996;119:2143–54.
165. Topakian R, Stieglbauer K, Nussbaumer K, et al. Cerebral vasculitis and stroke in Lyme neuroborreliosis. Two case reports and review of current knowledge. Cerebrovasc Dis 2008;26:455–61.
166. Miklossy J, Kuntzer T, Bogousslavsky J, et al. Meningovascular form of neuroborreliosis: similarities between neuropathological findings in a case of Lyme

disease and those occurring in tertiary neurosyphilis. Acta Neuropathol 1990; 80:568–72.

167. Schmiedel J, Gahn G, von Kummer R, et al. Cerebral vasculitis with multiple infarcts caused by Lyme disease. Cerebrovasc Dis 2004;17:79–81.

168. May EF, Jabbari B. Stroke in neuroborreliosis. Stroke 1990;21:1232–5.

169. Wilke M, Eiffert H, Christen HJ, et al. Primary chronic and cerebrovascular course of Lyme neuroborreliosis: case reports and literature review. Arch Dis Child 2000;83:67–71.

170. Chehrenama M, Zagardo MT, Koski CL. Subarachnoid hemorrhage in a patient with Lyme disease. Neurology 1997;48:520–3.

171. Uldry PA, Regli F, Bogousslavsky J. Cerebral angiopathy and recurrent strokes following *Borrelia burgdorferi* infection. J Neurol Neurosurg Psychiatry 1987;50: 1703–4.

172. Klingebiel R, Benndorf G, Schmitt M, et al. Large cerebral vessel occlusive disease in Lyme neuroborreliosis. Neuropediatrics 2002;33:37–40.

173. Heinrich A, Khaw A, Ahrens N, et al. Cerebral vasculitis as the only manifestation of *Borrelia burgdorferi* infection in a 17-year old patient with basal ganglia infarction. Eur Neurol 2003;50:109–12.

174. Cox MG, Wolfs TF, Lo TF, et al. Neuroborreliosis causing focal cerebral arteriopathy in a child. Neuropediatrics 2005;36:104–7.

175. Meurers B, Kohlhepp W, Gold R, et al. Histopathological findings in the central and peripheral nervous system in neuroborreliosis. J Neurol 1990;237:113–6.

176. Lebas A, Toulgoat F, Saliou G, et al. Stroke due to Lyme neuroborreliosis: changes in vessel wall contrast enhancement. J Neuroimaging 2012;22: 210–2.

177. Kleinschmidt-DeMasters BK, Gilden DH. Varicella-zoster virus infections of the nervous system: clinical and pathologic correlates. Arch Pathol Lab Med 2001;125:770–80.

178. Kleinschmidt-DeMasters BK, Amliee-Lefond C, Gilden DH. The patterns of varicella zoster virus encephalitis. Hum Pathol 1996;27:927–38.

179. Gilden DH, Kleinschmidt-DeMasters BK, Wellish M, et al. Varicella zoster virus, a cause of waxing and waning vasculitis: the *New England Journal of Medicine* case 5-1995 revisited. Neurology 1996;47:1441–6.

180. Eidelberg D, Sotrel A, Horoupian S, et al. Thrombotic cerebral vasculopathy associated with herpes zoster. Ann Neurol 1985;19:7–14.

181. Rosenblum WI, Hadfield MG. Granulomatous angiitis of the nervous system in cases of herpes zoster and lymphosarcoma. Neurology 1972;22:348–54.

182. Linnemann CC Jr, Alvira MM. Pathogenesis of varicella-zoster angiitis in the CNS. Arch Neurol 1980;37:329–40.

183. Melanson M, Chalk C, Georgevich L, et al. Varicella-zoster virus DNA in CSF and arteries in delayed contralateral hemiplegia: evidence for viral invasion of cerebral arteries. Neurology 1996;47:569–70.

184. Amlie-LeFond C, Kleinschmidt-DeMasters BK, Mahalingam R, et al. The vasculopathy of varicella-zoster virus encephalitis. Ann Neurol 1995;37:784–90.

185. Reshef E, Greenberg SB, Jankovic J. Herpes zoster ophthalmicus followed by contralateral hemiparesis: report of two cases and review of literature. J Neurol Neurosurg Psychiatry 1985;48:122–7.

186. Nagel MA, Traktinskiy I, Azarkh Y, et al. Varicella zoster virus vasculopathy. Analysis of virus-infected arteries. Neurology 2011;77:364–70.

187. Nagel MA, Traktinskiy I, Stenmark KR, et al. Varicella-zoster virus vasculopathy: immune characteristics of virus-infected arteries. Neurology 2013;80:62–8.

188. Schigenaga K, Okabe M, Etoh K. An autopsy case of *Aspergillus* infection of the brain. Kumamoto Med J 1975;28:135–44.
189. Davidson P, Robertson DM. A true mycotic (*Aspergillus*) aneurysm leading to fatal subarachnoid hemorrhage in a patient with hereditary hemorrhagic telangiectasia. Case report. J Neurosurg 1971;35:71.
190. Wollschlaeger G, Wollschlaeger PB, Lopez VF, et al. A rare cause of occlusion of the internal carotid artery. Neuroradiology 1970;1:32–8.
191. Nachega JB, Morroni C, Chaisson RE, et al. Impact of immune reconstitution inflammatory syndrome on antiretroviral therapy adherence. Patient Prefer Adherence 2012;6:887–91.
192. Sharer LR, Kapila R. Neuropathologic observations in acquired immunodeficiency syndrome (AIDS). Acta Neuropathol 1985;66:188–98.
193. McArthur JC, Haughey N, Gartner S, et al. Human immunodeficiency virus-associated dementia: an evolving disease. J Neurovirol 2003;9:205–21.
194. Price RW, Brew B, Sidtis J, et al. The brain in AIDS: central nervous system HIV-1 infection and AIDS dementia complex. Science 1988;239:586–92.
195. Bell JE, Busuttil A, Ironside JW, et al. Human immunodeficiency virus and the brain: investigation of virus load and neuropathologic changes in pre-AIDS subjects. J Infect Dis 1993;168:818–24.
196. Esiri MM, Scaravilli F, Millard PR, et al. Neuropathology of HIV infection in haemophiliacs: comparative necropsy study. BMJ 1989;299:1312–5.
197. van der Ven AJ, Van Oostenbrugge RJ, Kubat B, et al. Cerebral vasculitis after initiation antiretroviral therapy. AIDS 2002;16:2362–4.
198. Bleehan SS, Lovelace RE, Cotton RE. Mononeuritis multiplex in polyarteritis nodosa. Q J Med 1962;32:193–209.
199. Lovelace RE. Mononeuritis multiplex in polyarteritis nodosa. Neurology 1964;14:434–42.
200. Wees SJ, Sunwood LN, Oh SJ. Sural nerve biopsy in systemic necrotizing vasculitis. Am J Med 1981;71:525–32.
201. Kissel JT, Slivka AP, Warmolts JR, et al. The clinical spectrum of necrotizing angiopathy of the peripheral nervous system. Ann Neurol 1985;18:251–7.
202. Said G, Lacroix-Ciaudo C, Fujimura H, et al. The peripheral neuropathy of necrotizing arteritis: a clinicopathologic study. Ann Neurol 1988;23:461–5.
203. Collins MP, Dyck JB, Gronseth GS, et al. Peripheral Nerve Society Guideline on the classification, diagnosis, investigation, and immunosuppressive therapy of non-systemic vasculitic neuropathy: executive summary. J Peripher Nerv Syst 2010;15:176–84.
204. Mouthon L. Management of relapses in vasculitis. Presse Med 2013;42:619–22.
205. El-Chammas K, Keyes J, Thompson N, et al. Pharmacologic treatment of pediatric headaches: a meta-analysis. JAMA Pediatr 2013;167:250–8.
206. Tfelt-Hansen PC. Evidence-based guideline update: pharmacologic treatment for episodic migraine prevention in adults: report of the Quality Standards subcommittee of the American Academy of Neurology and the American Headache Society. Neurology 2013;80:869–70.
207. Loder E, Burch R, Rizzoli P. The 2012 AHS/AAN guidelines for prevention of episodic migraine: a summary and comparison with other recent clinical practice guidelines. Headache 2012;52:930–45.
208. Fauci AS, Haynes BF, Katz P, et al. Wegener's granulomatosis: prospective clinical and therapeutic experience with 85 patients over 21 years. Ann Intern Med 1983;98:76–85.

209. Guillevin L, Cordier JF, Lhote F, et al. A prospective, multicenter, randomized trial comparing steroids and pulse cyclophosphamide versus steroids and oral cyclophosphamide in the treatment of generalized Wegener's granulomatosis. Arthritis Rheum 1997;40:2187–98.

210. Haubitz M, Schellong S, Gobel U, et al. Intravenous pulse administration of cyclophosphamide versus daily oral treatment in patients with antineutrophilic cytoplasmic antibody-associated vasculitis and renal involvement: a prospective, randomized study. Arthritis Rheum 1998;41:1835–44.

211. Jones RB, Tervaert JW, Hauser T, et al, for the European Vasculitis Study Group. Rituximab versus cyclophosphamide in ANCA-associated renal vasculitis. N Engl J Med 2010;363:211–20.

212. Stone JH, Merkel PA, Spiera R, et al, for the RAVE-ITN Research Group. Rituximab versus cyclophosphamide for ANCA-associated vasculitis. N Engl J Med 2010;363:221–32.

213. Kindler V, Sappino AP, Grau GE, et al. The inducing role of tumor necrosis factor in the development of bactericidal granulomas during BCG infection. Cell 1989; 56:731–40.

214. Ludviksson BR, Sneller MC, Chua KS, et al. Active Wegener's granulomatosis is associated with HLA-DR+ CD4+ T cells exhibiting an unbalanced Th1-type cytokine pattern: reversal with IL-10. J Immunol 1998;160:3602–9.

215. Noronha IL, Kruger C, Andrassy K, et al. In situ production of TNF-alpha, IL-1 beta and IL-2R in ANCA-positive glomerulonephritis. Kidney Int 1993;43:682–92.

216. Wegener's Granulomatosis Etanercept Trial (WGET) Research Group. Etanercept plus standard therapy for Wegener's granulomatosis. N Engl J Med 2005;352:351–61.

217. Bartolucci P, Ramanoelina J, Cohen P, et al. Efficacy of the anti-TNF-α antibody infliximab against refractory systemic vasculitides: an open pilot study on 10 patients. Rheumatology 2002;41:1126–32.

218. de Groot K, Rasmussen N, Bacon PA, et al, for the European Vasculitis Study Group. Randomized trial of cyclophosphamide versus methotrexate for induction of remission in early systemic antineutrophil cytoplasmic antibody-associated vasculitis. Arthritis Rheum 2005;52:2461–9.

219. Dalakas MC. Intravenous immunoglobulin in autoimmune neuromuscular diseases. JAMA 2004;291:2367–75.

220. Martinez V, Cohen P, Pagnoux C, et al, for the French Vasculitis Study Group. Intravenous immunoglobulin for relapses of systemic vasculitides associated with antineutrophil cytoplasmic antibodies. Arthritis Rheum 2008;58:308–17.

221. Shick RM, Baggenstoss AH, Fuller BF, et al. Effects of cortisone and ACTH on periarteritis nodosa and cranial arteritis. Mayo Clin Proc 1950;25:492–4.

222. Langford CA. Perspectives on the treatment of giant cell arteritis. Presse Med 2013;42:609–12.

223. Ohigashi H, Haraguchi G, Konishi M, et al. Improved prognosis of Takayasu arteritis over the past decade. Circ J 2012;76:1004–11.

224. Kamisawa T, Okazaki K, Kawa S, et al. Japanese consensus guidelines for management of autoimmune pancreatitis: III. Treatment and prognosis of AIP. J Gastroenterol 2010;45:471–7.

225. Hoffman GS, Cid MC, Rendt-Zagar KE, et al. Infliximab for maintenance of glucocorticoid-induced remission of giant cell arteritis: a randomized trial. Ann Intern Med 2007;146:621–30.

226. Novikov P, Smitienko I, Moiseev S. Efficacy of long-term treatment with TNF inhibitors in patients with refractory Takayasu arteritis. Presse Med 2013;42:723.

227. Youngstein T, Peters J, Mason J. Biologic agents offer an effective long-term therapeutic option for refractory Takayasu arteritis. Presse Med 2013;42: 677–8.
228. Abisror N, Mekinian A, Lavigne C, et al. Tocilizumab in refractory Takayasu arteritis: case series and literature review [abstract]. Presse Med 2013;42:725–6.
229. Nesher G, Berkun Y, Mates M, et al. Low-dose aspirin and prevention of cranial ischemic complications in giant cell arteritis. Arthritis Rheum 2004;50:1332–7.
230. Lee MS, Smith SD, Galor A, et al. Antiplatelet and anticoagulant therapy in patients with giant cell arteritis. Arthritis Rheum 2006;54:3306–9.
231. Guillevin L, Cohen P, Mahr A, et al, the French Vasculitis Study Group. Treatment of polyarteritis nodosa and microscopic polyangiitis with poor prognosis factors: a prospective trial comparing glucocorticoids and six or twelve cyclophosphamide pulses in sixty-five patients. Arthritis Rheum 2003;49:93–100.
232. Guillevin L, Mahr A, Callard P, et al, for the French Vasculitis Study Group. Hepatitis B virus-associated polyarteritis nodosa: clinical characteristics, outcome, and impact of treatment in 115 patients. Medicine 2005;84:313–22.
233. Henegar C, Pagnoux C, Puechal X, et al, for the French Vasculitis Study Group. A paradigm of diagnostic criteria for polyarteritis nodosa. Arthritis Rheum 2008; 58:1528–38.
234. Hoffman GS, Kerr GS, Leavitt RY, et al. Wegener granulomatosis: an analysis of 158 patients. Ann Intern Med 1992;116:488–98.
235. Cordier JF. Eosinophilic granulomatosis with polyangiitis (Churg-Strauss). Presse Med 2013;42:507–10.
236. Little MA, Nightingale P, Verburgh CA, et al. Early mortality in systemic vasculitis: relative contribution of adverse events and active vasculitis. Ann Rheum Dis 2009;69:1036–43.
237. Jayne D. Rituximab for ANCA-associated vasculitis: the UK experience. Presse Med 2013;42:532–4.
238. Brihaye B, Aouba A, Pagnoux C, et al. Adjunction of rituximab to steroids and immunosuppressants for refractory/relapsing Wegener's granulomatosis: a study on 8 patients. Clin Exp Rheumatol 2007;25:523–7.
239. Charles P, Guillevin L. Rituximab for ANCA-associated vasculitides: the French experience. Presse Med 2013;42:534–6.
240. Jones RB, Ferraro AJ, Chaudhry AN, et al. A multicenter survey of rituximab for refractory antineutrophil cytoplasmic antibody-associated vasculitis. Arthritis Rheum 2009;60:2156–68.
241. Cartin-Ceba R, Golbin JM, Keogh KA, et al. Rituximab for remission induction and maintenance in refractory granulomatosis with polyangiitis (Wegener's): ten-year experience at a single center. Arthritis Rheum 2012;64:3770–8.
242. Holle JU, Dubrau C, Herlyn K, et al. Rituximab for refractory granulomatosis with polyangiitis (Wegener's granulomatosis): comparison of efficacy in granulomatous versus vasculitic manifestations. Ann Rheum Dis 2012;71:327–33.
243. Smith RM, Jones RB, Guerry MJ, et al. Rituximab for remission maintenance in relapsing antineutrophil cytoplasmic antibody-associated vasculitis. Arthritis Rheum 2012;64:3760–9.
244. Roubaud-Baudron C, Pagnoux C, Méaux-Ruault N, et al. Rituximab maintenance for granulomatosis with polyangiitis and microscopic polyangiitis. J Rheumatol 2012;39:125–30.
245. Smith R, Alberici F, Jones R, et al. Long term follow up of patients who received repeat dose rituximab as maintenance therapy for ANCA associated vasculitis (AAV). Presse Med 2013;42:775–6.

246. Jayne D, Smith R, Merkel P. An international, open label, randomised controlled trial comparing rituximab with azathioprine as maintenance therapy in relapsing ANCA-associated vasculitis (RITAZAREM). Presse Med 2013;42:768.

247. Miloslavsky E, Specks U, Merkel P, et al. Retreatment with rituximab in the RAVE trial. Presse Med 2013;42:778.

248. Terrier B, Cacoub P. Cryoglobulinemia vasculitis: an update. Curr Opin Rheumatol 2013;25:10–8.

249. Conlon KC, Urba WJ, Smith JW, et al. Exacerbation of symptoms of autoimmune disease in patients receiving alpha interferon therapy. Cancer 1990;65:2237–42.

250. Boonyapisit K, Katirji B. Severe exacerbation of hepatitis C-associated vasculitic neuropathy following treatment with interferon alpha: a case report and literature review. Muscle Nerve 2002;25:909–13.

251. Cacoub P, Terrier B, Saadoun D. Hepatitis C virus mixed cryoglobulinemia vasculitis: therapeutic options. Presse Med 2013;42:523–6.

252. Saadoun D, Pol S, Ziza JM, et al. Ribavirin/protease inhibitor combination in hepatitis C virus associated mixed cryoglobulinemia vasculitis/Peg-INFa. Presse Med 2013;42:694–5.

253. Weiss PF, Feinstein JA, Luan X, et al. Effects of corticosteroid on Henoch-Schonlein purpura: a systematic review. Pediatrics 2007;120:1079–87.

254. Noel N, Wechsler B, Le Thi Huong Boutin D, et al. Outcome of neuro-Behçet: analysis of a large cohort. Presse Med 2013;42:692.

255. Nanthapisal S, Eleftheriou D, Hong Y, et al. Behçet disease in children: the Great Ormond Street Hospital experience. Presse Med 2013;42:651.

256. Stone JH, Zeri Y, Deshpande V. IgG-4 related disease. N Engl J Med 2012;366: 539–51.

257. de Boyson H, Zuber M, Naggara O, et al. Primary angiitis of the central nervous system: description of the first 52 adult patients enrolled in the French COVAC cohort. Arthritis Rheum 2012;64(Suppl 10):S663.

258. Benseler SM, Silverman E, Aviv RI, et al. Primary central nervous system vasculitis in children. Arthritis Rheum 2006;54:1291–7.

259. Pagnoux C, de Boyson H. How to treat primary vasculitis of the central nervous system. Presse Med 2013;42:605–7.

260. Puéchal X, Gottenberg JE, Berthelot JM, et al. Rituximab therapy for systemic vasculitis associated with rheumatoid arthritis: results from the autoimmunity and rituximab registry. Arthritis Care Res 2012;64:331–9.

261. Buch MH, Smolen JS, Betteridge N, et al. Updated consensus statement on the use of rituximab in patients with rheumatoid arthritis. Ann Rheum Dis 2011;70: 909–20.

262. Puéchal X, Miceli-Richard C, Mejjad O, et al. Anti-tumor necrosis factor treatment in patients with refractory systemic vasculitis associated with rheumatoid arthritis. Ann Rheum Dis 2008;67:880–4.

263. Puechal X. Rheumatoid arthritis vasculitis. Presse Med 2013;42:527–30.

The Pseudotumor Cerebri Syndrome

Deborah I. Friedman, MD, MPH[a,b,*]

KEYWORDS

- Pseudotumor cerebri • Idiopathic intracranial hypertension • Papilledema
- Cerebrospinal fluid

KEY POINTS

- The pseudotumor cerebri syndrome (PTCS) may be primary (idiopathic intracranial hypertension, IIH) or arise from a secondary cause.
- PTCS is an important cause of new daily persistent headaches and may lead to permanent visual loss if untreated. Papilledema is the hallmark of PTCS and is required to make a definite diagnosis, emphasizing the importance of a funduscopic examination on all patients with new or unexplained headaches.
- PTCS affects boys and girls equally until puberty, when the incidence in girls increases markedly. IIH in adults is almost exclusively a disease of overweight women of child-bearing age.
- A high opening pressure on a lumbar puncture is not adequate to make the diagnosis of PTCS if papilledema is absent.
- Treatments for PTCS include treating the secondary cause (if present), weight loss, medications, and surgery. Repeated lumbar punctures are helpful to control the pressure urgently while awaiting surgery, during pregnancy, and for infrequent relapses.
- The main goal of treatment is to preserve or restore vision; careful ophthalmologic follow-up with perimetry is necessary.
- Headache treatment may be independent of therapies to address intracranial hypertension.

INTRODUCTION

The pseudotumor cerebri syndrome (PTCS) is a perplexing syndrome of increased intracranial pressure without a space-occupying lesion. The terminology for the disorder has changed over the years and the diagnostic criteria were revised to reflect

Disclosures: The author received grant funding from the National Eye Institute for the Idiopathic Intracranial Hypertension Treatment Trial and has no other relevant disclosures.
[a] Department of Neurology and Neurotherapeutics, University of Texas Southwestern Medical Center, 5323 Harry Hines Boulevard, MC-9036, Dallas, TX 75390-9036, USA; [b] Department of Ophthalmology, University of Texas Southwestern Medical Center, 5323 Harry Hines Boulevard, Dallas, TX 75390-9036, USA
* Department of Neurology and Neurotherapeutics, 5323 Harry Hines Boulevard, MC-9036, Dallas, TX 75390-9036.
E-mail address: Deborah.Friedman@UTSouthwestern.edu

Neurol Clin 32 (2014) 363–396
http://dx.doi.org/10.1016/j.ncl.2014.01.001
0733-8619/14/$ – see front matter © 2014 Elsevier Inc. All rights reserved.

advances in diagnostic technology and new insights into the disease process.[1] The classification and nomenclature depend on the presence or absence of an underlying cause. When the diagnostic criteria are followed, an alternative diagnosis is unlikely (**Box 1**). When no secondary cause is identified, the syndrome is termed "Idiopathic Intracranial Hypertension (IIH)." An accurate diagnosis is imperative to initiating appropriate treatment, which may incorporate medical or surgical modalities. The main goal of therapy is the preservation of vision.

EPIDEMIOLOGY

Incidence studies from various countries estimate the annual incidence of pseudotumor cerebri syndrome (PTCS) as 0.9/100,000 in the general population, rising to 3.5/100,000 in women 15 to 44 years and 19.3/100,000 in women ages 20 to 44 years who weigh 20% or more than their ideal body weight.[2–5] Some of the patients included in those studies had an identifiable secondary cause; the statistics are not strictly applicable to the idiopathic form. However, the incidence is rising, which may be attributed to improved recognition and the obesity epidemic.[6] After puberty, the disorder affects women 9 times as often as men. Boys and girls are equally affected before puberty.[7–10] When the diagnostic criteria are strictly applied in patients over the age of 18 years, the idiopathic form occurs almost exclusively in women. It rarely develops in patients over age 45 years.[11]

Box 1
Diagnostic criteria for PTCS

A diagnosis of PTCS is "definite" if the patient fulfills criteria A–E. The diagnosis is considered "probable" if criteria A–D are met but the measured CSF pressure is lower than specified for a "definite" diagnosis.

1. Required for diagnosis of the pseudotumor cerebri syndrome

   A. Papilledema

   B. Normal neurologic examination except for cranial nerve abnormalities

   C. Neuro-imaging: Normal brain parenchyma without evidence of hydrocephalus, mass, or structural lesion and no abnormal meningeal enhancement on MRI, with and without gadolinium, for typical patients (female and obese), and MRI, with and without gadolinium, and magnetic resonance venography for others. If MRI is unavailable or contraindicated, contrast-enhanced CT may be used.

   D. Normal CSF composition

   E. Elevated LP opening pressure (>250 mm CSF in adults and >280 mm CSF in children [250 mm CSF if the child is not sedated and not obese]) in a properly performed LP.

2. Diagnosis of PTCS without papilledema

   - In the absence of papilledema, a diagnosis of PTCS can be made if B–E are satisfied, and in addition, the patient has a unilateral or bilateral abducens nerve palsy.

   - In the absence of papilledema or sixth nerve palsy, a diagnosis of PTCS can be "suggested" but not made if B–E are satisfied, and in addition, at least 3 of the following neuroimaging criteria are satisfied:

      i. Empty sella

      ii. Flattening of the posterior aspect of the globe

      iii. Distention of the perioptic subarachnoid space with or without a tortuous optic nerve

      iv. Transverse venous sinus stenosis

SYMPTOMS
Headache

Almost all patients with PTCS have headache, which is the most common presenting symptom.[12–14] Occasionally patients are asymptomatic[13] and seek medical attention when papilledema is detected on a routine eye examination.[15] There are no specific distinguishing characteristics of the headache, which is often daily, bilateral, frontal, or retroocular.[13,16] It is usually moderate to severe in intensity and some patients describe increased severity on awakening. The headache may also be throbbing, with nausea, vomiting, and photophobia, resembling migraine. Neck and back pain are often prominent features.[13,17] It is not unusual for patients with PTCS to have coexisting migraine headaches, making the diagnosis difficult unless other signs are present.[18,19] PTCS is in the differential diagnosis of new daily persistent headache. The presence of chronic daily headaches raises the possibility of medication overuse headache (MOH), which occurs in PTCS patients, particularly in the chronic stages. Analgesic overuse may worsen an unrelated primary headache disorder and simulates "IIH without papilledema" (IIHWOP).[20]

Transient Visual Obscurations

Although not specific for PTCS, transient obscurations of vision are most commonly experienced in this disorder and are sometimes the presenting symptom. They likely are a manifestation of disc edema leading to transient ischemia of the optic nerve head.[21] Patients describe brief episodes of monocular or binocular visual loss that may be partial or complete. The obscurations are present in about 70% of PTCS patients, typically last seconds, and do not correlate with the degree of disc edema or visual loss.[22,23]

Pulsatile Tinnitus

Pulsatile tinnitus occurs in 60% of patients and 9% of controls.[16] Patients should be queried about this symptom because it is often not volunteered. The noises may be unilateral or bilateral, often described as a heartbeat or whooshing sound. They are often abolished with a lumbar puncture (LP) or jugular venous compression.[24] Intracranial noises have been attributed to transmission of intensified vascular pulsations via cerebrospinal fluid (CSF) under high pressure to the walls of the venous sinuses, converting laminar to turbulent flow.[25] Others postulate that the endolymphatic duct may transmit pressure sensations from the CSF to the endolymph of the membranous labyrinth.[26] Hearing loss or a "high-altitude" sensation are also described.[27,28]

Visual Loss

A small percentage of patients experience subjective visual loss as the initial symptom of PTCS.[22] They may report blurred vision, a dark spot temporally that correlates with enlargement of the physiologic blind spot, or tunnel vision. In severe cases, profound visual loss or complete blindness occurs. The tempo of visual loss is variable in PTCS, but rapid deterioration may occur over days in severe cases. Early loss of central vision is a worrisome sign.

Diplopia

Diplopia is a frequently reported symptom in PTCS, occurring in one-third to two-thirds of patients at presentation.[13,22] It is usually binocular and horizontal, resulting from a unilateral or bilateral abducens paresis. Binocular diplopia almost always resolves when the intracranial pressure is normalized. Monocular diplopia or distorted vision may arise from macular edema or exudates in the setting of severe papilledema.

Other Symptoms

Minor symptoms of PTCS include radicular pain, paresthesias, neck stiffness, arthralgias of the shoulders, wrists, and knees, ataxia, and facial palsy.[13,17,29–32] Depression and anxiety are more common in patients with PTCS than in obese or normal weight control subjects.[33] It is uncertain whether the depression results from having PTCS, or whether there is a common pathogenesis in some patients.[34] Occasionally depression is the initial symptom.[34] Complaints of impaired concentration and memory are common; cognitive decline may be related the disorder itself, chronic headaches, visual impairment, fear of blindness, depression, anger, and anxiety.[35]

SIGNS
Papilledema

The hallmark of PTCS is papilledema that may be asymmetric or occasionally unilateral.[36] If stereoscopic viewing and fluorescein angiography show no evidence of papilledema, prolonged intracranial pressure monitoring is occasionally used for diagnosis.[37] Although there is an association between visual loss and high-grade papilledema,[36,38] the appearance of the optic nerves does not predict visual outcome in an individual patient.[39] Early or mild papilledema may be difficult to detect with the direct ophthalmoscope, and stereoscopic viewing of the optic discs with indirect ophthalmoscopy is recommended. Stereoscopic fundus photography and fluorescein angiography may be helpful to determine the presence of subtle papilledema, but treatment should not be based on the appearance of the optic nerves alone. Rarely, increased intracranial pressure results in retinal choroidal folds with little to no papilledema.[40]

Because the severity of papilledema influences the overall treatment strategy, it is useful to have a standardized papilledema grading system. The Frisén scale describes papilledema in stages that are clinically meaningful in the acute and subacute stages (**Box 2**).[41] Early papilledema is characterized by disruption of the normal radial nerve fiber layer arrangement with grayish opacity accentuating the nerve fiber bundles. A subtle gray peripapillary halo is apparent with the indirect ophthalmoscope (**Figs. 1** and **2**). There may be concentric or retinochoroidal folds. As the papilledema grade increases, the borders of the optic disc become indistinct, with progressive elevation of the disc margins. The nerve head diameter increases and the edematous nerve fiber layer obscures one or more segments of major blood vessels leaving the disc (**Figs. 3** and **4**). With severe papilledema, the optic nerve protrudes, the peripapillary halo becomes more demarcated, and the optic cup is obliterated (**Figs. 5** and **6**). Hyperemia, vessel tortuosity, hemorrhages, exudates, nerve fiber layer infarcts (cotton wool spots), and optic nerve pallor are often observed but are too variable to use for staging purposes (**Fig. 7**).[41] Papilledema will not develop in the setting of optic atrophy, which is an important consideration when considering recurrence.

It is important to differentiate true papilledema from pseudopapilledema caused by optic disc drusen, tilted optic discs, or a myelinated nerve fiber layer (**Figs. 8–10**). Stereoscopic viewing of the fundus can usually distinguish these entities. Optic disc drusen may also cause transient visual obscurations[21] and can easily be confused with PTCS, particularly with direct ophthalmoscopy. Rarely, optic nerve drusen and PTCS coexist.[42] This diagnostic dilemma is resolved with ultrasonography of the optic

Box 2
Papilledema grading system (Frisén scale)

Stage 0: Normal optic disc

A. Blurring of nasal, superior, and inferior poles in inverse proportion to disc diameter

B. Radial nerve fiber layer (NFL) without NFL tortuosity

C. Rare obscuration of a major vessel, usually on the upper pole

Stage 1: Very early papilledema

A. Obscuration of the nasal border of the disc

B. No elevation of disc borders

C. Disruption of the normal radial NFL arrangement with grayish opacity accentuating nerve fiber bundles

D. Normal temporal disc margin

E. Subtle grayish halo with temporal gap (best seen with indirect ophthalmoscope)

F. Concentric or radial retinochoroidal folds

Stage 2: Early papilledema

A. Obscuration of all borders

B. Elevation of the nasal border

C. Complete peripapillary halo

Stage 3: Moderate papilledema

A. Obscuration of all borders

B. Elevation of all borders

C. Increased diameter of the optic nerve head

D. Obscuration of one or more segments of major blood vessels leaving the disc

E. Peripapillary halo: irregular outer fringe with fingerlike extensions

Stage 4: Marked papilledema

A. Elevation of entire nerve head

B. Obscuration of all borders

C. Peripapillary halo

D. Total obscuration on the disc of a segment of a major blood vessel

Stage 5: Severe papilledema

A. Dome-shaped protrusions, representing anterior expansion of the optic nerve head

B. Peripapillary halo is narrow and smoothly demarcated

C. Total obscuration of a segment of a major blood vessel may or may not be present

D. Obliteration of the optic cup

From Frisén L. Swelling of the optic nerve head: a staging scheme. J Neurol Neurosurg Psychiatry 1982;45:13–8; with permission.

nerves. Drusen are visualized as highly reflective areas on the optic nerve head, whereas the 30° tilt test demonstrates a distended optic nerve sheath with papilledema. High-resolution computed tomography (CT) scanning of the orbits often demonstrates calcified drusen that may be buried behind the optic nerve papilla.

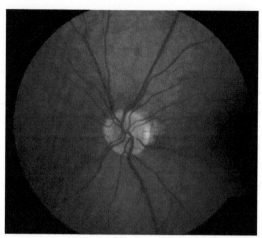

Fig. 1. Normal (stage 0) optic nerve. There is no peripapillary halo, obscuration of a major vessel crossing the disc margin, or disruption of the retinal nerve fiber layer. This patient has no physiologic cup, a normal variant. (*Courtesy of* IIHTT Photography Reading Center, Rochester, NY.)

Loss of spontaneous venous pulsations is often used to gauge intracranial pressure. Spontaneous venous pulsations typically disappear if CSF pressure if greater than 250 mm, and their presence generally indicates that the CSF pressure at the time is 190 mm or less.[43,44] However, because many normal individuals lack spontaneous venous pulsations, it is not a reliable sign unless venous pulsations were previously observed in a particular patient.

Papilledema may not be present very early in the course of the disease or there is pre-existing optic atrophy. Gliotic changes in the retinal nerve fiber layer may preclude the development of papilledema in patients having a relapse of the disease.

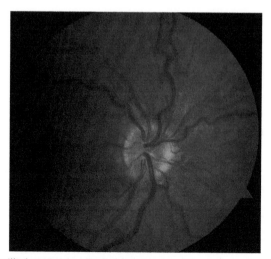

Fig. 2. Stage 1 papilledema. Note the C-shaped halo with a temporal gap. There is disruption of the normal retinal nerve fiber layer and a normal temporal disc margin. (*Courtesy of* IIHTT Photography Reading Center, Rochester, NY.)

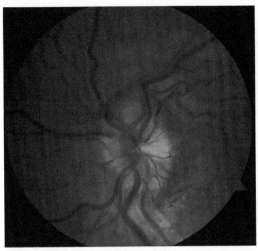

Fig. 3. Elevation of the nasal optic disc border with no major vessel obscuration and a circumferential peripapillary halo are characteristics of stage 2 papilledema. (*Courtesy of* IIHTT Photography Reading Center, Rochester, NY.)

Visual Acuity and Optic Nerve Function Tests

Early papilledema is typically associated with normal or near-normal Snellen visual acuity. In severe cases of pseudotumor cerebri, the acuity may deteriorate rapidly as the optic nerve becomes ischemic. Approximately 15% of patients have visual acuities worse than 20/20 at the initial visit; it is this author's experience that decreased visual acuity at presentation often portends a poor prognosis.[13,22] Because Snellen

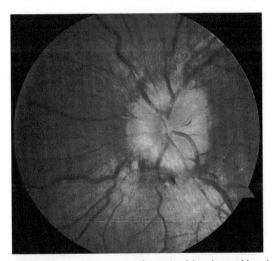

Fig. 4. Obscuration of one or more segments of a major blood vessel leaving the disc margin and elevation of all optic disc borders are seen in stage 3 papilledema. The outer fringe of the peripapillary halo is irregular with fingerlike extensions. (*Courtesy of* IIHTT Photography Reading Center, Rochester, NY.)

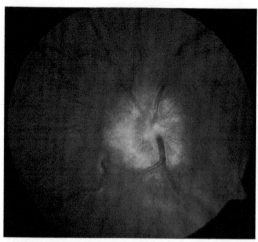

Fig. 5. Stage 4 papilledema. There is total obscuration of a major vessel on the optic disc with elevation of the entire optic nerve head and a complete peripapillary halo. (*Courtesy of* IIHTT Photography Reading Center, Rochester, NY.)

visual acuity is not sensitive to visual loss found on perimetry, it should not be used as the sole indicator of visual function.[39]

Contrast sensitivity is a sensitive and early indicator of optic nerve dysfunction in PTCS. Low-, middle-, and high-frequency loss has been reported.[45,46] However, contrast sensitivity has not proved to be as useful as perimetry in the assessment patients with PTCS. Color vision testing is insensitive for visual loss.[13] There is no role for visual-evoked potentials in this disorder; they are unreliable and remain normal until substantial vision is lost.[45] The presence of a relative afferent pupillary defect indicates asymmetric visual loss and is uncommonly present, as the optic neuropathy of PTCS is most often symmetric.[22,39]

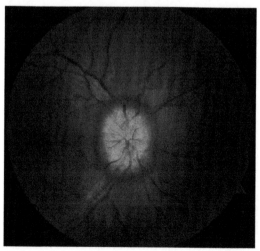

Fig. 6. Partial obscuration of all vessels leaving the disc and at least one vessel on the disc with diffuse optic nerve elevation and a complete peripapillary halo define stage 5 papilledema. (*Courtesy of* IIHTT Photography Reading Center, Rochester, NY.)

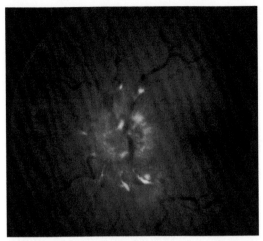

Fig. 7. Stage 4 papilledema with retinal exudates. (*Courtesy of* IIHTT Photography Reading Center, Rochester, NY.)

Perimetry

The most useful test for evaluating visual function in patients with PTCS is perimetry. The visual field defects are similar to those in other causes of papilledema and are characteristic of optic nerve dysfunction. Goldmann or automated threshold perimetry is required for adequate assessment. One study showed enlargement of the blind spot, representing papilledema, in 96% of patients by Goldmann perimetry and 92% of patients with automated perimetry.[39]

Other visual field defects include inferonasal loss and generalized constriction (**Figs. 11** and **12**). Occasionally it is difficult to distinguish genuine visual field constriction

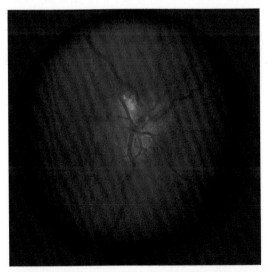

Fig. 8. The "lumpy-bumpy" irregular contour of optic disc drusen may simulate papilledema. (*Courtesy of* Valerie Biousse, MD, Atlanta, GA.)

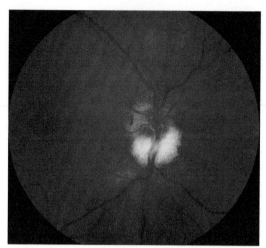

Fig. 9. Myelinated optic nerve fibers. The optic disc is surrounded inferiorly by myelinated, feathery nerve fibers. (*Courtesy of* Anil D. Patel, MD, FRCSC, FACS, Oklahoma City, OK.)

from functional (nonorganic) visual loss.[47,48] Central, paracentral, arcuate, and altitudinal scotomas may occur. The visual field loss may be severe, leading to blindness.[22] The most frequently detected visual field abnormalities in 50 PTCS patients prospectively evaluated with automated and Goldmann perimetry were blind spot enlargement, generalized field constriction, and nasal defects.[13]

Ocular Motility Abnormalities

Unilateral or bilateral lateral rectus palsy is a nonlocalizing sign of increased intracranial pressure. It typically produces binocular, horizontal diplopia, and an esotropia may be detected. Vertical diplopia from a skew deviation or fourth nerve palsy is uncommon.[49–51] Global ophthalmoparesis is rare and generally indicates the presence

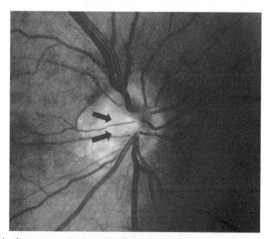

Fig. 10. Tilted optic discs may mimic optic disc edema. The nasal portion of the optic disc is markedly elevated compared with the temporal portion with temporal peripapillary atrophy. (*arrows*) Temporal margin of the optic disc.

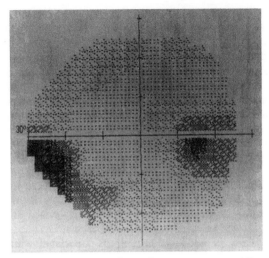

Fig. 11. Automated threshold perimetry (Humphrey Instruments, Allergan-Humphrey, San Leandro, CA, USA) of the central 24° shows an enlarged blind spot and inferonasal depression in a patient with pseudotomor cerebri and mild papilledema. (*From* Friedman DI. Pseudotumor cerebri. Neurosurg Clin North Am 1999;10:612; with permission.)

of an underlying disorder such as venous sinus occlusive disease.[52,53] The ocular motor paresis resolves when the intracranial pressure is lowered.[52]

Neuroimaging

Neuroimaging is mandatory before the performance of an LP to exclude a space-occupying lesion or ventriculomegaly. Although early studies with CT described small

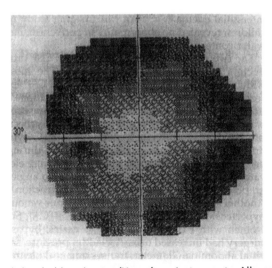

Fig. 12. Automated threshold perimetry (Humphrey Instruments, Allergan-Humphrey, San Leandro, CA, USA) of the central 24° reveals a diffuse reduction in sensitivity with marked generalized constriction of the visual field. Nonphysiological visual field loss may cause a similar pattern of visual field loss and must be excluded. (*From* Friedman DI. Pseudotumor cerebri. Neurosurg Clin North Am 1999;10:613; with permission.)

"slit-like" ventricles,[54] a subsequent study showed no difference in ventricular size between patients and controls.[55] Other reported abnormalities include dilated optic nerve sheaths, an empty sella (**Fig. 13**), and enlargement of the subarachnoid space.[56,57] Sellar contents may revert to a normal appearance with correction of the intracranial pressure.[58] The optic nerve can be clearly differentiated from the sheath on high-resolution orbital magnetic resonance imaging (MRI) with dilation of the perineuronal subarachnoid space.[57,59] Protrusion of the optic papilla into the posterior aspect of the globe and flattening of the posterior sclera may be seen.[57,59,60] A small percentage of patients also have a Chiari I malformation that may be coincidental.[61]

MRI is the preferred imaging study in patients with suspected PTCS. If there is concern about a meningeal process or a subtle intraparenchymal lesion producing increased intracranial pressure, contrast enhancement is needed. A normal plain CT scan can be misleading. If MRI is not possible because of availability or the patient's weight, a CT scan with contrast is recommended.

Cerebral venous sinus abnormalities are often detected in PTCS patients. If the patient is taking oral contraceptives, is postpartum, or has a known coagulopathy, then a magnetic resonance venogram is indicated to search for a cerebral venous thrombosis.[62] However, magnetic resonance venography and catheter angiography sometimes fail to detect subtle cerebral venous thrombosis.[63,64] Venous sinus stenosis may be present in the absence of thrombosis. Elliptic-centric-ordered 3-dimensional gadolinium-enhanced magnetic resonance venography increases the ability to detect intracranial sinovenous stenosis.[65] The transverse sinuses are typically affected with smooth-walled stenosis, or flow voids from enlarged arachnoid granulations.[66] Transverse sinus stenosis is most commonly a result of increased ICP, reversing with LP or shunting, but it may be a primary finding.[66,67] "Atypical" patients, including men, children, and slim women, should be thoroughly evaluated for an underlying cause. Contrast-enhanced MRI and magnetic resonance venography are recommended in these cases; digital subtraction angiography with venous phase imaging may also be necessary.

CSF Examination

The spinal fluid examination is critical for diagnosing PTCS. No patient should be diagnosed presumptively without a LP. There are several confounding conditions that may simulate PTCS: (1) patients with optic disc drusen or other congenital optic disc anomalies with or without chronic daily headaches; (2) central nervous system

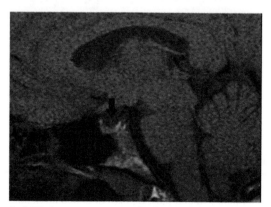

Fig. 13. Sagittal brain MRI shows an empty sella (*arrow*).

infections or malignancy producing increased intracranial pressure; (3) infiltrative optic neuropathies. The LP is crucial to document elevated CSF pressure and assure normal CSF contents.

The accepted value of CSF pressure for diagnosing PTCS in adults is greater than 250 mm of water in adults; values of 201 to 249 are nondiagnostic. The CSF pressure required for diagnosis in children and adolescents is 280 mm CSF (250 mm CSF if the child is not sedated and not obese).[68] As spinal fluid pressure fluctuates, the LP may need to be repeated if the clinical suspicion is high but the pressure is normal.[69] Occasionally prolonged intracranial monitoring is needed.[37]

Many patients with PTCS are obese, making the procedure of LP technically challenging. The patient's pressure must be measured in the lateral decubitus position with the legs relaxed. An 18- to 20-gauge spinal needle is preferred for resilience and optimal CSF flow. The clinician should be aware that pressures recorded in the sitting position are not accurate. Measurements in the prone position (ie, under fluoroscopy) are acceptable as long as the base of the manometer is at the level of the right atrium. Alternatively, the subarachnoid space may be entered with the patient in the sitting or prone position and the patient then carefully repositioned into the lateral decubitus position. If a patient is nervous or in pain during the procedure, which may require several attempts, the intracranial pressure will increase; a Valsalva maneuver can double the measured pressure.[70–72] Administration of an anxiolytic agent, such as diazepam or zolpidem tartrate, before the LP is often very helpful. Sedation and general anesthesia are to be avoided, as the decreased respiratory rate and resulting hypercapnia increase the CSF pressure.[73] The spinal fluid should be analyzed for glucose, protein, cell count, bacterial, fungal, and tuberculosis cultures, and cytology during the diagnostic evaluation. A therapeutic, "large-volume" spinal tap (removal of more than 20 cc of fluid) is sometimes used, although of uncertain value. Patients with PTCS are not protected against postspinal headaches.

PATHOPHYSIOLOGY

Over one hundred years after its original description by Quincke, the pathogenesis of PTCS is still uncertain.[74] Any proposed mechanism must explain the (1) lack of ventriculomegaly, (2) predilection of IIH in young, obese women, and (3) induction of PTCS by various medications, including tetracyclines and vitamin A.

Interstitial cerebral edema, increasing brain compliance and preventing hydrocephalus, was originally postulated based on a brain specimen obtained during subtemporal decompression,[75] but contradictory evidence emerged with the subsequent review of the original histologic slides and evaluation of postmortem tissue of 2 additional patients with PTCS who died of other causes. The original findings were thought to be a fixation artifact.[76]

Either increased CSF production or decreased CSF absorption could produce PTCS. The most widely accepted theory postulates impaired CSF absorption at the level of the arachnoid granulations[77] or the olfactory lymphatics.[78] Impaired CSF absorption also occurs in the presence of intracranial venous hypertension and is proposed as a unifying hypothesis of PTCS.[79,80] Cerebral venous sinus thrombosis may present solely as PTCS without impaired consciousness or lateralizing signs.[81–83] Transverse sinus stenosis, a frequent finding in IIH, has also been detected by magnetic resonance venogram in patients with chronic daily headaches, no papilledema, and normal to elevated CSF pressure.[84] Venous manometry and cervical spinal fluid pressure were recorded simultaneously in PTCS and found to have a reciprocal relationship.[80] Elevated cerebral venous sinus pressure would explain the lack of ventriculomegaly in PTCS, because the total fluid volume within the cranial vault remains constant when either component (CSF or blood) is altered. Conversely, cerebral venous hypertension may be the response to elevated CSF pressure rather than the cause of it.[85] The near-instantaneous lowering of cerebral venous pressure with CSF removal may explain why some patients are "cured" after their diagnostic LP.

Central obesity leading to raised intra-abdominal filling pressure, increased cardiac filling pressure, and decreased venous return from the brain causing increased intracranial pressure was proposed but unsubstantiated.[86]

Because the choroid plexus, the site of CSF production, is largely regulated by the sympathetic nervous system and neuroendocrine signaling, neurotransmitter abnormalities could result in abnormal spinal fluid production.[87–91] Serotonin and norepinephrine are important in this regard. The choroid plexus contains the highest density of serotonin $5\text{-}HT_{1C}$ receptors in the brain, with levels 10-fold higher than other brain regions.[92,93] CSF production by the choroid plexus can be affected by varying the levels of serotonin and norepinephrine in the central nervous system in animal studies. Pharmacologically increasing the levels of serotonin norepinephrine produces a decline in CSF production,[88,89,94] raising the possibility that patients with IIH have abnormal norepinephrine and serotonin regulation.[95] Abnormally low serotonin levels might account for the increased CSF pressure (via increased production) as well as the high incidence of depression, anxiety, and obesity among these patients.

Understanding the mechanism whereby exogenous agents produce PTCS may provide additional insights into the pathogenesis of the disorder. For example, vitamin A intoxication is a well-established cause of PTCS. Its mechanism of action in this regard is uncertain but may be related to a toxic effect on cell membranes when the capacity of retinal binding protein is exceeded.[96] Aquaporins are a family of regulatory membrane water channel proteins that participate in the secretion and reabsorption of CSF.[97–99] Aquaporin subtypes 1 and 4 are of major interest in the pathogenesis of IIH, although no definite association has been found to date.[100] In addition to its effects on the kidneys, the mineralocorticoid aldosterone is also active on epithelial cells of the choroid plexus, serving to enhance the activity of the Na^+/K^+-ATPase exchanger on the luminal membrane.[101] Enhanced Na^+ passage into the CSF results in increased CSF production. As yet there is no direct evidence of increased CSF production in cases of hyperaldosteronism, although aldosterone is found in the CSF in levels correlating to plasma aldosterone and has a known effect on the regulation of CSF volume.[101,102] Familial cases of IIH suggest a genetic component, which is being further explored in the IIHTT.[103,104]

Atypical Cases

Because there is no specific diagnostic test for PTCS, exceptions to the diagnostic criteria are reported. "IIH without papilledema," previously mentioned, is perhaps the most common.[20,105–107] The largest series of IIHWOP included 25 patients in a large headache center with refractory chronic daily headaches, normal neuroimaging, and an elevated CSF pressure.[20] Review of the data presented indicates that 80% of the patients were overusing analgesics. Various analgesics may affect CSF pressure. Alternatively, the patients may have been tense, in pain, or performing a Valsalva maneuver during the LP that would elevate their CSF pressure.[70] Among 353 IIH patients seen at a neuro-ophthalmology center, only 5.7% of patients had IIHWOP.[47] Compared with patients with papilledema, they tended to have lower CSF pressures, higher rates of nonphysiologic ("functional") visual loss, a longer duration of symptoms before diagnosis, and a poor response to conventional PTCS treatments.[47]

"Normal-pressure" PTCS has been reported in a patient who had otherwise typical signs and symptoms of PTCS, including papilledema.[108] The 2013 diagnostic criteria allow for a diagnosis of "probable" PTCS in such cases. Seven patients with clinical features of IIH, elevated CSF pressure, and CSF pleocytosis showed no evidence of another systemic process after a 3- to 10-year follow-up interval; the cause of the pleocytosis is uncertain.[109]

Headache and elevated LP opening pressure are inadequate to make the diagnosis of PTCS, because they are nonspecific. Of 168 patients who had an LP in the emergency department to evaluate a chief complaint of headaches, 28 had an opening pressure measured.[70] It ranged from 85 to 370 mm of CSF. Pressures greater than 200 mm water were found in 14 patients, 10 of whom had a pressure greater than 250 mm water. None had other features of IIH, and all patients were discharged from the emergency department with a diagnosis of benign headache disorder. A more recent study using evoked acoustic emissions to measure CSF pressure noninvasively in patients with migraine found significantly increased pressure during a migraine attack compared with the interictal period.[110] Thus, elevated CSF pressure may be a marker of headache in some patients and an isolated CSF pressure measurement is not sufficient to make or exclude a diagnosis of PTCS; the results of the LP must be combined with the other clinical features.

Associated Conditions and Differential Diagnosis

There are many conditions associated with PTCS, some fairly well substantiated and others in isolated case reports. These conditions are listed in **Box 3**. Weight gain and obesity are the only risk factors that have been demonstrated in case-control studies.[111,112] The major differential diagnoses are meningeal invasion of tumor and venous sinus thrombosis.

Many women with PTCS also have orthostatic edema, a benign condition characterized by abnormal sodium or water retention in the upright posture.[113] Elevated arginine vasopressin levels have been found in both disorders.[114–117] Most subjects in the IIHTT were at high risk for obstructive sleep apnea using a standard screening questionnaire (Wall M, and the IIHTT Study Group, submitted for publication.).

TREATMENT

PTCS is best managed using a team approach (**Fig. 14**). The neurologist is generally in the best position to direct the management of the patient in collaboration with the ophthalmologist, neurosurgeon, and primary care physician. **Fig. 11** provides an algorithm of general management principles. If the major problem is headache and the patient has good vision, then medical management is appropriate. The goal is to treat the symptoms and the visual function, rather than basing therapy solely on the appearance of the optic nerves. The IIHTT is a multicenter, randomized, double-masked placebo-controlled trial of a supervised dietary program plus acetazolamide or matching placebo tablets for the treatment of patients with IIH and mild visual loss (perimetric mean deviation −2 to −7 dB).[104] The results of the IIHTT will be released in 2014, providing the first evidence-based recommendations for treatment.

MEDICAL MANAGEMENT
Diet and Weight Loss

Weight loss is advocated for obese patients. In one study, 8 morbidly obese women with IIH achieved weight loss (58 ± 5 kg) by gastric surgery.[118] They all had resolution of papilledema and improvement in headaches and pulsatile tinnitus with long-term

---

Box 3
Associated conditions

Obstruction to venous drainage
Cerebral venous sinus thrombosis[62,81,83]
   Aseptic (hypercoagulable state)[173]
   Septic (middle ear or mastoid infection)
Bilateral radical neck dissection with jugular vein ligation
Jugular vein tumor[187,188]
Superior vena cava syndrome
Brachiocephalic vein thrombosis[188]
Increased right heart pressure
Following embolization of arteriovenous malformation[189]
Endocrine disorders
Addison disease[190]
Hypoparathyroidism
Obesity, recent weight gain[111]
Orthostatic edema[113]
Exogenous agents
Amiodarone[191,192]
Cytarabine[192]
Chlordecone (kepone)
Corticosteroids (particularly withdrawal)[124,193,194]
Cyclosporine[195]
Growth hormone[196–200]
Leuprorelin acetate (LH-RH analogue)[201]
Levothyroxine (children)[202,203]
Lithium carbonate[204]
Naladixic acid[205,206]
Levonorgestrel (Norplant)[184,207,208]
Sulfa antibiotics
Tetracycline and related compounds[209–218]
   Minocycline[219–222]
   Doxycycline[223]
Vitamin A[211,224–226]
   Vitamin supplements, liver
   Cis-retinoic acid (Accutane)[211,227–231]
   All-*trans*-retinoic acid (for acute promyelocytic leukemia)[232–235]
Infectious or Postinfectious
HIV infection[236–238]
Lyme disease[239]

Following childhood varicella[240,241]

Other medical conditions

Antiphospholipid antibody syndrome[242–244]

Behçet disease[245–247]

Occult craniosynostosis[248]

Polycystic ovary syndrome[249]

Sarcoidosis[250]

Obstructive sleep apnea[251–253]

Systemic lupus erythematosis[254,255]

Turner syndrome[256]

follow-up. Postoperative CSF pressures normalized when measured between 4 months and 6 years after surgery. Another retrospective analysis of 58 women with IIH showed that papilledema grade and visual fields improved more rapidly in those losing at least 2.5 kg over a period of 3 months.[119] The final visual acuity and visual field were independent of weight loss. Headache and CSF pressure were not quantified in this study. A study of 15 female patients treated with acetazolamide and weight loss correlated a 6% weight loss with resolution of their papilledema and the authors questioned the effectiveness of acetazolamide in this cohort.[120] Because IIH is frequently associated with orthostatic fluid retention,[113] salt and fluid restriction are also recommended.

Medications

Traditional therapy uses diuretics, particularly carbonic anhydrase inhibitors. Carbonic anhydrase, present in the choroid plexus, has a major role in the secretion of CSF. One study showed that acetazolamide was effective in 75% of patients with PTCS.[121] The effective dose is 1 to 4 g daily in divided doses. Almost all patients taking acetazolamide experience paresthesias, an unpleasant taste with carbonated beverages, altered taste of food, and a low serum bicarbonate level. Severe reactions include allergic rash, aplastic anemia, and renal stones. Acetazolamide and most other diuretics contain a sulfonamide moiety that differs from that of sulfa antibiotics. Thus, sulfa allergy is not a contraindication to acetazolamide treatment.[122] Methazolamide may be considered in patients who cannot tolerate acetazolamide.

Furosemide reduces CSF secretion in the choroid plexus in addition to its loop diuretic effect. Other diuretics, including thiazides, spironolactone, and triamterene, have been tried with varying success.[123] Spironolactone and triamterene can be used in the setting of acetazomide allergy. Diuretics before a planned period of recumbency are usually helpful in controlling the symptoms of orthostatic edema.[113]

Corticosteroids will rapidly decrease the intracranial pressure but are not suitable for chronic use. Their side effects of weight gain and fluid retention are undesirable and counterproductive. Moreover, patients may experience rebound intracranial hypertension as the dose is tapered.[124] Corticosteroids are generally reserved for the short-term, urgent treatment of patients with visual loss, used in conjunction with a surgical procedure.[125]

The headaches of PTCS can often be managed with medications and techniques that are used in the treatment of migraine. Many of the prophylactic headache

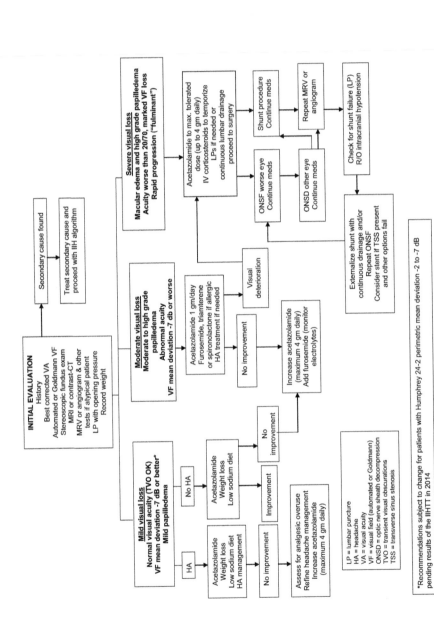

Fig. 14. General treatment algorithm for PTCS. Monitoring of vision with best-corrected acuity and perimetry is imperative because patients may transition between categories.

medications have undesirable side effects in IIH and patients must be monitored carefully while taking them. For example, tricyclic antidepressants and sodium valproate often cause weight gain. Calcium channel blockers carry the potential side effect of peripheral edema. β-Blockers may induce or worsen depression and add to the lethargy caused by acetazolamide. Topiramate is useful for headache prevention and often produces weight loss that is a desirable side effect in most patients with PTCS. In a retrospective review of 24 patients using topiramate during their course of treatment of PTCS, 4 patients did not tolerate it, 15 experienced weight loss, and 10 had improvement in their headaches.[126] An open-label study comparing acetazolamide and topiramate for treatment of IIH found improvement in both groups with respect to visual field change, and no significant differences between groups.[127] The role of topiramate as a primary treatment of PTCS is unsubstantiated. Nonsteroidal anti-inflammatory medications may be useful on an intermittent basis. However, patients often self-medicate with over-the-counter pain relievers and may confuse the clinical picture with a superimposed MOH.[20] Indomethacin lowers CSF pressure[128] and does not produce MOH. The triptans and dihydroergotamine may be helpful in patients with concomitant migraine headaches.[19]

Repeated LPs are occasionally useful, particularly if patients have infrequent exacerbations of their symptoms. Because they are painful and technically difficult to perform on obese individuals, they are not routinely recommended.

SURGICAL TREATMENT

Surgery is indicated for visual loss or worsening of vision that is attributable to papilledema. The 2 surgical treatments are optic nerve sheath fenestration (ONSF) and shunting. These procedures are not recommended to treat headache alone. The decision to perform one or the other depends on the availability of an orbital surgeon and the status of the patient. Because reported cases include patients who had shunt surgery for intractable headaches, rather than visual loss, it is difficult to compare the efficacy of the 2 procedures for restoring vision. Either procedure may fail, necessitating the use of the other.[129–131] There have been no prospective, randomized trials of surgical treatments. A comprehensive review of the literature supported ONSF as the preferred treatment of visual loss from IIH, perhaps because visual outcomes were better documented with this procedure.[132]

ONSF

ONSF performed by a lateral or medial orbital approach or through a lid crease incision, involves fenestrating the optic nerve sheath or opening a "window" in the sheath of an edematous optic nerve.[133] Most neuro-ophthalmologists consider ONSF the treatment of choice for patients with failing vision. Its mechanism is not well understood. Some consider it a filtering procedure,[134] while others contend that the resultant perineuronal scarring shifts the pressure gradient posteriorly from the lamina cribrosa to the myelinated portion of the optic nerve.[133,135] The procedure likely increases blood flow to the optic nerve as demonstrated by color Doppler imaging preoperatively and postoperatively.[136,137] Patients in whom vision improved postoperatively had improvement in color Doppler parameters. ONSF should also be considered when severe papilledema extends into the macula. Macular exudates may improve after ONSD.[138] Pigment mottling and macular scars often persist following surgery, although they are often visually insignificant.[138]

Because headaches are sometimes relieved after ONSF, it is postulated that ONSF produces a global decrease in ICP in some cases,[139] presuming continuity between the perineural subarachnoid space and the intracranial subarachnoid space. There is likely much individual variation in this regard. The optic nerve sheath diameter and CSF pressure had a linear relationship within the 15- to 30-mg Hg range in humans participating in CSF absorption studies, with different slopes across subjects. In measures greater than 30 mm Hg, the optic nerve sheath diameter remained constant.[140]

ONSF is generally effective, but sometimes requires revision.[141,142] ONSF tends to be more effective in acute papilledema than chronic papilledema[142] and is not indicated once the papilledema has resolved. Studies show that bilateral improvement in vision often occurs after a unilateral procedure.[143,144] The complications of ONSF include failure, ischemic optic neuropathy, transient diplopia, and transient blindness.[145]

CSF Shunting

Because the ventricles are not enlarged in PTCS, lumboperitoneal shunting was previously preferred over ventriculoperitoneal (VP) shunting. Shunts are often quite effective in the short term but some patients require multiple revisions.[146–149] One study reviewed the efficacy of lumboperitoneal and VP from 6 institutions, where 37 patients underwent a total of 73 lumboperitoneal shunts and 9 VP shunts.[150] Only 14 patients were "cured" after a single surgical procedure. The shunt failure rate was high, and 27 shunts were replaced within 2 months.

Another retrospective review of 30 patients showed 82% overall improvement of symptoms (headache, diplopia, transient visual obscurations) with resolution of symptoms in 29%.[151] Most patients had improvement or stabilization of the visual field. There was a high revision rate (126 revisions; range 0–38 revisions per patient). There was no association between early shunt durability and the long-term need for multiple revisions; patients requiring more than 3 revisions were more likely to need additional shunt procedures.

Overall, the lumboperitoneal shunt failure rate is approximately 50% in PTCS.[147,149,150,152,153] The most common reasons for revision are shunt obstruction, intracranial hypotension, and lumbar radiculopathy. Visual deterioration may be the only sign of shunt failure and may occur even if the shunt is functioning.[154,155] Other complications include infection, abdominal pain, CSF leak, hindbrain herniation headaches, and migration of the peritoneal catheter.[149,156,157] Intracerebral hematoma occurs rarely.[158] Cisterna magna shunting avoids the problems of low-pressure headaches and radiculopathy but is a more extensive procedure with a significant failure rate.[159] There is renewed enthusiasm for VP shunts, which may be inserted quite accurately using stereotactic techniques.[153,160] The effect of shunting on CSF production is unknown.

Bariatric surgery may be an option for the long-term management of morbidly obese patients but is not helpful for acute management.[118] It may also confer additional health benefits in these patients who face considerable life-long medical morbidity from their obesity.

Venous Sinus Stenting

The discovery of transverse sinus stenosis in association with IIH prompted endovascular stenting as a treatment for the disorder. Numerous case series have been reported, with variable criteria for stenting and generally positive results.[161–166] Unfortunately, considerable morbidity has also occurred including subdural hematoma, epidural hematoma, anaphylaxis, hearing loss, and death.[167] Given that transverse sinus stenosis does not seem to affect the clinical course of IIH,[168,169] stenting should be reserved for patients with severe or fulminant disease who have exhausted other surgical methods.

SPECIAL CIRCUMSTANCES
Pregnancy

Although IIH may develop or worsen in pregnancy, its occurrence rate in pregnancy is similar to age-matched nonpregnant controls.[87] There is no increased risk of fetal loss in these patients, and therapeutic abortion is not indicated.[87] The diagnostic criteria of IIH during pregnancy is no different than for the general population. The management of active PTCS in a pregnant woman can be challenging, but most patients do well, with little or no permanent visual loss.[170] Most patients can be managed conservatively with careful neuro-ophthalmic follow-up and repeated LPs. Acetazolamide may be used after 20 weeks' gestation.[171] Thiazide diuretics and tricyclic antidepressants are generally avoided. If vision deteriorates, corticosteroids may be used. There is no contraindication to ONSF or shunting during pregnancy, although there is a theoretical risk of LP shunt malfunction from peritoneal catheter obstruction with the enlarging uterus.[172] PTCS arising in the postpartum period or following fetal loss raises the suspicion of cerebral venous thrombosis.[173]

Children and Adolescents

PTCS occurs with equal frequency in boys and girls before puberty.[7,8,174] In adolescents, girls are more often affected than boys.[7] Obesity is not as prevalent in young children as in adolescents and adults, and a secondary cause of intracranial hypertension is identifiable in approximately 50% of cases.[9,175,176] The most commonly predisposing conditions are otitis media, viral infection, medications, and closed head trauma.[177] It is possible that antibiotic use is underestimated as a precipitating factor, because all children with otitis media and many with viral infections are treated with antibiotics. The presenting signs of PTCS in young children are stiff neck, strabismus, irritability, apathy, somnolence, dizziness, and ataxia.[175,178] If the fontanelles are open and patent, papilledema may be absent.[174,178] Focal signs including lateral rectus palsy, facial palsy, and torticollis seem to be more common in children than adults.[178–181] If the precipitating cause is addressed, the disorder is generally benign and short-lived. However, permanent visual loss may occur, particularly if there is an associated dural venous sinus thrombosis.[179] The treatment is similar to management in adults.[174,182,183]

PTCS with an Identified Secondary Cause

Withdrawal of the causative agent or treatment of the underlying cause is imperative but neither guarantees rapid reversion of CSF pressure to normal nor reversal of symptoms and signs.[184] Medical and surgical treatments are used as clinically indicated to prevent permanent visual loss.

Fulminant PTCS

There is a small subgroup of patients who experience a rapid onset of symptoms and precipitous visual decline. They often have significant visual field loss, central visual acuity loss, and marked papilledema at presentation.[185] Macular edema or ophthalmoparesis may also be present. A progressive or "malignant" course requires rapid and aggressive treatment. A multidisciplinary physician team and one or more surgical procedures are usually required. Other therapeutic measures include intravenous corticosteroids, intravenous acetazolamide, and insertion of a lumbar drain. Cerebral venous sinus thrombosis is an important diagnostic consideration in these patients.

EVALUATION, ADJUSTMENT, AND RECURRENCE

Although headaches may persist indefinitely, most patients with PTCS have a monophasic course illness with remission. Re-evaluation and visual monitoring are most frequent in the acute to subacute stages. Depending on the visual status and tempo of visual decline, daily or weekly monitoring may be needed in the acute phases. As the patient's vision stabilizes and the papilledema remits, the interval between monitoring visits may be gradually extended, and many neuro-ophthalmologists advocate life-long yearly monitoring once the disorder remits. Retinal nerve fiber layer gliosis may prevent the resolution of optic disc elevation in some patients. IIH may recur with weight gain[186] and unwitting exposure to a provoking medication may incite recurrence in patients with medication-induced IIH. Papilledema may not be robust with a recurrence and may be absent following ONSF or with optic atrophy.

SUMMARY

IIH is officially considered a "rare" disorder by the National Institutes of Health but the incidence is rising. A primary care physician, an urgent care facility, or the emergency department is often the patient's first point of contact in the medical system. Even those with visual symptoms may not see an ophthalmologist or optometrist initially, particularly if their pain is severe. There is considerable variability in the presentation, making it imperative to measure the visual acuity and perform fundoscopy in all patients with headaches, particularly if they fit the typical demographic for IIH. Evaluation by an ophthalmologist is imperative to assess the vision, perimetry, and status of the optic nerve appearance at diagnosis and throughout the course of disease. Medical and surgical treatment options are used, depending on the visual status of the patient, the tempo of visual loss, and the availability of the appropriate surgical specialist. In some circumstances, patients who present with visual acuity loss or pronounced visual field loss may be best managed at a tertiary center with access to a neuro-ophthalmologist and specialty surgical care. Most patients with PTCS have a good outcome but a small percentage is left with legal or complete blindness and the associated devastating consequences.

The IIHTT is an important step not only in determining evidence-based guidelines for treating patients with mild vision loss but also in understanding the disease process. The published results will be available in 2014. The IIH Study Group is proposing a prospective, randomized surgical trial to provide evidence-based guidelines for treating patients with moderate to severe vision loss. It is hoped that during the next decade, significant advances will be made toward the understanding and treatment of this disorder.

REFERENCES

1. Friedman DI, Liu G, Digre KB. Diagnostic criteria for the pseudotumor cerebri syndrome in adults and children. Neurology 2013;81(13):1159–65.
2. Durcan FJ, Corbett JJ, Wall M. The incidence of pseudotumor cerebri. Population studies in Iowa and Louisiana. Arch Neurol 1988;45:875–7.
3. Radhakrishanan K, Ahlskog JE, Cross SA, et al. Idiopathic intracranial hypertension (pseudotumor cerebri). Descriptive epidemiology in Rochester, Minn, 1976-1990. Arch Neurol 1993;50(1):78–80.

4. Kesler A, Gadoth N. Epidemiology of idiopathic intracranial hypertension in Israel. J Neuroophthalmol 2001;21(1):12–4.
5. Radhakrishanan K, Sridharan R, Askhok PP, et al. Pseudotumor cerebri: incidence and pattern in north-eastern Libya. Acta Neurol 1986;25:117–24.
6. Jacobs DA, Corbett JJ, Balcer LJ. Annual incidence of idiopathic intracranial hypertension (IIH) in the Philadelphia area. Paper presented at: North American Neuro-Ophthalmology Society. Orlando, March 31, 2004.
7. Gordon K. Pediatric pseudotumor cerebri: descriptive epidemiology. Can J Neurol Sci 1997;24:219–21.
8. Scott IU, Siatkowski RM, Eneyni M, et al. Idiopathic intracranial hypertension in children and adolescents. Am J Ophthalmol 1997;124(2):253–5.
9. Balcer LJ, Liu GT, Forman S, et al. Idiopathic intracranial hypertension: relation of age and obesity in children. Neurology 1999;52:870–2.
10. Ko MW, Liu GT. Idiopathic intracranial hypertension. Horm Res Paediatr 2011; 74:381–9.
11. Bandyopadhyay S, Jacobson DM. Clinical features of late life-onset pseudotumor cerebri fulfilling the Modified Dandy Criteria. J Neuroophthalmol 2002;22:9–11.
12. Celebisoy N, Secil Y, Akyurekli O. Pseudotumor cerebri: etiological factors, presenting features and prognosis in the western part of Turkey. Acta Neurol Scand 2002;106(6):367–70.
13. Wall M, George D. Idiopathic intracranial hypertension. A prospective study of 50 patients. Brain 1991;114:155–80.
14. Wall M, Kupersmith MJ, Kieburtz KD, et al.The Idiopathic Intracranial Hypertension Treatment Trial: Clinical Profile at Baseline. JAMA Neurology, in press.
15. Weig SG. Asymptomatic idiopathic intracranial hypertension in young children. J Child Neurol 2002;17(3):239–41.
16. Giuseffi V, Wall M, Spiegel PZ, et al. Symptoms and disease associations in idiopathic intracranial hypertension (pseudotumor cerebri): a case-control study. Neurology 1991;41:239–44.
17. Round R, Keane JR. The minor symptoms of increased intracranial pressure: 101 patients with benign intracranial hypertension. Neurology 1988;38:1461–4.
18. Ramadan NM. Intracranial hypertension and migraine. Cephalalgia 1993;13:210–1.
19. Friedman DI, Rausch EA. Headache diagnoses in patients with treated idiopathic intracranial hypertension. Neurology 2002;58:1551–3.
20. Wang S-J, Silberstein SD, Patterson S, et al. Idiopathic intracranial hypertension without papilledema. A case-control study in a headache center. Neurology 1998;51:245–9.
21. Sadun AA, Currie J, Lessell S. Transient visual obscurations with elevated optic discs. Ann Neurol 1984;16:489–94.
22. Corbett JJ, Savino PJ, Thompson HS, et al. Visual loss in pseudotumor cerebri. Follow-up of 57 patients from five to 41 years and a profile of 14 patients with permanent severe visual loss. Arch Neurol 1982;39:461–74.
23. Rush JA. Pseudotumor cerebri: clinical profile and visual outcome in 63 patients. Mayo Clin Proc 1980;55:541–6.
24. Meador KJ, Swift TR. Tinnitus from intracranial hypertension. Neurology 1984; 34:1258–61.
25. Sismanis A. Otologic manifestations of benign intracranial hypertension syndrome: diagnosis and management. Laryngoscope 1987;97:1–17.
26. Fishman RA. Anatomical aspects of the cerebrospinal fluid. In: Fishman R, editor. Cerebrospinal fluid in diseases of the nervous system. Philadelphia: W.B. Sanders Co; 1992. p. 20–1.

27. Sismanis A, Hughes GB, Abedi E, et al. Otologic symptoms and findings of the pseudotumor cerebri syndrome: a preliminary report. Otolaryngol Head Neck Surg 1985;93:398–402.

28. Dorman PJ, Campbell MJ. Hearing loss as a false localising sign in raised intracranial pressure. J Neurol Neurosurg Psychiatry 1995;58:516.

29. Bortoluzzi M, Di Lauro L, Marini G. Benign intracranial hypertension with spinal and radicular pain. J Neurosurg 1982;57:833–6.

30. Selky AK, Dobyns WB, Yee RD. Idiopathic intracranial hypertension and facial diplegia. Neurology 1994;44:357.

31. Groves MD, McCutcheon IE, Ginsberg LE, et al. Radicular pain can be a symptom of elevated intracranial pressure. Neurology 1999;52:1093–5.

32. Murray RS, Tait VF, Thompson JA. Spinal and radicular pain in pseudotumor cerebri. Pediatr Neurol 1986;2(2):106–7.

33. Kleinschmidt JJ, Digre KB, Hanover R. Idiopathic intracranial hypertension. Relationship to depression, anxiety, and quality of life. Neurology 2000;54: 319–24.

34. Ross DR, Coffey CE, Massey EW, et al. Depression and benign intracranial hypertension. Psychosomatics 1985;26(5):387–93.

35. Kaplan CP, Miner ME, McGregor JM. Pseudotumor cerebri: risk for cognitive impairment? Brain Inj 1997;11(4):293–303.

36. Wall M, White WN II. Asymmetric papilledema in idiopathic intracranial hypertension. Prospective interocular comparison of sensory visual function. Invest Ophthalmol Vis Sci 1998;39:132–42.

37. Spence JD, Amacher AL, Willis NR. Benign intracranial hypertension without papilledema: role of 24-hour cerebrospinal fluid pressure monitoring in diagnosis and management. Neurosurgery 1980;34:1509–11.

38. Orcutt JC, Page NG, Sanders MD. Factors affecting visual loss in benign intracranial hypertension. Ophthalmology 1984;91:1303–12.

39. Wall M, George D. Visual loss in pseudotumor cerebri: incidence and defects related to visual field strategy. Arch Neurol 1987;44:170–5.

40. Griebel SR, Kosmorsky GS. Choroidal folds associated with increased intracranial pressure. Am J Ophthalmol 2000;129:513–6.

41. Frisén L. Swelling of the optic nerve head: a staging scheme. J Neurol Neurosurg Psychiatry 1982;45:13–8.

42. Shuper A, Snir M, Barash D, et al. Ultrasonography of the optic nerves: clinical application in children with pseudotumor cerebri. J Pediatr 1997;131:734–40.

43. Walsh TJ, Garden JW, Gallangher B. Obliteration of retinal venous pulsations. Am J Ophthalmol 1969;67:954–6.

44. Jacks AS, Miller NR. Spontaneous retinal venous pulsation: aetiology and significance. J Neurol Neurosurgy Psychiatry 2003;74:7–9.

45. Verplanck M, Kaufman DI, Parsons T, et al. Electrophysiology versus psychophysics in the detection of visual loss in pseudotumor cerebri. Neurology 1988;38:1789–92.

46. Wall M. Contrast sensitivity in pseudotumor cerebri. Ophthalmology 1986;93: 4–7.

47. Digre KB, Nakamoto BK, Warner JE, et al. A comparison of idiopathic intracranial hypertension with and without papilledema. Headache 2009;49(2):185–93.

48. Ney JJ, Volpe NJ, Liu GT, et al. Functional visual loss in idiopathic intracranial hypertension. Ophthalmology 2009;116(9):1801–3.

49. Baker RS, Buncic JR. Vertical ocular motility disturbances in pseudotumor cerebri. J Clin Neuroophthalmol 1985;5:41–4.

50. Frohman LP, Kupersmith MJ. Reversible vertical ocular deviations associated with raised intracranial pressure. J Clin Neuroophthalmol 1985;5:158–63.
51. Merikangas JR. Skew deviation in pseudotumor cerebri. Ann Neurol 1978;4:583.
52. Friedman DI, Forman S, Levi L, et al. Unusual ocular motility disturbances with increased intracranial pressure. Neurology 1998;50:1893–6.
53. Snyder DA, Frankel M. An unusual presentation of pseudotumor cerebri. Ann Ophthalmol 1979;11:1823–7.
54. Weisberg LA. Computed tomography in benign intracranial hypertension. Neurology 1985;35:1075–8.
55. Jacobson DM, Karanjia PN, Olson KA, et al. Computed tomography ventricular size has no predictive value in diagnosing pseudotumor cerebri. Neurology 1990;40:1454–5.
56. Maralani PJ, Hassanlou M, Torres C, et al. Accuracy of brain imaging in the diagnosis of idiopathic intracranial hypertension. Clin Radiol 2012;67:656–63.
57. Brodsky MC, Vaphiades M. Magnetic resonance imaging in pseudotumor cerebri. Ophthalmology 1998;105:1686–93.
58. Zagardo MT, Call WS, Kelman SE, et al. Reversible empty sella in idiopathic intracranial hypertension: an indicator of successful therapy? AJNR Am J Neuroradiol 1996;17:1953–6.
59. Gass A, Barker GJ, Riordan-Eva P, et al. MRI of the optic nerve in benign intracranial hypertension. Neuroradiology 1996;38:769–73.
60. Jinkins JR, Zthale S, Xiong A, et al. MR of the optic papilla protrusion in patients with high intracranial pressure. AJNR Am J Neuroradiol 1996;17:665–8.
61. Sinclair N, Asaad N, Johnston I. Pseudotumor cerebri occurring in association with the Chiari malformation. J Clin Neurosci 2002;9(1):99–101.
62. Lam BL, Schatz NJ, Glaser JS, et al. Pseudotumor cerebri from cranial venous obstruction. Ophthalmology 1992;99:706–12.
63. Cremer PD, Thompson EO, Johnston IH, et al. Pseudotumor cerebri and cerebral venous hypertension. Neurology 1996;47:1602.
64. King JO, Mitchell PJ, Thomson KR, et al. Cerebral venography and manometry in idiopathic intracranial hypertension. Neurology 1995;45:2224–8.
65. Farb RI, Vanek I, Scott JN, et al. Idiopathic intracranial hypertension. The prevalence and morphology of sinovenous stenosis. Neurology 2003;60:1418–24.
66. Baryshnik DB, Farb RI. Changes in the appearance of venous sinuses after treatment of disordered intracranial pressure. Neurology 2004;62:1445–6.
67. Rohr A, Dörner L, Stingele R, et al. Reversibility of venous sinus obstruction in idiopathic intracranial hypertension. AJNR Am J Neuroradiol 2007;28:656–9.
68. Avery RA, Shah SS, Licht DJ, et al. Reference range of cerebrospinal fluid opening pressure in children undergoing diagnostic lumbar puncture. N Engl J Med 2010;363(9):891–3.
69. Ecker A. Irregular fluctuation of elevated cerebrospinal fluid pressure. AMA Arch Neurol Psychiatry 1955;74:641–9.
70. Khandhar S, Friedman DI. Cerebrospinal fluid measurements in patients experiencing severe, benign headaches. Headache 2003;43(5):553–4.
71. Neville L, Egan RA. Frequency and amplitude of elevation of cerebrospinal fluid resting pressure by the Valsalva maneuver. Can J Ophthalmol 2005;40:775–7.
72. Bø SH, Davidsen EM, Benth JŠ. Cerebrospinal fluid opening pressure measurements in acute headache patients and in patients with either chronic or no pain. Acta Neurol Scand 2010;122(Suppl 190):6–10.
73. Eidlitz-Markus T, Stiebel-Kalish H, Rubin Y, et al. CSF pressure measurement during anesthesia: an unreliable technique. Paediatr Anaesth 2005;15(12):1078–82.

74. Quinckne H. Uber meningitis serosa and verewandte zustande. Deutsche Zeitschrift für Nervenheilkunde 1897;9:149–68 [in German].
75. Sahs AL, Joynt RJ. Brain swelling of unknown cause. Neurology 1956;6: 791–803.
76. Wall M, Dollar JD, Sadun AA, et al. Idiopathic intracranial hypertension. Lack of histological evidence for cerebral edema. Arch Neurol 1995;52:141–5.
77. Johnston I. The definition of a reduced CSF absorption syndrome: a reappraisal of benign intracranial pressure and related conditions. Med Hypotheses 1975;1: 10–4.
78. Johnston M, Zakharov A, Papaiconomou C, et al. Evidence of connections between cerebrospinal fluid and nasal lymphatic vessels in humans, non-human primates and other mammalian species. Cerebrospinal Fluid Res 2004;1(2):1–13.
79. Karahalios DG, Rekate HL, Khayata MH, et al. Elevated intracranial venous pressure as a universal mechanism in pseudotumor cerebri of varying etiologies. Neurology 1996;46:198–202.
80. King JO, Mitchell PJ, Thomson KR, et al. Manometry combined with cervical puncture in idiopathic intracranial hypertension. Neurology 2002;58:26–30.
81. Biousse V, Ameri A, Bousser MG. Isolated intracranial hypertension as the only sign of cerebral venous thrombosis. Neurology 1999;53:1537–42.
82. Purvin VA, Trobe JD, Kosmorsky G. Neuro-ophthalmic features of cerebral venous obstruction. Arch Neurol 1995;52:880–5.
83. Daif A, Awada A, Al-Rajeh S, et al. Cerebral venous thrombosis in adults: a study of 40 cases from Saudi Arabia. Stroke 1995;26:1193–5.
84. Quattrone A, Bono F, Oliveri R, et al. Cerebral venous thrombosis and isolated intracranial hypertension without papilledema in CDH. Neurology 2001;57:31–6.
85. Corbett JJ, Digre KB. Idiopathic intracranial hypertension. An answer to, "the chicken or the egg?". Neurology 2002;58:5–6.
86. Sugarman HJ, DeMaria EJ, Felton WL, et al. Increased aintra-abdominal pressure and cardiac filling pressure in obesity-associated pseudotumor cerebri. Neurology 1997;49:507–11.
87. Digre KB, Varner MW, Corbett JJ. Pseudotumor cerebri and pregnancy. Neurology 1984;34:721–9.
88. Lindvall M, Edvinsson L, Owman C. Reduced cerebrospinal fluid formation through cholinergic mechanisms. Neurosci Lett 1978;9:77–82.
89. Lindvall M, Edvinsson L, Owman C. Effect of sympathomimetic drugs and corresponding receptor antagonists on the rate of cerebrospinal fluid production. Exp Neurol 1979;64:132–45.
90. Lindvall M, Owman C. Autonomic nerves in the mammalian choroid plexus and their influence on the formation of cerebrospinal fluid. J Cereb Blood Flow Metab 1981;1:245–66.
91. Nilsson C, Lindvall-Axelsson M, Owman C. Sympathetic nervous control of cerebrospinal fluid production from the choroid plexus. Science 1978;201:176–8.
92. Hoffman BJ, Mezey E. Distribution of the serotonin 5-HT$_{1C}$ receptor mRNA in the adult rat brain. FEBS Lett 1989;247:453–62.
93. Pazos A, Baker RS, Khorram D, et al. The binding of serotonergic ligands to the porcine choroid plexus: characterization of a new type of serotonin recognition site. Eur J Pharmacol 1985;106:539–46.
94. Lindvall-Axelsson M, Nilsson C, Owman C, et al. Involvement of 5-HT$_{1C}$ receptors in the production of CSF from the choroid plexus. In: Seylaz JM, MacKenzie ET, editors. Neurotransmission and cerebrovascular function I. Amsterdam: Elsevier; 1989. p. 237–40.

95. Friedman DI, Ingram P, Rogers MA. Low tyramine diet in the treatment of idiopathic intracranial hypertension. A pilot study. Neurology 1998;50:A5.
96. Fishman R. Polar bear liver, vitamin A, aquaporins, and pseudotumor cerebri. Ann Neurol 2002;52(5):531–3.
97. Wintour EM. Water channels and urea transporters. Clin Exp Pharmacol Physiol 1997;24(1):1–9.
98. King LS, Agre P. Pathophysiology of the aquaporin water channels. Annu Rev Physiol 1996;58:619–48.
99. Nielsen S, Nagelhus EA, Amiry-Moghaddam M, et al. Specialized membrane domains for water transport in glial cells: high-resolution immunogold cytochemistry of aquaporin-4 in rat brain. J Neurosci 1997;17(1):171–80.
100. Kerty E, Heuser K, Indahl UG, et al. Is the brain water channel aquaporin-4 a pathogenetic factor in idiopathic intracranial hypertension? Results from a combined clinical and genetic study in a Norwegian cohort. Acta Ophthalmol 2013; 91(1):88–91.
101. Weber KT. Aldersteronism revisited: perspectives on less well-recognized actions of aldosterone. J Lab Clin Med 2003;142:71–82.
102. Kageyama Y, Suzuki H, Saruta T. Presence of aldeosterone-like immunoreactivity in cerebrospinal fluid in normotensive subjects. Acta Endocrinol (Copenh) 1992;126:501–4.
103. Corbett JJ. The first Jacobson lecture: familial idiopathic intracranial hypertension. J Neuroophthalmol 2008;24:337–47.
104. Wall M. Idiopathic intracranial hypertension and the idiopathic intracranial hypertension treatment trial. J Neuroophthalmol 2013;33(1):1–3.
105. Huff AL, Hupp SL, Rothrock JF. Chronic daily headache with migrainous features due to papilledema-negative idiopathic intracranial hypertension. Cephalalgia 1996;16:451–2.
106. Marcelis J, Silberstein SD. Idiopathic intracranial hypertension without papilledema. Arch Neurol 1991;48:392–9.
107. Mathew NT, Ravishankar K, Sanin LC. Coexistence of migraine and idiopathic intracranial hypertension without papilledema. Neurology 1996;46:1226–30.
108. Green JP, Newman NJ, Stowe ZN, et al. "Normal pressure" pseudotumor cerebri. J Neuroophthalmol 1997;17(4):279–90.
109. Barkana T, Levin N, Steiner I, et al. Pseudo-pseudotumor cerebri: Idiopathic intracranial hypertension with pleocytosis. Paper presented at: American Academy of Ophthalmology/Pan American Association of Ophthalmology. Orlando, October 20, 2002.
110. van Oosterhout WP, Gagaouzova BS, Terwindt GM, et al. Transient intracranial pressure changes during migraine attack. Cephalalgia 2013;33(11):956.
111. Ireland B, Corbett JJ. The search for causes of idiopathic intracranial hypertension. Arch Neurol 1990;47:315–20.
112. Wall M, Giuseffi V, Rojas PB. Symptoms and disease associations in pseudotumor cerebri: a case-control study. Neurology 1989;39:210.
113. Friedman DI, Streeten DH. Idiopathic intracranial hypertension and orthostatic edema may share a common pathogenesis. Neurology 1998;50:1099–104.
114. Seckl J, Lightman S. Cerebrospinal fluid neurohypophysial peptides in benign intracranial hypertension. J Neurol Neurosurg Psychiatry 1988;51:1538–41.
115. Sorenson PS, Gjerris F, Hammer M. Cerebrospinal fluid vasopressin and increased intracranial pressure. Neurology 1982;3:1255–9.
116. Sorenson PS, Hammer M, Gjerris F. Cerebrospinal fluid vasopressin in benign intracranial hypertension. Ann Neurol 1984;15:435–40.

117. Thibonnier MJ, Marchetti JP, Corvol PJ, et al. Abnormal regulation of antidiuretic hormone in idiopathic edema. Am J Med 1979;67:67–73.
118. Sugerman HJ, Felton WL, Salvant JB, et al. Effects of surgically induced weight loss on idiopathic intracranial hypertension in morbid obesity. Neurology 1995; 45:1655–9.
119. Kupersmith MJ, Gamell L, Turbin R, et al. Effects of weight loss on the course of idiopathic intracranial hypertension in women. Neurology 1998;50:1094–8.
120. Johnson LN, Krohel GB, Madsen RW, et al. The role of weight loss and acetazol-amide in the treatment of idiopathic intracranial hypertension (pseudotumor cer-ebri). Ophthalmology 1998;105:2313–7.
121. Tomsak RL, Niffenegger AS, Remler BF. Treatment of pseudotumor cerebri with Diamox (acetazolamide). J Clin Neuroophthalmol 1988;18:93–8.
122. Lee AG, Anderson R, Kardon RH, et al. Presumed "sulfa allergy" in patients with intracranial hypertension treated with acetazolamide or furosemide: cross-reactivity, myth or reality? Am J Ophthalmol 2004;138(1):114–8.
123. Corbett JJ, Thompson HS. The rational management of idiopathic intracranial hypertension. Arch Neurol 1989;46:1049–51.
124. Liu GT, Kay MD, Bienfang DC, et al. Pseudotumor cerebri associated with corti-costeroid withdrawal in inflammatory bowel disease. Am J Ophthalmol 1994; 117:352–7.
125. Liu GT, Glaser JS, Schatz N. High-dose methylprednisolone and acetazolamide for visual loss in pseudotumor cerebri. Am J Ophthalmol 1994;118:88–96.
126. Friedman DI, Eller PE. Topiramate for treatment of idiopathic intracranial hyper-tension. Headache 2003;43(5):592.
127. Celebisoy N, Gokcay F, Sirin H, et al. Treatment of idiopathic intracranial hyper-tension: topiramate vs acetazolamide, an open-label study. Acta Neurol Scand 2007;116(5):322–7.
128. Godoy DA, Rabinstein AA, Biestro A, et al. Effects of indomethacin test on intracranial pressure and cerebral hemodynamics in patients with refractory intracranial hypertension: a feasibility study. Neurosurgery 2012;71(2):245–57 [discussion: 257–8].
129. Wilkes BN, Siatkowski RM. Progressive optic neuropathy in idiopathic intracra-nial hypertension after optic nerve sheath fenestration. J Neuroophthalmol 2009;29(4):281–3.
130. Ramsey CN 3rd, Proctor BL, Baker RS, et al. Prevention of visual loss caused by shunt failure: a potential role for optic nerve sheath fenestration. Report of three cases. J Neurosurg 2006;104(Suppl 2):149–51.
131. Kelman SE, Sergott RC, Cioffi GA, et al. Modified optic nerve decompression in patients with functioning lumboperitoneal shunts and progressive visual loss. Ophthalmology 1991;98:1449–53.
132. Feldon SE. Visual outcomes comparing surgical techniques for management of severe idiopathic intracranial hypertension. Neurosurg Focus 2007;23(5):E6.
133. Keltner JL. Optic nerve sheath decompression. How does it work? Has its time come? Arch Ophthalmol 1988;206:1365–9.
134. Tsai JC, Petrovich MD, Sadun AA. Histological and ultratructural examination of optic nerve sheath decompression. Br J Ophthalmol 1995;79:182–5.
135. Hamed LM, Tse DT, Glaser JS, et al. Neuroimaging of the optic nerve after fenestration for management of pseudotumor cerebri. Arch Ophthalmol 1992; 110:636–9.
136. Mittra RA, Sergott RC, Flaharty PM, et al. Optic nerve decompression improves hemodynamic parameters in papilledema. Ophthalmology 1993;100:987–97.

137. Lee SY, Shin DH, Spoor TC, et al. Bilateral retinal venous caliber decrease following unilateral optic nerve sheath decompression. Ophthalmic Surg 1995;6:25–8.

138. Carter SR, Seiff SR. Macular changes in pseudotumor cerebri before and after optic nerve fenestration. Ophthalmology 1995;102:937–41.

139. Ngyun R, Carta A, Geleris A, et al. Long-term effect of optic sheath decompression on intracranial pressure in pseudotumor cerebri. Invest Ophthalmol Vis Sci 1997;38:S388.

140. Hansen H, Helmke K. Validation of optic nerve sheath response to changing cerebrospinal fluid pressure: ultrasound findings during intrathecal infusion. J Neurosurg 1997;87(1):34–40.

141. Pearson PA, Baker RS, Khorram D, et al. Evaluation of optic nerve sheath fenestration in pseudotumor cerebri using automated perimetry. Ophthalmology 1991;98:99–105.

142. Spoor TC, Ramocki JM, Madion MP, et al. Treatment of pseudotumor cerebri by primary and secondary optic nerve sheath decompression. Am J Ophthalmol 1991;112:177–85.

143. Alsuhaibani AH, Carter KD, Nerad JA, et al. Effect of optic nerve sheath fenestration on papilledema of the operated and the contralateral nonoperated eyes in idiopathic intracranial hypertension. Ophthalmology 2011;118(2):412–4.

144. Sergott RC, Savino PJ, Bosley TM. Modified optic nerve sheath decompression provides long-term visual improvement for pseudotumor cerebri. Arch Ophthalmol 1988;106:1384–90.

145. Flynn WJ, Westfall CT, Weisman JS. Transient blindness after optic nerve sheath fenestration. Am J Ophthalmol 1994;117:678–9.

146. Cornblath WT, Miller NR. Pseudotumor cerebri treated with lumbo-peritoneal shunt. Ann Neurol 1989;26:183.

147. Johnston I, Besser M, Morgan M. Cerebrospinal fluid diversion in the treatment of benign intracranial hypertension. J Neurosurg 1988;69:195–202.

148. Sinclair AJ, Kuruvath S, Sen D, et al. Is cerebrospinal fluid shunting in idiopathic intracranial hypertension worthwhile? A 10-year review. Cephalalgia 2011; 31(16):1627–33.

149. Eggenberger ER, Miller NR, Vitale S. Lumboperitoneal shunt for the treatment of pseudotumor cerebri. Neurology 1996;46:1524–30.

150. Rosenberg ML, Corbett JJ, Smith C, et al. Cerebrospinal diversion procedures for pseudotumor cerebri. Neurology 1993;43:1071–2.

151. Burgett RA, Purvin VA, Kawasaki A. Lumboperitoneal shunting for pseudotumor cerebri. Neurology 1997;49:734–9.

152. Mauriello JA, Shaderowfsky P, Gizzi M, et al. Management of visual loss after optic nerve sheath decompression in patients with pseudotumor cerebri. Ophthalmology 1995;102:441–5.

153. Howard J, Appen R. Ventriculoperitoneal shunting for pseudotumor cerebri. Invest Ophthalmol Vis Sci 2002;43 [E-abstract 2461].

154. Lee AG. Visual loss as the manifesting symptoms of ventriculoperitoneal shunt malfunction. Am J Ophthalmol 1996;122:127–9.

155. Liu GT, Volpe NJ, Schatz NJ, et al. Severe sudden visual loss caused by pseudotumor cerebri and lumboperitoneal shunt failure. Am J Ophthalmol 1996;122: 129–31.

156. Alleyne CH Jr, Shutter LA, Colohan AR. Cranial migration of a lumboperitoneal shunt catheter. South Med J 1996;89:634–46.

157. Miller NR. Bilateral visual loss and simultagnosia after lumboperitoneal shunt for pseudotumor cerebri. J Neuroophthalmol 1997;17:36–8.

158. Turkoglu E, Kazanci B, Karavelioglu E, et al. Intracerebral hematoma following lumboperitoneal shunt insertion: a rare case report. Turk Neurosurg 2011; 21(1):94–6.
159. Johnston IH, Sheridan MM. CSF shunting from the cisterna magna: a report of 16 cases. Br J Neurosurg 1993;7:39–44.
160. Abu-Serieh B, Ghassempour K, Duprez T, et al. Stereotactic ventriculoperitoneal shunting for refractory idiopathic intracranial hypertension. Neurosurgery 2007; 60(6):1039–43 [discussion: 1043–4].
161. Owler BK, Parker G, Halmagyi GM, et al. Pseudotumor cerebri syndrome: venous sinus obstruction and its treatment with stent placement. J Neurosurg 2003;98:1045–55.
162. Higgins JN, Cousins C, Owler BK, et al. Idiopathic intracranial hypertension: 12 cases treated by venous sinus stenting. J Neurol Neurosurg Psychiatry 2003;74: 1662–6.
163. Ahmed R, Wilkinson MJ, Parker G, et al. Management of idiopathic intracranial hypertension (IIH) with stenting of transverse sinus stenosis. Vancouver (Canada): North American Neuro-Ophthalmology Society; 2011.
164. Arac A, Lee M, Steinberg GK, et al. Efficacy of endovascular stenting in dural venous sinus stenosis for the treatment of idiopathic intracranial hypertension. Neurosurg Focus 2009;27(5):E14.
165. Donnet A, Metellus P, Levrier O, et al. Endovascular treatment of idiopathic intra-cranial hypertension: clinical and radiologic outcome of 10 consecutive pa-tients. Neurology 2008;70(8):641–7.
166. Puffer RC, Mustafa W, Lanzino G. Venous sinus stenting for idiopathic intracra-nial hypertension: a review of the literature. J Neurointerv Surg 2013;5(5):483–6.
167. Friedman DI. Cerebral venous pressure, gastric bypass surgery and dural venous sinus stenting in idiopathic intracranial hypertension. J Neuroophthalmol 2006;26: 61–4.
168. Riggeal BD, Bruce BB, Saindane AM, et al. Clinical course of idiopathic intra-cranial hypertension with transverse sinus stenosis. Neurology 2013;80(3): 289–95.
169. Bono F, Quattrone A, Bruce BB, et al. Clinical course of idiopathic intracranial hypertension with transverse sinus stenosis. Neurology 2013;81(7):695.
170. Huda-Baron R, Kupersmith MJ. Idiopathic intracranial hypertension in preg-nancy. J Neurol 2002;249(8):1078–81.
171. Lee AG, Pless M, Falardeau J, et al. The use of acetazolamide in idiopathic intra-cranial hypertension during pregnancy. Am J Ophthalmol 2005;139(5):855–9.
172. Shapiro S, Yee R, Brown H. Surgical management of pseudotumor cerebri in pregnancy: case report. Neurosurgery 1995;37:829–31.
173. McDonnell GV, Patterson VH, McKinstry S. Cerebral venous thrombosis ocurring during an ectopic pregnancy and complicated by intracranial hypertension. Br J Clin Pract 1997;51:194–7.
174. Lessell S. Pediatric pseudotumor cerebri (idiopathic intracranial hypertension). Surv Ophthalmol 1992;37:155–66.
175. Cinciripini GS, Donahue S, Borchert MS. Idiopathic intracranial hypertension in prepubertal pediatric patients: characteristics, treatment and outcome. Am J Ophthalmol 1999;127:178–82.
176. Kesler A, Fattal-Valevski A. Idiopathic intracranial hypertension in the pediatric population. J Child Neurol 2002;17(10):745–8.
177. Dhiravibulya K, Ouvrier R, Johnston I, et al. Benign intracranial hypertension in childhood; a review of 23 patients. J Paediatr Child Health 1991;27:204–7.

178. Baker RS, Baumann RJ, Buncic JR. Idiopathic intracranial hypertension (pseudotumor cerebri) in pediatric patients. Pediatr Neurol 1989;5:5–11.
179. Baker RS, Carter DC, Hendrock EB, et al. Visual loss in pseudotumor cerebri of childhood: a follow-up study. Arch Ophthalmol 1985;103:1681–6.
180. Phillips PH, Repka MX, Lambert SR. Pseudotumor cerebri in children. J AAPOS 1998;2(1):33–8.
181. Speer C, Pearlman J, Phillips PH, et al. Fourth cranial nerve palsy in pediatric patients with pseudotumor cerebri. Am J Ophthalmol 1999;127(2):236–7.
182. Schoeman JF. Childhood pseudotumor cerebri: clinical and intracranial pressure response to acetazolamide and furosemide treatment in a case series. J Child Neurol 1994;9:130–4.
183. Rangwala LM, Liu GT. Pediatric idiopathic intracranial hypertension. Surv Ophthalmol 2007;52(6):597–617.
184. Friedman DI, Gordon LK, Egan RA, et al. Doxycycline and intracranial hypertension. Neurology 2004;62:2297–9.
185. Thambisetty M, Lavin PJ, Newman NJ, et al. Fulminant idiopathic intracranial hypertension. Neurology 2007;68(3):229–32.
186. Ko MW, Chang SC, Ridha MA, et al. Weight gain and recurrence in idiopathic intracranial hypertension: a case-control study. Neurology 2011;76(18):1564–7.
187. Kikuchi M, Kudo S, Wada M, et al. Retropharyngeal rhabdomyosarcoma mimicking pseudotumor cerebri. Pediatr Neurol 1999;21:496–9.
188. Molina JC, Martinez-Vea A, Riu S, et al. Pseudotumor cerebri: an unusual complication of brachiocephalic vein thrombosis associated with hemodialysis catheters. Am J Kidney Dis 1998;31:E3.
189. Kollar DC, Johnston IH. Pseudotumor after arteriovenous malformation embolisation. J Neurol Neurosurg Psychiatry 1999;67:249–52.
190. Condulis N, Germain G, Charest N, et al. Pseudotumor cerebri: a presenting manifestation of Addison's disease. Clin Pediatr 1997;36:711–4.
191. Bourruat FX, Regli F. Pseudotumor cerebri as a complication of amiodarone therapy. Am J Ophthalmol 1993;116(6):776–7.
192. Fort JA, Smith LD. Pseudotumor cerebri secondary to intermediate-dose cytarabine HCl. Ann Pharmacother 1999;33:576–8.
193. Greer M. Benign intracranial hypertension. II. Following corticosteroid therapy. Neurology 1963;13:439–41.
194. Walker AE, Adamkiewitz JJ. Pseudotumor cerebri associated with prolonged corticosteroid therapy. JAMA 1964;188(9):779–84.
195. Cruz OA, Fogg SG, Roper-Hall G. Pseudotumor cerebri associated with cyclosporine use. Am J Ophthalmol 1996;122:436.
196. Blethen SL. Complications of growth hormone therapy in children. Curr Opin Pediatr 1995;7:466–71.
197. Grancois I, Castells I, Silberstein J, et al. Empty sella, growth hormone deficiency and pseudotumour cerebri: effect of initiation, withdrawal and resumption of growth hormone therapy. Eur J Pediatr 1997;156:69–70.
198. Koller EA, Stadel BV, Malozowski SN. Papilledema in 15 renally compromised patients treated with growth hormone. Pediatr Nephrol 1997;11:451–4.
199. Malozozwski S, Tanner LA, Wysowski DK, et al. Benign intracranial hypertension in children with growth hormone deficiency treated with growth hormone. J Pediatr 1995;126:996–9.
200. Rogers AH, Rogers GL, Bremer DL, et al. Pseudotumor cerebri in children receiving recombinant human growth hormone. Ophthalmology 1999;106:1186–90.

201. Boot JH. Pseudotumor cerebri as a side effect of leuprorelin acetate. Ir J Med Sci 1996;165:60.
202. Campos SP, Olitsky S. Idiopathic intracranial hypertension after L-thyroxine therapy for acquired hypothyroidism. Clin Pediatr 1995;34:334–7.
203. Raghavan S, DiMartino-Nardi J, Saenger P, et al. Pseudotumor cerebri in an infant after L-thyroxine therapy for transient neonatal hypothyroidism. J Pediatr 1997;130:478–80.
204. Saul RF, Hamburger HA, Selhorst JB. Pseudotumor cerebri secondary to lithium carbonate. JAMA 1985;253:2869–70.
205. Cohen DN. Intracranial hypertension and papilledema associated with nalidixic acid therapy. Am J Ophthalmol 1973;76:680–2.
206. Mukherjee A, Dutta B, Lahiri M, et al. Benign intracranial hypertension after nalidixic acid overdose in infants. Lancet 1990;335:1602.
207. Wysowski DK, Green L. Serious adverse events in Norplant users reported to the Food and Drug Administration's MedWatch spontaneous reporting system. Obstet Gynecol 1995;85:538–42.
208. Alder J, Fraunfelder F, Edwards R, et al. Levonorgestrel implants and intracranial hypertension. N Engl J Med 1995;332(25):1720–1.
209. Gardner K, Cox T, Digre K. Idiopathic intracranial hypertension associated with tetracycline use in fraternal twins: case report and review. Neurology 1995;45:6–10.
210. Giles CL, Soble AR. Intracranial hypertension and tetracycline therapy. Am J Ophthalmol 1971;72:981–2.
211. Lee AG. Pseudotumor cerebri after treatment with tetracycline and isotretinoin for acne. Cutis 1995;55:165–8.
212. Meacock DJ, Hewer RL. Tetracycline and benign intracranial hypertension. Br Med J 1981;282:1240.
213. Minutello JS, Dimayuga RG, Carter J. Pseudotumor cerebri, a rare adverse reaction to tetracycline therapy. J Periodontol 1988;58:848–51.
214. Maroon JC, Mealy J Jr. Benign intracranial hypertension. Sequel to tetracycline therapy in a child. JAMA 1971;216(9):1479–80.
215. Quinn AG, Singer SB, Bunic JR. Pediatric tetracycline-induced pseudotumor cerebri. J AAPOS 1999;3(1):53–7.
216. Ohlrich GD, Ohlrich JG. Papilloedema in an adolescent due to tetracycline. Med J Aust 1977;1:334–5.
217. Pierog SH, Al-Salihi FL, Cinotti D. Pseudotumor cerebri - a complication of tetracycline treatment of acne. J Adolesc Health Care 1986;7:139–40.
218. Stuart BH, Litt IF. Tetracycline-induced intracranial hypertension in an adolescent: a complication of systemic acne therapy. J Pediatr 1978;92(4):679–80.
219. Chiu AM, Chuenkongkaew WL, Cornblath WT, et al. Minocycline treatment and pseudotumor cerebri syndrome. Am J Ophthalmol 1998;126:116–21.
220. Moskowitz T, Leibowitz E, Ronen M, et al. Pseudotumor cerebri induced by vitamin A combined with minocycline. Ann Ophthalmol 1993;25:306–8.
221. Donnet A, Dufour H, Graziani N, et al. Minocycline and benign intracranial hypertension. Biomed Pharmacother 1992;46:171–2.
222. Beran RG. Pseudotumor cerebri associated with minocycline therapy for acne. Med J Aust 1980;1:323–4.
223. Lochhead J, Elston JS. Doxycycline induced intracranial hypertension. BMJ 2003;326:641–2.
224. Alemeyehu W. Pseudotumor cerebri (toxic effect of the "magic bullet"). Ethiop Med 1995;33:265–70.

225. Feldman MH, Schlezinger NS. Benign intracranial hypertension associated with hypervitaminosis A. Arch Neurol 1970;22:1–7.
226. Lombaert A, Carton H. Benign intracranial hypertension due to A-hypervitaminosis in adults and adolescents. Eur Neurol 1976;14:340–50.
227. Fraunfelder FW, Fraunfelder FT, Edwards R. Ocular side effects possibly associated with isotretinoin usage. Am J Ophthalmol 2001;132(2):299–305.
228. Bigby M, Stern RS. Adverse reactions to isotretinoin. A report for the Adverse Reaction Reporting System. J Am Acad Dermatol 1988;18:543–52.
229. Roytman M, Frumkin A, Boyn TG. Pseudotumor cerebri caused by isotretinoin. Cutis 1988;42:399–400.
230. Lebowitz MA, Berson DS. Ocular effects of oral retinoids. J Am Acad Dermatol 1988;19:209–11.
231. Fraunfelder FW, Fraunfelder FT, Corbett JJ. Isotretinoin usage and intracranial hypertension. Ophthalmology 2004;111:1248–50.
232. Tallman MS, Andersen JW, Schiffer CA, et al. Clinical description of 44 patients with acute promyelocytic leukemia who developed the retinoic acid syndrome. Blood 2000;95(1):90–5.
233. Viraben R, Mathieu C, Fontan B. Benign intracranial hypertension during etretinate therapy for mycosis fungoides. J Am Acad Dermatol 1985;13(3):515–7.
234. Bonnetblanc JM, Hugon J, Dumas M, et al. Intracranial hypertension with etretinate. Lancet 1983;2(8356):974.
235. Visani G, Manfroi S, Tosi P, et al. All-trans-retinoic acid and pseudotumor cerebri. Leuk Lymphoma 1996;23:437–42.
236. Javeed N, Shaikh J, Jayaram S. Recurrent pseudotumor cerebri in an HIV-positive patient. AIDS 1995;9:817–9.
237. Prevett MC, Plant GT. Intracranial hypertension and HIV associated meningoradiculitis. J Neurol Neurosurg Psychiatry 1997;62:407–9.
238. Schwartz S, Husstedt IW, Georgiadis D, et al. Benign intracranial hypertension in an HIV-infected patient: headache as the only presenting sign. AIDS 1995;9: 657–8.
239. Kan L, Sood SK, Maytal J. Pseudotumor cerebri in Lyme disease: a case report and literature review. Pediatr Neurol 1998;18:439–41.
240. Konrad D, Kuster H, Hunzinker UA. Pseudotumor cerebri after varicella. Eur J Pediatr 1998;157:904–6.
241. Lahat E, Leshem M, Barzilai A. Pseudotumor cerebri complicating varicella in a child. Acta Paediatr 1998;87:1310–1.
242. Sussman J, Leach M, Greaves M, et al. Potentially pro-thrombotic abnormalities of coagulation in benign intracranial hypertension. J Neurol Neurosurg Psychiatry 1997;62:229–33.
243. Kesler A, Ellis MG, Reshef T, et al. Idiopathic intracranial hypertension and anti-cardiolipin antibodies. J Neurol Neurosurg Psychiatry 2000;68:379–80.
244. Leker RR, Steiner I. Anticardiolipin antibodies are frequently present in patients with idiopathic intracranial hypertension. Arch Neurol 1998;55:817–20.
245. Kalbian VV, Challis MT. Behcet's disease: report of twelve cases with three manifesting as papilledema. Am J Med 1970;49:823–9.
246. Teh LS, O'Connor GM, O'Sullivan MM, et al. Recurrent papilloedema and early onset optic atrophy in Behcet's syndrome. Ann Rheum Dis 1990;49:410–1.
247. Graham EM, Al-Akshar R, Sanders MD, et al. Benign intracranial hypertension in Behcet's syndrome. J Neuroophthalmol 1980;1(1):73–6.
248. Martinez-Lage JF, Alamo L, Poza M. Raised intracranial pressure in minimal forms of cranial synostosis. Childs Nerv Syst 1999;15:11–5.

249. Au Eong KG, Hariharan S, Chua EC, et al. Idiopathic intracranial hypertension, empty sella turcica and polycyctic ovary syndromes – a case report. Singapore Med J 1997;38:129–30.
250. Pelton RW, Lee AG, Orengo-Nania SD, et al. Bilateral optic disk edema caused by sarcoidosis mimicking pseudotumor cerebri. Am J Ophthalmol 1999;127: 229–30.
251. Wolin MJ, Brannon WL, Kay MD, et al. Disk edema in an overweight woman (clinical conference). Surv Ophthalmol 1995;39:307–14.
252. Miller JJ, Thomas D, Lynn JL, et al. Sleep disorders: a risk factor for pseudotumor cerebri (PTC). Invest Ophthalmol Vis Sci 2000;41(4):S313.
253. Purvin VA, Kawasaki A, Yee RD. Papilledema and obstructive sleep apnea syndrome. Arch Ophthalmol 2000;118(12):1626–30.
254. Green L, Vinker S, Amital H, et al. Pseudotumor cerebri in systemic lupus erythematosis. Semin Arthritis Rheum 1995;25:103–8.
255. Horoshovski D, Amital H, Katz M, et al. Pseudotumor cerebri in SLE. Clin Rheumatol 1995;14:708–10.
256. Sybert VP, Bird TD, Salk DJ. Pseudotumor cerebri and Turner syndrome. J Neurol Neurosurg Psychiatry 1985;48:164–6.

Spontaneous CSF Leaks
Low CSF Volume Syndromes

Bahram Mokri, MD

KEYWORDS

- Spontaneous CSF leak • Spontaneous intracranial hypotension (SIH)
- CSF hypovolemia • Orthostatic headaches • Diffuse patchy meningeal enhancement
- Acquired Chiari malformation • Epidural blood patch • Radioisotope cisternography

KEY POINTS

- Spontaneous intracranial hypotension nearly always results from spontaneous cerebro-spinal fluid (CSF) leaks, typically at the spine level and only rarely from the skull base.
- The triad of orthostatic headaches, diffuse patchy meningeal enhancement, and low CSF pressure, although a diagnostic hallmark, may or may not be encountered because the variability in clinical presentations, imaging observations, and CSF findings is indeed substantial.
- The core pathogenetic factor is a decreased volume of CSF rather than its pressure.
- The anatomy of the leak may be complex. A preexisting dural weakness, usually in connection with an abnormality of the connective tissue matrix sometimes along with triv-ial traumas, may play an etiologic role.
- Slow-flow and fast-flow CSF leaks each present challenges on locating the actual site of the leak.
- Epidural blood patch (EBP) has emerged as the treatment of choice when conservative measures have failed. However, expect considerable variability in response to this treat-ment, and recall that the efficacy of EBP in spontaneous CSF leaks is substantially less than its efficacy in postlumbar puncture leaks.
- Surgery may be helpful in well-selected cases, when less invasive measures have failed and when the site of the leak has been definitely identified.

INTRODUCTION

About 2 decades ago, the first report on pachymeningeal gadolinium enhancement in spontaneous intracranial hypotension (SIH) appeared in the literature.[1] This relatively short interval has witnessed enormous progress while a much larger number of pa-tients are now identified and a far broader clinical spectrum is recognized.[2]

Funding Source: None.
Conflict of Interest: Dr B. Mokri reports no disclosures.
Department of Neurology, Mayo Clinic, 200 First Street Southwest, Rochester, MN 55905, USA
E-mail address: bmokri@mayo.edu

It is now known that almost all cases of SIH result from spontaneous cerebrospinal fluid (CSF) leaks, typically at the level of the spine. Spontaneous (nontraumatic) leaks at the level of the skull base occur only rarely.

A substantial variability in clinical, imaging, and CSF findings is also recognized, such as consistently normal CSF opening pressures in some of the patients, absent pachymeningeal enhancement or even essentially normal head magnetic resonance imaging (MRI) in some other patients, and yet absent headache in occasional patients. Decreased CSF volume (CSF hypovolemia), rather than decreased CSF opening pressure, seems to be the core pathogenetic factor as the independent variable, whereas CSF opening pressure, MRI findings, and clinical features seem to be variables dependent on the CSF volume.[3] The term *SIH* no longer seems broad enough to embrace all of these variables. Alternative terms, such as *CSF volume depletion*, *CSF hypovolemia*, or *spontaneous CSF leak*, have appeared in the literature and have been used interchangeably.[4,5]

Spontaneous CSF leak should not be equated with postdural puncture headaches. There are often substantial differences in the clinical features, response to treatment, and outcome in the two. In spontaneous CSF leak, the dural defect is often not a simple hole or rent. Many patients have a preexisting dural defect and display focal areas of dural attenuation, meningeal diverticula, or even focal zones of absent dura with nude arachnoid. These areas may weep CSF with variable rates or sometimes intermittently.

CSF DYNAMICS

The choroid plexus forms more than 75% of the CSF; the rest is secreted by the brain capillaries into the neuropil and enters the ventricles through the ependyma.[6] The rate of CSF formation in adults is 0.35 mL/min or about 500 mL/24 hr. CSF is absorbed by arachnoid villi into the cerebral venous sinuses and veins via a valvelike mechanism called bulk flow.[7,8] Normally, a minor portion of the CSF is absorbed into the cerebral vessels by simple diffusion. Recent studies suggest that a portion of the CSF is absorbed via the lymphatics of the region of the cribriform plate to the nasal submucosa.[9]

Although the rate of CSF formation is fairly constant, its volume is not. Based on old autopsy data, the total volume of the CSF was estimated to be about 500 mL. This figure has been, and continues to be, repeated in the literature. Tremendous variability in the size of the ventricles and the subarachnoid and cisternal spaces, especially in the young versus old, is obvious in modern head imaging. MRI volumetric studies point to substantial variations. The mean +/− standard deviation of cranial CSF for both sexes and for all people aged 24 to 80 years was noted to be 157 ± 59 SD; the number was smaller for women versus men and much smaller for young versus old patients.[10] Spinal CSF volume from T11-T12 to the sacral terminus was calculated to be 49.9 ± 12.1 SD[11]; the number is significantly smaller for obese versus nonobese patients.

In the horizontal position, the CSF pressure at lumbar, cisternal, and presumably intracranial or vertex levels are equal, measuring about 65 to 195 mm of water. In the vertical position, these pressures diverge. The vertex pressure becomes negative, whereas the lumbar pressure increases. Along the CSF axis, somewhere between the spinous processes of C7 and T5, there is a point referred to as the *hydrostatic independent point* where the CSF pressure remains unchanged whether patients are upright or supine.[12] The relationship between the CSF pressure and volume is exponential.[13] In experimental low-pressure headaches in human patients, it has been shown that withdrawal of approximately 10% of CSF will decrease the already negative vertex pressure by more than 40%.[14]

CAUSE

Spontaneous CSF leaks typically take place at the spinal dural sac at any level but more commonly at the thoracic level.[15] Posttraumatic and postsurgical CSF leaks (motor vehicle accidents [MVAs]; severe falls; blows to the head; cranial or spinal surgeries; ears, nose, and throat [ENT] surgeries) are not uncommon. However, spontaneous CSF leaks from the skull base are rare. Some of the patients with spontaneous CSF leaks may report occasional flow of clear fluid from the nose. It should not come as a surprise if such fluids do not prove to be CSF. A CSF leak leads to CSF volume depletion (CSF hypovolemia), which is also the pathogenetic core in overdraining CSF shunts and postsurgical CSF leaks. Reduced total body volume (true hypovolemic state) should also be expected to cause reduced CSF volume.

When the cause is discussed (**Box 1**), it is the spontaneous group that presents the real challenge. The exact cause of a spontaneous CSF leak often remains unclear. A preexisting dural weakness can lead to a CSF leak or sometimes render the dura more vulnerable to the effect of a trivial trauma. A minority of the patients may report a history of a previous trivial trauma (coughing, lifting, pushing, routine sport activities, and so forth). Evidence for a preexisting weakness of the dural sac has gained momentum. Dural abnormalities, meningeal diverticula, and CSF leaks have been noted in Marfan syndrome.[16–18] Stigmata of connective tissue disorder are seen in a minority of the patients with spontaneous CSF leaks.[19] Single or multiple meningeal diverticula are noted frequently in patients with spontaneous CSF leaks and in certain heritable disorders of connective tissue.[20–23] Dural ectasia is a common feature of Marfan

---

Box 1
Cause of CSF hypovolemia or CSF leaks

1. True hypovolemic state (reduced total body water)

2. CSF shunt overdrainage

3. Traumatic CSF leaks

   a. Overt injuries (MVAs, sports injuries, brachial plexus avulsions)

   b. Iatrogenic (postdural puncture, postepidural catheterization)

   c. Postsurgical (cranial or spinal surgeries, ENT surgeries)

4. Spontaneous CSF leaks

   a. Unknown cause

   b. Preexisting dural sac weakness

   c. Meningeal diverticula

   d. Evidences disorders of connective tissue matrix

     • Marfan syndrome or marfanoid features

     • Joint hypermobility

     • Retinal detachment at young age

     • Abnormalities of elastin and fibrillin in dermal fibroblast cultures

     • Familial occurrence of spontaneous CSF leaks

5. Trivial trauma (perhaps in the setting of preexisting dural weakness)

6. Herniated disks, spondylotic spurs

syndrome.[24,25] Familial occurrence of spontaneous CSF leak in the setting of familial joint hypermobility and aortic aneurysms is yet another testimony on the role of dural weakness based on a disorder of connective tissue matrix in some of the spontaneous CSF leaks (**Fig. 1**).[26] Uncommonly, a spondylotic spur or herniated disk may penetrate the dura and cause a CSF leak.[27–29] Sometimes, with brachial plexus avulsions, a tear in a nerve root sleeve may lead to CSF leakage.[30]

CLINICAL MANIFESTATIONS
Headache

The most common clinical manifestation is orthostatic headache, a headache in the upright position relieved in recumbency.[31–33] The interval from change in posture (erect or recumbent) to the appearance of headache or relief from it is classically assumed to be a few minutes; but in many patients, it is much longer. The headache may be throbbing, but often it is not and is described as a pressure sensation that can range from dull to very severe. It is often, but not always, bilateral and can be frontal, fronto-occipital, holocephalic, or occipital. At this juncture, 2 points need emphasizing: (1) Not all patients with an orthostatic headache have CSF leaks, although

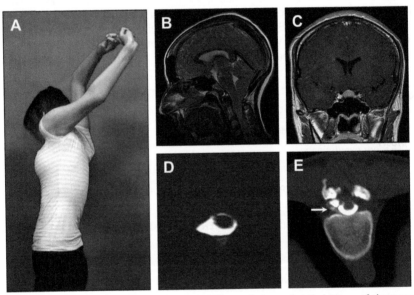

Fig. 1. (A) Young woman with joint hypermobility and strong family history of the same as well as aortic aneurysms presented with orthostatic headaches. (B) Head MRI on sagittal view shows descent of the cerebellar tonsils, flattened anterior pons, near obliteration of prepontine cistern, and crowded posterior fossa. (C) Coronal gadolinium enhance shows little for abnormal gadolinium enhancement, but there is pituitary engorgement and obliteration of the perichiasmatic cistern. Lower imaging panels: (D) Axial, heavily T2-weighted spine MRI that shows a meningeal diverticulum. (E) Hyperdynamic computed tomography myelography shows this to be a leaking meningeal diverticulum (arrow). Patient had a younger and an older sister; both had joint hypermobility and leaking meningeal diverticula, both were also seen in the past by the author,[26] and both had responded to surgical treatment of the meningeal diverticula, as did this patient. (From Mokri B. Unpublished data, with permission of Mayo Foundation; and Courtesy of Mayo Clinic, Rochester, MN, with permission.)

the large majority does. (2) Not all headaches related to CSF leaks are orthostatic. The variability is indeed substantial (**Box 2**). Sometimes, especially with chronicity, the orthostatic features of a typically orthostatic headache may dampen; and it may gradually transform into a lingering chronic daily headache.

Manifestations Other than Headaches

The clinical manifestations of SIH-CSF hypovolemia apart from headaches are listed in **Box 3**. Of these, neck and interscapular pain, cochleovestibular manifestations, and perhaps nausea are far more common than others. The level of the spine pain may not necessarily correspond to the level of the leak, and indeed it often does not.

Mechanisms of Clinical Manifestations

One consequence of a decrease in CSF volume is sinking of the brain. This outcome leads to traction or distortion of the anchoring or supporting pain-sensitive structures of the brain[34,35] and, therefore, to the headaches that are orthostatic or have some orthostatic features. The dilatation of intracranial venous structures also plays a likely role in the pathogenesis of headaches in CSF hypovolemia.

Traction, distortion, or compression of some of the cranial nerves, some of the structures or lobes of the brain, brainstem, mesencephalon, and diencephalon are thought to be responsible for the various cranial nerve palsies as well as many central nervous system manifestations seen in this disorder.[34] Cochleovestibular manifestations (tinnitus, hearing change, dizziness) may be related to traction on the eighth cranial nerve; but an alternative and perhaps a more plausible mechanism is altered pressure in the perilymphatic fluid or of the inner ear.[36] Galactorrhea, which may occur only rarely, and an increase in prolactin have been attributed to traction on or distortion of the pituitary stalk.[37] Dilatation of epidural venous plexus or traction and distortion of nerve roots are thought to be the cause of radicular symptoms.[38]

Diagnosis

For CSF examination, expect considerable variability in CSF findings (**Table 1**).

Box 2
Headache in intracranial hypotension (CSF leak–CSF hypovolemia)

- Orthostatic headaches (present in upright position, relieved in recumbency)
- Neck or interscapular pain or a lingering nonorthostatic headache preceding the orthostatic headache (by days or weeks)
- Orthostatic headache gradually evolving into lingering nonorthostatic chronic daily headaches (transformed orthostatic headaches)
- Nonorthostatic chronic daily headaches from start
- Exertional headaches[84]
- Acute thunderclaplike onset of orthostatic headaches[85]
- Second-half-of-the-day headaches (often with some orthostatic features)[85]
- Paradoxic orthostatic headaches (present in recumbency, relieved when upright)[86]
- Intermittent headaches of intermittent leaks
- The acephalgic form (where patients have no headache and present with other clinical manifestations of the CSF leak – CSF hypovolemia)

Box 3
Nonheadache manifestations of CSF leak–CSF hypovolemia

- Neck or interscapular pain (common), low back pain (much less common)
- Cochleovestibular manifestations, including tinnitus, change in hearing (muffled, distant, distorted, or echoed hearing, even hearing loss), and dizziness (vertigo, woozy, or lightheaded feelings)
- Nausea, less commonly emesis, often orthostatic
- Diplopia, often horizontal and caused by unilateral or bilateral sixth cranial nerve palsy,[15] less commonly third and fourth cranial nerve palsies[87]
- Visual complaints including blurred vision, photophobia, superior binasal visual field defect[88]
- Facial numbness or numb feeling, unilateral or bilateral
- Galactorrhea[37]
- Labyrinthine hydrops[36]
- Radicular upper limb symptoms[38]
- Stupor, diencephalic compression[89]
- Coma[90]
- Parkinsonism, ataxia, bulbar weakness[91]
- Frontotemporal dementia[92]
- Encephalopathy[93]
- Gait unsteadiness[94]
- Trouble with sphincter control
- Bibrachial amyotrophy[80]
- Cognitive difficulties
- Chorea[95]

Radioisotope Cisternography

Indium-111 is the radioisotope of choice. It is introduced intrathecally via a lumbar puncture, and its dynamic is followed by sequential scanning at various intervals of up to 24 or even 48 hours. Normally by 24 hours, but often even earlier, abundant radioactivity can be detected over the cerebral convexities.[39–41] In CSF leaks, the radioactivity typically does not extend much beyond the basal cisterns; therefore, at 24 hours or even 48 hours, there is paucity of activity over the cerebral convexities (**Fig. 2**). This abnormality is the most common cisternographic abnormality in CSF leaks. The detection of parathecal activity pointing to the level or approximate site of the leak, although more desirable, is less common. Meningeal diverticula or dilated nerve root sleeves, if large enough, may appear as foci of parathecal activity that may not be reliably distinguishable from sites of a CSF leak (**Fig. 3**). Computed tomography myelography (CTM) typically enables the differentiation. Early appearance of radioactivity in the kidneys and the urinary bladder (in less than 4 hours vs 6–24 hours) is another fairly common finding, indicating that intrathecally introduced radioisotope has been extravasated and has entered the systemic circulation, with subsequent renal clearance and early appearance in the urinary bladder. This cisternographic abnormality, however, is not always a very reliable indication of a CSF leak because

Table 1
CSF findings in spontaneous CSF leaks

Opening pressure	It is often low, occasionally atmospheric, or rarely even negative. It is sometimes within normal limits even on repeated taps despite active CSF leak.[96] Sometimes in the same patient, variable CSF opening pressures may be recorded in different occasions. This variability may be related to variability in the rate of the flow of the leak.
Color	It is often clear, occasionally xanthochromic, and sometimes blood tinged. Note that difficult and traumatic taps are not unusual when CSF opening pressure is very low. Engorgement of the epidural venous plexus is also a contributory factor.
Protein concentration	It may be normal or high. Values of up to 100 mg/dL are not uncommon, and protein concentrations as high as 1000 mg/dL have been rarely observed.[15]
Leukocyte count	It may be normal, but a lymphocytic pleocytosis of up to 50 cells per square millimeter is not uncommon, and higher counts are not rare. Counts as high as 222 cells per square millimeter have been documented.[15,97]
Erythrocyte count	It may be normal or elevated (sometimes considerably, in connection with traumatic taps).
Cytology and microbiology	It is normal/negative.
Glucose concentration	It is never low.

inadvertent partial extradural injection of the radioisotope or, more commonly, extravasation of the intrathecally introduced radioisotope through the dural puncture site may also lead to an early appearance of radioactivity in the urinary bladder. Furthermore, the early appearance of radioactivity in the urinary bladder should not be misinterpreted as evidence of increased CSF reabsorption[39,40] because the radioisotope in CSF leaks hardly reaches the cerebral convexities to be reabsorbed.

Head CT

The usual head CT is of limited value in the evaluation of spontaneous CSF leaks. Infrequently, it may show subdural fluid collections or increased tentorial enhancement.[35]

Head MRI

Head MRI subnormalities are listed in **Box 4.**

Diffuse pachymeningeal enhancement without leptomeningeal enhancement is the most common MRI abnormality. This abnormality is typically linear, uninterrupted, non-nodular, bilateral, and both supratentorial and infratentorial. It may vary from thick to quite thin (**Fig. 4**).[15,42–44]

The descent or sinking or sagging of the brain and brainstem is manifested by the descent of the cerebellar tonsils, often below the foramen magnum, sometimes mimicking type 1 Chiari malformation.[45] (**Fig. 5**), decrease in size of prepontine and perichiasmatic cisterns (see **Fig. 4**), inferior displacement and flattening of the optic chiasm, and crowding of the posterior fossa (see **Figs. 4** and **5**). The descent and distortion of the brainstem may be manifested by an increase in the anteroposterior diameter of the pons and by the downward displacement of the iter below the incisural line. The iter is the cephalad opening of the aqueduct of Sylvius seen on midline

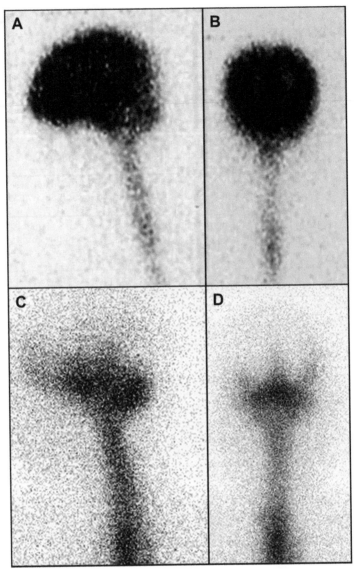

Fig. 2. Indium-111 radioisotope cisternography 24-hour images. (*A, B*) Normal study: (*A*) lateral view, (*B*) anteroposterior view. Note that there is plenty of radioactivity over the cerebral convexities at 24 hours. (*C, D*) Patient with active CSF leak: (*C*) lateral view, (*D*) posteroanterior view. Note paucity of radioactivity over the cerebral convexities at 24 hours.

sagittal image. The incisural line is the line drawn in midsagittal view between the anterior tuberculum sellae to the point of the junction of the straight sinus, inferior sagittal sinus, and the great vein of Galen.[44] Sometimes the descent of the brainstem and iter may be apparent while the cerebellar tonsils are still above the foramen magnum.

Subdural fluid collections may be bilateral or unilateral and are typically noted over the cerebral convexities (**Fig. 6**). They are often, but not always, thin and without compression of the underlying brain or effacement of the underlying sulci. These

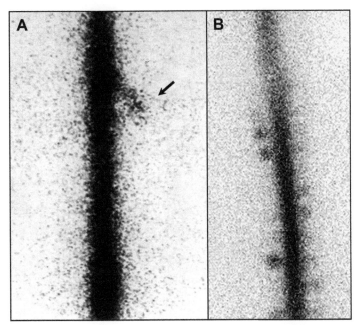

Fig. 3. (*A*) Parathecal activity (*arrow*). This activity may be seen in association with focal CSF leaks, dilated nerve root sleeves, or meningeal diverticula. Differentiation typically calls for additional studies, such as computed tomography myelography (CTM). (*B*) Multiple areas of parathecal activity often related to multiple dilated nerve root sleeves, multiple meningeal diverticula, or both. In this case, no active leak was detected on detailed CTM. Although such lesions may sometimes cause CSF leaks, such a cisternographic appearance should not be automatically labeled as a CSF leak or, worse, multiple areas of a CSF leak.

Box 4
Head MRI abnormalities in spontaneous CSF leak–CSF hypovolemia

1. Diffuse pachymeningeal enhancement

2. Descent or sinking or sagging of the brain

   a. Descent of the cerebellar tonsils (may mimic Chiari I malformation)

   b. Descent of brainstem or mesencephalon (occasionally without descent of cerebellar tonsils)

   c. Distortion and increase in anteroposterior diameter of the brainstem, flattening of anterior pons

   d. Descent of the iter below the incisural line

   e. Obliteration of some of the basal cisterns (ie, prepontine, perichiasmatic)

   f. Crowding of the posterior fossa

   g. Flattening of the optic chiasm

3. Subdural fluid collections (typically hygromas, infrequently hematomas)

4. Engorgement/enlargement of pituitary (may mimic pituitary tumor or hyperplasia)

5. Engorged cerebral venous sinuses

6. Decrease in size of the ventricles (sometimes referred to as ventricular collapse)

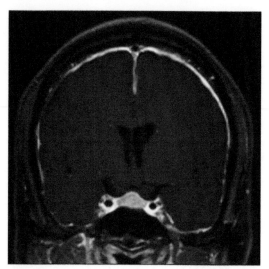

Fig. 4. Head MRI, T1-weighted gadolinium-enhanced coronal view at the level of the sella. Note diffuse pachymeningeal enhancement, enlarged pituitary, flattened optic chiasm, and near obliteration of the perichiasmatic cistern.

collections are usually hygromas but may show various signal intensity depending on the fluid protein concentration. Subdural hematomas can form and can become large enough to compress and shift the brain and become symptomatic. This, however, occurs uncommonly.

Pituitary engorgement and enlargement may mimic pituitary hyperplasia or tumor.[46,47] It may assume a domed appearance with the descended and flattened optic chiasm draped on it (see **Fig. 3**).

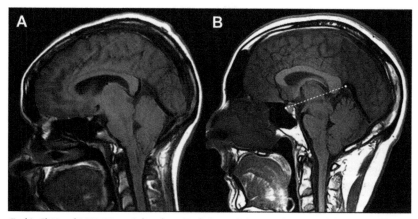

Fig. 5. (*A, B*) Head MRI, T1-weighted sagittal views. (*A*) Note descent of the cerebellar tonsils below the foramen magnum resembling Chiari I, crowded posterior fossa, increase in anteroposterior diameter of the brainstem, and decrease in prepontine cistern. (*B*) Descent of the cerebellar tonsils and flattening of the anterior pons. Also note descent of the iter (cephalad opening of the aqueduct of Sylvius) below the incisural line (*dashed line*) (see text) pointing to the descent of the brainstem.

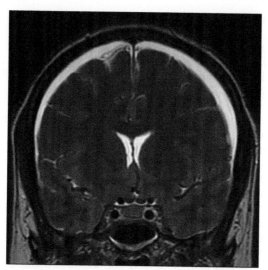

Fig. 6. Head MRI, T2-weighted unenhanced coronal view. Bilateral subdural fluid collections. Also note enlarged pituitary and obliteration of parasellar-perichiasmatic cistern caused by sinking of the brain.

Engorgement of cerebral venous sinuses (**Fig. 7**)[48] as well as decreased ventricular size (ventricular collapse) may be obvious, but often is not so obvious, and can best be appreciated in retrospect when images of the symptomatic phase are compared with postrecovery images.

In MR study of the brain in CSF leaks, this author has been helped most by T1-weighted gadolinium-enhanced coronal images at the level of the sella and by T1-weighted midline sagittal images. The latter can show the descent of the cerebellar tonsils and brainstem and its related distortions and crowding of the posterior fossa. The former can show a variety of abnormalities, including diffuse pachymeningeal enhancement, subdural fluid collections, pituitary engorgement, flattening of optic chiasm, decrease in perichiasmatic cistern; additionally, particularly when prerecovery and postrecovery images are compared, engorgement of cerebral venous sinuses

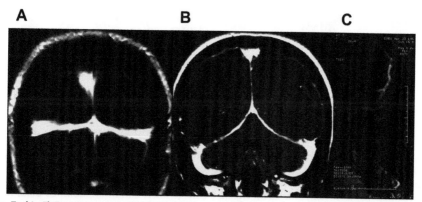

Fig. 7. (*A, B*) Engorgement of cerebral venous sinuses and (*C*) epidural venous plexus. Also note the very thin pachymeningeal enhancement.

may become more apparent and a previously unrecognized ventricular collapse may come to attention. These imaging changes are reflected schematically in the drawings of **Fig. 8**. This statement reflects personal preference and is not at all intended to diminish the high value of a complete study and other sequences but to simply emphasize that head MRI for evaluation of the CSF leaks should serve the clinician best when it includes T1 sagittal and T1 gadolinium enhanced coronal images.

Spine MRI abnormalities are listed in **Box 5**.

Extradural (or extra-arachnoid) fluid collections are fairly common.[15,49–51] These collections may be focal or extend along several spinal levels (**Fig. 9**). They only uncommonly enable the determination of the exact site of the CSF leak. Also uncommon, although not rare, is the detection of extravasated fluid into the paraspinal soft tissues. This fluid often occurs across fewer levels and may point to the site or the approximate site of the leak. Heavily T2-weighted spine MRI or the so-called heavily T2-weighted MR myelography[52] provides cleaner and nicer images but, in the author's experience, has not been notably superior to the usual but high-quality spine MRIs and certainly, for the detection of the site of the CSF leakage, has not been a substitute for CTM. It should be noted that in patients with typical clinical and head MRI findings, the real question is not if there is extradural fluid but, instead, where the fluid is leaking from. To answer this question, CTM and its versions (dynamic and hyperdynamic CTM) remain the dependable method of choice (see **Fig. 1**).

Meningeal diverticula (single but often multiple that may vary in size) and also dilated nerve root sleeves are fairly common in spontaneous CSF leaks. Spinal dural enhancement,[43] engorgement of epidural venous plexus, and engorgement of intradural spinal veins may be seen.[53]

Mechanism of MRI Abnormalities

In exploring the mechanism of MRI abnormalities in the setting of decreased CSF volume, the principles of the Monro-Kellie doctrine have to be considered. According to

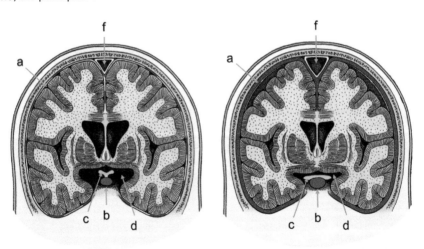

Fig. 8. Gadolinium-enhanced head MRI (see text). Left (normal). Right (during active CSF leak). (*a*) pachymeninges. (*b*) pituitary gland. (*c*) optic chiasm. (*d*) prechiasmatic cistern. (*f*) superior sagittal sinus indicating extraarachnoid fluid collections in blue, over the cerebral convexities. Contrast with images on **Fig. 12** (*A, D*). (*From* Mokri B. Unpublished data, with permission of Mayo Foundation; and *Courtesy of* Mayo Clinic, Rochester, MN, with permission.)

> **Box 5**
> **Spine MRI abnormalities in spontaneous CSF leaks-CSF hypovolemia**
>
> - Extra-arachnoid fluid collections that may be focal or frequently extend along several spinal levels
> - Extra-dural extravasation of fluid toward paraspinal soft tissues
> - Meningeal diverticula, single or multiple; various sizes at various levels
> - Spinal dural enhancement
> - Engorgement of epidural venous plexus
> - Engorgement of intradural spinal veins

this doctrine, "with intact skull, the sum of volumes of brain plus CSF plus intracranial blood is constant."[54] Therefore, an increase or decrease in one will result in a decrease or increase in one or both of the remaining two. In the case of a decrease in CSF volume, given the fact that the brain is basically nonexpandable, it is an increase in the intracranial blood volume that has to compensate for a decrease in CSF volume (**Fig. 10**). Therefore, an intracranial venous hypervolemia occurs with such changes as dilatation of cerebral venous sinuses, engorgement of the pituitary, and diffuse meningeal engorgement. Because leptomeninges have blood-brain barriers and pachymeninges do not, it is only the pachymeninges that enhance with gadolinium.[55] Another volume compensatory mechanism is the collection of subdural fluids.

Similarly, spinal pachymeningeal enhancement can be seen on spine MRI. However, at the spine level, in contrast to the skull, there is an epidural space containing adipose and soft connective tissue as well as the epidural venous plexus. In CSF hypovolemia, a relatively mild collapse of the dural sac may take place that, in turn, leads to the dilatation of the epidural venous plexus. Engorgement of the intradural veins may also be encountered.[53]

Other consequences of CSF volume loss include a decrease in the size of the ventricles sometimes referred to as ventricular collapse and the descent of the brain with such MRI changes as the descent of the cerebellar tonsils; crowding of the posterior fossa; decrease in the size of some of the basal cisterns (ie, prepontine or perichiasmatic cisterns); descent of the brainstem and iter, which is not uncommonly accompanied by deformity; and an increase in the anteroposterior diameter of the brainstem.

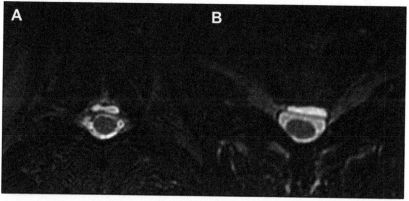

Fig. 9. Spine MRI, axial views (*A*, *B*). Elongated ventral extra-arachnoid fluid collection. This collection had extended across several spinal levels.

Mechanisms of MRI Abnormalities in CSF Volume Depletion

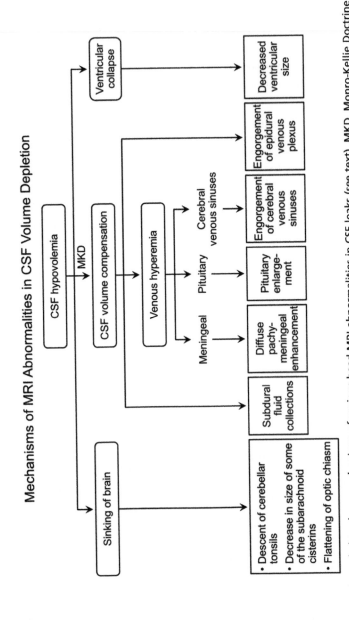

Fig. 10. Diagram intended to show mechanisms of various head MRI abnormalities in CSF leaks (see text). MKD, Monro-Kellie Doctrine.

Myelography/CTM

This study may show several abnormalities and also provides an opportunity to measure CSF opening pressure. The following abnormalities may be detected:

- Extra-arachnoid fluid, which may be quite focal or could extend across several vertebral levels or even several spinal levels, such as from cervical all the way to the lumbar level
- Meningeal diverticula, single or multiple, various sizes, different levels, may or may not be the site of CSF leakage even when large
- Extradural egress of contrast extending into the paraspinal soft tissues

The rate of the CSF leak may vary from patient to patient and, in the same patient, from one encounter to the next. CTM is more reliable than other imaging studies for locating the exact site of the CSF leakage (see **Fig. 9**). When an attempt is made to locate the site of the CSF leak, the two extremes of rapid flow or slow flow each present substantial challenges.

In rapid-flow leaks, after the initial myelogram and by the time patients are taken for the CT scanning, enough contrast has been extravasated epidurally to extend across several vertebral levels making it virtually impossible to determine the actual site of the CSF leakage. This obstacle is overcome by proceeding with high-speed CT scanning of the spine right after the intrathecal injection of the contrast and bypassing the myelographic phase. This technique, known as *dynamic CTM*,[56] and its variations, as well as digital subtraction myelography,[57] have been very helpful in locating the site of the leakage in high-flow leaks.

In slow-flow CSF leaks, several maneuvers have been tried including

- Another CT scanning can be obtained after a delayed period of three to four hours.
- Positive pressure myelography which involves intrathecal injection of fluid to elevate CSF pressure from low to normal levels before injection of contrast in order to increase the likelihood of CSF-contrast extravasation. The results have been variable and not enough to generate strong enthusiasm.
- Gadolinium myelography is essentially a spine MRI after intrathecal injection of gadolinium.[58] This maneuver is sometimes helpful in detecting the site of a slow-flow CSF leak but not as much as initially hoped. This maneuver is an off-label use of gadolinium and should be considered only when the diagnosis of a CSF leak is highly suspected[59] and when the site of the CSF leak has not been detected by other diagnostic techniques, such as CTM.

Overall, locating the site of the CSF leak in slow-flow CSF leaks often remains problematic and sometimes quite frustrating for patients and the physicians.

Treatment

The treatment modalities advocated for patients with spontaneous CSF leaks are listed in **Table 2**. Fortunately, the leak stops in some of the patients regardless of any treatments.

Bed rest has traditionally been recommended. Nevertheless, because many of the patients have significant orthostatic symptoms, at least initially, they tend to stay recumbent much of the time anyway.

Another traditionally recommended measure is hydration, which is often an overhydration because many patients are not dehydrated. Its effectiveness has not been clearly established. The efficacy of caffeine and theophylline has been demonstrated

Table 2 Treatment of spontaneous CSF leaks	
Conservative measures	• Bed rest (Typically, patients with substantial orthostatic headaches tend to remain reclined much of the time anyway.) • Coffee • Hydration or, more accurately, overhydration because the large majority are not dehydrated • Time (might be the most important element)
Medications	• Analgesics (It is often, but not always, impractical because the effect of analgesics in the upright position may be only partial and many patients become completely or substantially headache free in recumbency.) • Caffeine • Theophylline • Corticosteroids
Abdominal binder	• Binders • Corsets
Epidural injections	• Homologous blood epidural blood patch: targeted, distant, bilevel, multilevel, blind (at lumbar level) • Fibrin glue (fibrin sealant) • Fibrin glue and blood
Surgical repair of the leak	• Surgical closure (not always possible) • Reinforcement with muscle and/or fibrin sealant
Other measures in special situations	• Epidural saline infusions (uncertain, unpredictable efficacy or durability; risk of infection) • Intrathecal fluid injection (for quick CSF volume replacement) in rare instances of progressing obtundation, stupor, or coma from descent and compromise of brainstem and midbrain • Epidural infusion of dextran (rarely practiced) • Intravenous saline infusions

in some studies[60]; but this efficacy often, although not always, is nonimpressive and of doubtful durability.

Some patients may report various degrees of symptom control from corticosteroids, but a few points need emphasizing:

- Not all patients respond to corticosteroids and indeed most may not.
- Even when effective, the effect is often partial and of doubtful durability.
- Considering the potential side effects of corticosteroid therapy, especially for extended periods of time, such treatment does not seem to be a long-term solution.

Intrathecal fluid infusions or epidural infusions of crystalloids (eg, saline) or colloids (eg, dextran) produce varying results[61–65] but can be considered with limited expectations and for a limited period in patients who fail repeated epidural blood patches (EBP) and when surgery is not an option. There is, however, concern about the possibility of the introduction of infection in prolonged infusions as well as the probability of catheter failures.

EBP is the treatment of choice in patients who fail an initial trial of conservative management.[66,67] The effect of EBP is twofold: (1) an early (sometimes almost immediate) effect related simply to volume replacement resulting from dural tamponade and (2) a latent effect, which results from sealing the leak. In spontaneous CSF leaks, the success rate with each EBP is approximately 30%.[67] Many patients require more than one EBP. The success rate is significantly more impressive for postlumbar puncture headaches whereby the first EBP gives relief in the vast majority and a second one in nearly all cases. This difference is likely a consequence of one or more of the following factors:

- In postlumbar puncture headaches, the level of the EBP is typically the same as the level of the leak, whereas in spontaneous CSF leaks, the EBP may be distant from the actual site of the leak.
- The anatomy of the leak in many patients with spontaneous CSF leaks is more complicated than a simple hole or rent produced by spinal tap needles.
- In spontaneous CSF leaks, the dural defect commonly is in the anterior aspect of the dural sac or in the nerve root sleeve or the axilla of the nerve root sleeve.
- Spontaneous CSF leaks may take place from multiple sites at different levels, and some patients who have spontaneous CSF leaks may fail even multiple EBPs.

Sometimes epidural injection of fibrin glue[68,69] may be carried out translaminar or transforaminal, depending on the situation at hand. Sometimes a combination of epidural injection of fibrin glue and homologous blood is considered. Epidural injections of blood or fibrin glue may be single level, bilevel, or even multilevel. They may be targeted, distant from the site of the leak, or could be blind EBPs (when the site of CSF leak has not been determined). These injections are typically placed at the lumbar level.

In well-selected cases, surgery is effective and is considered for those patients who fail conservative measures and less invasive treatments such as EBPs[15,70] or when the anatomy of the leak has been such that the success of nonsurgical approaches has been predicted to be remote. The surgery is not always straightforward because the anatomy of the leak is not always simple.[71] The surgeon may encounter the extravasated CSF but may not be able to locate the site of the leak and, therefore, may have to pack the area with blood-soaked gelatin sponge muscle, or fibrin glue and hope for the best. The margins of dural defect may be so markedly attenuated that they may not yield to suturing. Sometimes the site of the leak and the dural defect is in the anterior aspect of the dura or the leak may be from a meningeal diverticulum or a defect or diverticulum of a nerve root sleeve. Each of these may have varying anatomic configurations and provide the surgeon with unpredicted challenges. It is essential, however, to try to locate the site of the CSF egress before surgery and to realize that a meningeal diverticulum, even when large, may not necessarily be the actual site of the CSF leakage. With careful selection, surgical results can be fulfilling.

COMPLICATIONS OF CSF LEAKS
Subdural Hematomas

These hematomas may complicate subdural hygroma or may be subdural hematomas right from the start. They may be thin and asymptomatic but can be large, become symptomatic, and compress the underlying brain. Symptomatic and expanding subdurals require surgical intervention.[72,73] Careful postoperative monitoring is important, watching for manifestations of increased sagging of the brain. Surgical creation of a skull defect will violate the Monro-Kellie principle and may lead to increased sinking of the brain (**Fig. 11**).[74] It is wise to address the treatment of CSF leakage at some point along with the treatment of the subdural hematoma.

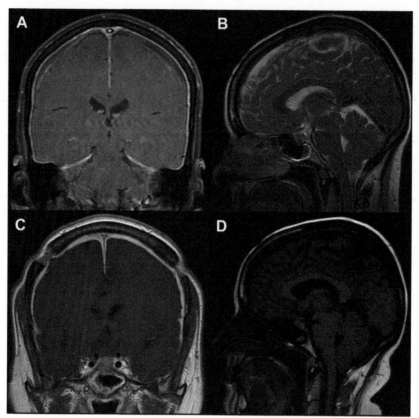

Fig. 11. Coronal (*A*) and sagittal (*B*) head MRIs in a patient with CSF leak and bilateral sub-dural collections. (*A*) Bilateral subdurals and diffuse pachymeningeal gadolinium enhancement. (*B*) Low-lying cerebellar tonsils. Patient had been subjected to bilateral burr hole evacuation of subdurals (*C*), but the leak had not been addressed. Note further descent of the cerebellar tonsils (*D*). (*From* Mokri B. Unpublished data, with permission of Mayo Foundation; and *Courtesy of* Mayo Clinic, Rochester, MN, with permission.)

Rebound Intracranial Hypertension

This complication is sometimes noted after a CSF leak has been successfully treated surgically or by EBP. Sometimes patients may present with recurrence of headache, although typically not an orthostatic headache, and sometimes even papilledema may be noted (**Fig. 12**).[75] This phenomenon is often a self-limiting phenomenon but may frustratingly take a long time to resolve. Acetazolamide is frequently helpful to decrease the symptoms. The true incidence of this rebound intracranial hypertension is likely higher than thought because some of the patients may be asymptomatic or minimally symptomatic.

Cerebral Venous Sinus Thrombosis

In patients with CSF leaks, change in headache characteristics within a short period of time may raise this possibility[76]; but fortunately, its incidence is very low. When cerebral venous sinus thrombosis develops, it calls for anticoagulation therapy.

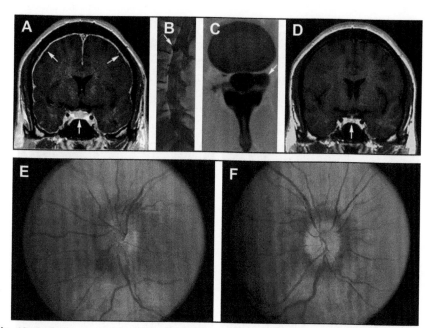

Fig. 12. Patient presented with orthostatic headaches. (*A*) Head MRI shows diffuse pachy-meningeal enhancement (*upper arrows*) and enlargement of pituitary (*lower arrow*) and flattened optic chiasm. (*B, C*) CTM identifies leaking meningeal diverticulum (*arrow*). Surgical repair is followed by resolution of the orthostatic headaches and reversal of the head MRI abnormalities. (*D*) Also noted is mildly smaller size of the ventricles (on [*A*]), in retrospect pointing to presence of ventricular collapse, which also subsequently reversed (*B*). The *arrow* (*D*) points to reversal of pituitary enlargement and flattening of optic chiasm. The ventricular collapse is often subtle and is recognized retrospectively. Sometimes, however, it is quite obvious. This patient's extra-arachnoid/subdural symptoms resolved after surgery but later presented with a different type of headache and bilateral papilledema (*E, F*) as the result of rebound intracranial hypertension. (*From* Mokri B. Unpublished data, with permission of Mayo Foundation; and *Courtesy of* Mayo Clinic, Rochester, MN, with permission.)

Superficial Siderosis

This complication is a rare and remote complication of spinal CSF leaks.[77–79] It is frequently associated with elongated extra-arachnoid fluid collections, often ventral to the cord and along several vertebral levels.

Bibrachial Amyotrophy

Another rare complication of CSF leaks, also often associated with elongated extra-arachnoid fluid collections, is painless bilateral weakness and atrophy of some of the upper limb myotomes. This complication often begins on one side before becoming bilateral. It may involve shoulder girdle myotomes, proximal upper limb myotomes, or distal upper limb myotomes (**Fig. 13**). It may mimic motor neuron disease.[80]

RECURRENCE OF CSF LEAKS

These recurrences are not rare and may occur with variable frequency and at variable intervals from a previous leak. There is paucity of reliable data regarding the incidence

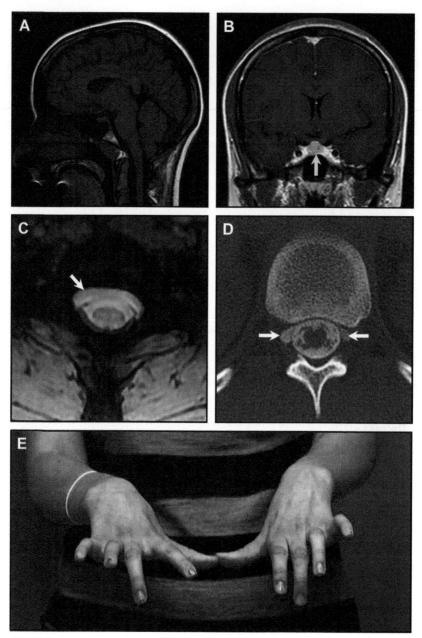

Fig. 13. Bibrachial amyotrophy in spontaneous CSF leak. Head MRIs: (*A*) sagittal view shows descent of cerebellar tonsils and brainstem, (*B*) enhanced coronal view shows enlarged pituitary (*arrow*) and obliteration of parasellar-perichiasmatic cistern. (*C*) Spine MRI shows ventral extra-arachnoid/extradural fluid collections (*arrow*) also seen in (*D*) CTM (*arrows*). The extra-arachnoid ventral fluid collection had extended across several cervical and thoracic levels. (*E*) The related bilateral distal upper limb muscle atrophy. The atrophic muscles were quite weak. She could not hold a pencil. (*From* Mokri B. Unpublished data, with permission of Mayo Foundation; and *Courtesy of* Mayo Clinic, Rochester, MN, with permission.)

of such recurrences, and information based on essentially surgical referrals may not be applicable to the entire group. Although not formally studied or proven, possibly those with stigmata of the disorders of the connective tissue matrix might be at a somewhat higher risk of recurrence.

ORTHOSTATIC HEADACHES WITHOUT CSF LEAK

As addressed earlier in the article, not all headaches of spontaneous CSF leaks are orthostatic. Similarly, not all orthostatic headaches are caused by CSF leaks. They have been noted in association with other conditions including

- Postural orthostatic tachycardia syndrome[81]
- After surgery for Chiari malformation
- The syndrome of the trephined[82]
- Increased compliance of dural sac[83]
- Occasional cases of colloid cyst of the third ventricle[31]

SUMMARY AND LESSONS OF THE PAST 2 DECADES

Schaltenbrand[31] described the spontaneous occurrence of the syndrome of intracranial hypotension in 1939, and he pointed out that the syndrome itself had been described in the French literature about 2 decades earlier. However, much of our current knowledge of this entity has been acquired in the past 2 decades, essentially in connection with the availability of MRI and its enormous impact on the recognition of this entity. The following are some of what has been recognized:

- SIH almost always results from spontaneous CSF leaks. The old theories of decreased CSF production or increased CSF absorption have never been substantiated.
- Decreased CSF volume (CSF hypovolemia) rather than decreased CSF pressure (CSF hypotension) is the core pathophysiologic factor as an independent variable, whereas CSF pressures, clinical manifestations, and imaging findings are variables that depend on the CSF volume.
- Most spontaneous CSF leaks occur at the spinal level, frequently on preexisting zones of dural weakness. As opposed to posttraumatic leaks, the spontaneous ones only rarely occur at the level of skull base, such as the cribriform plate.
- A significant minority of patients displays clinical stigmata of heritable disorders of the connective tissue matrix. These stigmata likely play an etiologic role in the formation of meningeal diverticula or zones of dural weakness and CSF leaks.
- Although the triad of orthostatic headaches, low CSF pressure, and diffuse pachymeningeal enhancement on head MRI is the hallmark of the diagnosis, expect substantial variability in just about every aspect of this entity, including CSF opening pressure (which may be normal), the clinical manifestations including headaches (broad clinical features, various headache types), and the imaging abnormalities (ie, absent pachymeningeal enhancement).
- The anatomy of spontaneous CSF leaks can be complex. One should not expect a simple hole or rent or equate the spontaneous CSF leak with the leaks that may occur after dural puncture or epidural catheterization.
- The rate of CSF leak can vary. Slow-flow and fast-flow CSF leaks each present diagnostic challenges when attempts are made to locate the site of the CSF leakage. Novel imaging techniques have helped enormously with locating the site of the fast-flow leaks, but the slow-flow leaks continue to remain challenging.

- EBP has emerged as the treatment of choice for those who fail the initial conservative measures. It can be targeted or distant, single level, bilevel, or, in selected cases, multilevel. Epidural fibrin glue injection also has utility in selected cases. Combined fibrin glue and EBP have been tried by some, but it is not a routine approach and needs particular considerations.
- It is expected that surgery is aimed at stopping the leak when less invasive measures, such as EBP, have failed or when the anatomy of the leak is such that the chance of nonsurgical success is predicted to be very slim. It is essential to determine the site of the leak before surgery is undertaken.

REFERENCES

1. Mokri B, Krueger BR, Miller GM. Meningeal gadolinium enhancement in low-pressure headaches. Ann Neurol 1991;30:294–5.
2. Mokri B, Posner JB. Spontaneous intracranial hypotension: the broadening clinical and imaging spectrum of CSF leaks. Neurology 2000;55(12):1771–2.
3. Mokri B. Spontaneous cerebrospinal fluid leaks: from intracranial hypotension to cerebrospinal fluid hypovolemia–evolution of a concept. Mayo Clin Proc 1999; 74(11):1113–23.
4. Miyazawa K, Shiga Y, Hasegawa T, et al. CSF hypovolemia vs intracranial hypotension in "spontaneous intracranial hypotension syndrome". Neurology 2003; 60(6):941–7.
5. Chung SJ, Lee JH, Im JH, et al. Short- and long-term outcomes of spontaneous CSF hypovolemia. Eur Neurol 2005;54(2):63–7.
6. Rowland LP, Fink ME, Rubin L. Cerebrospinal fluid blood brain barrier, brain edema and hydrocephalus. In: Kundel ER, Schwartz JS, Jessel TM, editors. Principles of neural science. 3rd edition. New York: Elsevier; 1991. p. 1050–60.
7. Tripathi BJ, Tripathi RC. Vacuolar transcellular channels as a drainage pathway for cerebrospinal fluid. J Physiol 1947;239:195–206.
8. Tripathi RC. Ultrastructure of the arachnoid mater in relation to outflow of cerebrospinal fluid. A new concept. Lancet 1973;2(7819):8–11.
9. Johnston M. The importance of lymphatics in cerebrospinal fluid transport. Lymphat Res Biol 2003;1(1):41–4 [discussion: 45].
10. Matsumae M, Kikinis R, Morocz IA, et al. Age-related changes in intracranial compartment volumes in normal adults assessed by magnetic resonance imaging. J Neurosurg 1996;84(6):982–91.
11. Hogan QH, Prost R, Kulier A, et al. Magnetic resonance imaging of cerebrospinal fluid volume and the influence of body habitus and abdominal pressure. Anesthesiology 1996;84(6):1341–9.
12. Magnaes B. Body position and cerebrospinal fluid pressure. Part 2: clinical studies on orthostatic pressure and the hydrostatic indifferent point. J Neurosurg 1976;44(6):698–705.
13. Miller JD. Volume and pressure in the craniospinal axis. Clin Neurosurg 1975;22: 76–105.
14. Kunkle EC, Ray BS, Wolff HG. Experimental studies on headache: analysis of headache associated with changes in intracranial pressure. Arch Neurol Psychiatr 1943;49:323–58.
15. Mokri B, Piepgras DG, Miller GM. Syndrome of orthostatic headaches and diffuse pachymeningeal gadolinium enhancement. Mayo Clin Proc 1997;72(5): 400–13.

16. Davenport RJ, Chataway SJ, Warlow CP. Spontaneous intracranial hypotension from a CSF leak in a patient with Marfan's syndrome. J Neurol Neurosurg Psychiatr 1995;59(5):516-9.

17. Fukutake T, Sakakibara R, Mori M, et al. Chronic intractable headache in a patient with Marfan's syndrome. Headache 1997;37(5):291-5.

18. Schrijver I, Schievink WI, Godfrey M, et al. Spontaneous spinal cerebrospinal fluid leaks and minor skeletal features of Marfan syndrome: a microfibrillopathy. J Neurosurg 2002;96(3):483-9.

19. Mokri B, Maher CO, Sencakova D. Spontaneous CSF leaks: underlying disorder of connective tissue. Neurology 2002;58(5):814-6.

20. Raftopoulos C, Pierard GE, Retif C, et al. Endoscopic cure of a giant sacral meningocele associated with Marfan's syndrome: case report. Neurosurgery 1992;30(5):765-8.

21. Harkens KL, el-Khoury GY. Intrasacral meningocele in a patient with Marfan syndrome. Case report. Spine (Phila Pa 1976) 1990;15(6):610-2.

22. Cilluffo JM, Gomez MR, Reese DF, et al. Idiopathic ("congenital") spinal arachnoid diverticula. Clinical diagnosis and surgical results. Mayo Clin Proc 1981; 56(2):93-101.

23. Schievink WI, Torres VE. Spinal meningeal diverticula in autosomal dominant polycystic kidney disease. Lancet 1997;349(9060):1223-4.

24. Fattori R, Nienaber CA, Descovich B, et al. Importance of dural ectasia in phenotypic assessment of Marfan's syndrome. Lancet 1999;354(9182):910-3.

25. Pyeritz RE, Fishman EK, Bernhardt BA, et al. Dural ectasia is a common feature of the Marfan syndrome. Am J Hum Genet 1988;43(5):726-32.

26. Mokri B. Familial occurrence of spontaneous spinal CSF leaks: underlying connective tissue disorder. Headache 2008;48(1):146-9.

27. Vishteh AG, Schievink WI, Baskin JJ, et al. Cervical bone spur presenting with spontaneous intracranial hypotension. Case report. J Neurosurg 1998;89(3):483-4.

28. Eross EJ, Dodick DW, Nelson KD, et al. Orthostatic headache syndrome with CSF leak secondary to bony pathology of the cervical spine. Cephalalgia 2002;22(6):439-43.

29. Winter SC, Maartens NF, Anslow P, et al. Spontaneous intracranial hypotension due to thoracic disc herniation. Case report. J Neurosurg 2002;96(Suppl 3): 343-5.

30. Hebert-Blouin MN, Mokri B, Shin AY, et al. Cerebrospinal fluid volume-depletion headaches in patients with traumatic brachial plexus injury. J Neurosurg 2013; 118(1):149-54.

31. Schaltenbrand G. Normal and pathological physiology of the cerebrospinal fluid circulation. Lancet 1953;1(6765):805-8.

32. Marcelis J, Silberstein SD. Spontaneous low cerebrospinal fluid pressure headache. Headache 1990;30(4):192-6.

33. Rando TA, Fishman RA. Spontaneous intracranial hypotension: report of two cases and review of the literature. Neurology 1992;42(3 Pt 1):481-7.

34. Fay T. Mechanism of headache. Arch Neurol Psychiatr 1937;37:471-4.

35. Mokri B, Schievink WI. Headache associated with abnormalities in intracranial structure or function: low-cerebrospinal-fluid-pressure headache. In: Silberstein SD, Lipton RB, Dodick DW, editors. Wolff's headache and other head pain. 8th edition. New York: Oxford University Press; 2007. p. 513-31.

36. Portier F, de Minteguiaga C, Racy E, et al. Spontaneous intracranial hypotension: a rare cause of labyrinthine hydrops. Ann Otol Rhinol Laryngol 2002; 111(9):817-20.

37. Yamamoto M, Suehiro T, Nakata H, et al. Primary low cerebrospinal fluid pressure syndrome associated with galactorrhea. Intern Med 1993;32(3):228–31.
38. Albayram S, Wasserman BA, Yousem DM, et al. Intracranial hypotension as a cause of radiculopathy from cervical epidural venous engorgement: case report. AJNR Am J Neuroradiol 2002;23(4):618–21.
39. Molins A, Alvarez J, Sumalla J, et al. Cisternographic pattern of spontaneous liquoral hypotension. Cephalalgia 1990;10(2):59–65.
40. Weber WE, Heidendal GA, de Krom MC. Primary intracranial hypotension and abnormal radionuclide cisternography. Report of a case and review of the literature. Clin Neurol Neurosurg 1991;93(1):55–60.
41. Bai J, Yokoyama K, Kinuya S, et al. Radionuclide cisternography in intracranial hypotension syndrome. Ann Nucl Med 2002;16(1):75–8.
42. Spelle L, Boulin A, Tainturier C, et al. Neuroimaging features of spontaneous intracranial hypotension. Neuroradiology 2001;43(8):622–7.
43. Lin WC, Lirng JF, Fuh JL, et al. MR findings of spontaneous intracranial hypotension. Acta Radiol 2002;43(3):249–55.
44. Pannullo SC, Reich JB, Krol G, et al. MRI changes in intracranial hypotension. Neurology 1993;43(5):919–26.
45. Atkinson JL, Weinshenker BG, Miller GM, et al. Acquired Chiari I malformation secondary to spontaneous spinal cerebrospinal fluid leakage and chronic intracranial hypotension syndrome in seven cases. J Neurosurg 1998;88(2):237–42.
46. Mokri B, Atkinson JL. False pituitary tumor in CSF leaks. Neurology 2000;55(4):573–5.
47. Alvarez-Linera J, Escribano J, Benito-Leon J, et al. Pituitary enlargement in patients with intracranial hypotension syndrome. Neurology 2000;55(12):1895–7.
48. Bakshi R, Mechtler LL, Kamran S, et al. MRI findings in lumbar puncture headache syndrome: abnormal dural-meningeal and dural venous sinus enhancement. Clin Imaging 1999;23(2):73–6.
49. Rabin BM, Roychowdhury S, Meyer JR, et al. Spontaneous intracranial hypotension: spinal MR findings. AJNR Am J Neuroradiol 1998;19(6):1034–9.
50. Yousry I, Forderreuther S, Moriggl B, et al. Cervical MR imaging in postural headache: MR signs and pathophysiological implications. AJNR Am J Neuroradiol 2001;22(7):1239–50.
51. Chiapparini L, Farina L, D'Incerti L, et al. Spinal radiological findings in nine patients with spontaneous intracranial hypotension. Neuroradiology 2002;44(2):143–50 [discussion: 151–2].
52. Wang YF, Lirng JF, Fuh JL, et al. Heavily T2-weighted MR myelography vs CT myelography in spontaneous intracranial hypotension. Neurology 2009;73(22):1892–8.
53. Burtis MT, Ulmer JL, Miller GA, et al. Intradural spinal vein enlargement in craniospinal hypotension. AJNR Am J Neuroradiol 2005;26(1):34–8.
54. Mokri B. The Monro-Kellie hypothesis: applications in CSF volume depletion. Neurology 2001;56(12):1746–8.
55. Fishman RA, Dillon WP. Dural enhancement and cerebral displacement secondary to intracranial hypotension. Neurology 1993;43(3 Pt 1):609–11.
56. Luetmer PH, Mokri B. Dynamic CT myelography: a technique for localizing high-flow spinal cerebrospinal fluid leaks. AJNR Am J Neuroradiol 2003;24(8):1711–4.
57. Hoxworth JM, Trentman TL, Kotsenas AL, et al. The role of digital subtraction myelography in the diagnosis and localization of spontaneous spinal CSF leaks. AJR Am J Roentgenol 2012;199(3):649–53.

58. Yoo HM, Kim SJ, Choi CG, et al. Detection of CSF leak in spinal CSF leak syndrome using MR myelography: correlation with radioisotope cisternography. AJNR Am J Neuroradiol 2008;29(4):649–54.
59. Akbar JJ, Luetmer PH, Schwartz KM, et al. The role of MR myelography with intrathecal gadolinium in localization of spinal CSF leaks in patients with spontaneous intracranial hypotension. AJNR Am J Neuroradiol 2012;33(3):535–40.
60. Vilmig ST, Titus F. Low cerebrospinal fluid pressure. In: Olesen J, Tfelt-Hansen P, Welch KM, editors. The headache. New York: Oxford University Press; 2001. p. 417–33.
61. Rice GG, Dabbs CH. The use of peridural and subarachnoid injections of saline solution in the treatment of severe postspinal headache. Anesthesiology 1950; 11(1):17–23 illust.
62. Usubiaga JE, Usubiaga LE, Brea LM, et al. Effect of saline injections on epidural and subarachnoid space pressures and relation to postspinal anesthesia headache. Anesth Analg 1967;46(3):293–6.
63. Gibson BE, Wedel DJ, Faust RJ, et al. Continuous epidural saline infusion for the treatment of low CSF pressure headache. Anesthesiology 1988;68(5):789–91.
64. Aldrete JA. Persistent post-dural-puncture headache treated with epidural infusion of dextran. Headache 1994;34(5):265–7.
65. Binder DK, Dillon WP, Fishman RA, et al. Intrathecal saline infusion in the treatment of obtundation associated with spontaneous intracranial hypotension: technical case report. Neurosurgery 2002;51(3):830–6 [discussion: 836–7].
66. Duffy PJ, Crosby ET. The epidural blood patch. Resolving the controversies. Can J Anaesth 1999;46(9):878–86.
67. Sencakova D, Mokri B, McClelland RL. The efficacy of epidural blood patch in spontaneous CSF leaks. Neurology 2001;57(10):1921–3.
68. Crul BJ, Gerritse BM, van Dongen RT, et al. Epidural fibrin glue injection stops persistent postdural puncture headache. Anesthesiology 1999;91(2):576–7.
69. Gerritse BM, van Dongen RT, Crul BJ. Epidural fibrin glue injection stops persistent cerebrospinal fluid leak during long-term intrathecal catheterization. Anesth Analg 1997;84(5):1140–1.
70. Schievink WI, Morreale VM, Atkinson JL, et al. Surgical treatment of spontaneous spinal cerebrospinal fluid leaks. J Neurosurg 1998;88(2):243–6.
71. Cohen-Gadol AA, Mokri B, Piepgras DG, et al. Surgical anatomy of dural defects in spontaneous spinal cerebrospinal fluid leaks. Neurosurgery 2006; 58(4 Suppl 2). p. ONS-238–45; [discussion: ONS-245].
72. de Noronha RJ, Sharrack B, Hadjivassiliou M, et al. Subdural haematoma: a potentially serious consequence of spontaneous intracranial hypotension. J Neurol Neurosurg Psychiatr 2003;74(6):752–5.
73. Mizuno J, Mummaneni PV, Rodts GE, et al. Recurrent subdural hematoma caused by cerebrospinal fluid leakage. Case report. J Neurosurg Spine 2006; 4(2):183–5.
74. Kelley GR, Johnson PL. Sinking brain syndrome: craniotomy can precipitate brainstem herniation in CSF hypovolemia. Neurology 2004;62(1):157.
75. Mokri B. Intracranial hypertension after treatment of spontaneous cerebrospinal fluid leaks. Mayo Clin Proc 2002;77(11):1241–6.
76. Berroir S, Grabli D, Heran F, et al. Cerebral sinus venous thrombosis in two patients with spontaneous intracranial hypotension. Cerebrovasc Dis 2004;17(1): 9–12.
77. Kumar N, Lane JI, Piepgras DG. Superficial siderosis: sealing the defect. Neurology 2009;72(7):671–3.

78. Kumar N, McKeon A, Rabinstein AA, et al. Superficial siderosis and CSF hypovolemia: the defect (dural) in the link. Neurology 2007;69(9):925–6.

79. Cohen-Gadol AA, Krauss WE, Spinner RJ. Delayed central nervous system superficial siderosis following brachial plexus avulsion injury. Report of three cases. Neurosurg Focus 2004;16(5):E10.

80. Deluca GC, Boes CJ, Krueger BR, et al. Ventral intraspinal fluid-filled collection secondary to CSF leak presenting as bibrachial amyotrophy. Neurology 2011; 76(16):1439–40.

81. Mokri B, Low PA. Orthostatic headaches without CSF leak in postural tachycardia syndrome. Neurology 2003;61(7):980–2.

82. Mokri B. Orthostatic headaches in the syndrome of the trephined: resolution following cranioplasty. Headache 2010;50(7):1206–11.

83. Leep Hunderfund AN, Mokri B. Orthostatic headache without CSF leak. Neurology 2008;71(23):1902–6.

84. Mokri B. Spontaneous CSF leaks mimicking benign exertional headaches. Cephalalgia 2002;22(10):780–3.

85. Schievink WI, Wijdicks EF, Meyer FB, et al. Spontaneous intracranial hypotension mimicking aneurysmal subarachnoid hemorrhage. Neurosurgery 2001; 48(3):513–6 [discussion: 516–7].

86. Leep Hunderfund AN, Mokri B. Second-half-of-the-day headache as a manifestation of spontaneous CSF leak. J Neurol 2012;259(2):306–10.

87. Brady-McCreery KM, Speidel S, Hussein MA, et al. Spontaneous intracranial hypotension with unique strabismus due to third and fourth cranial neuropathies. Binocul Vis Strabismus Q 2002;17(1):43–8.

88. Horton JC, Fishman RA. Neurovisual findings in the syndrome of spontaneous intracranial hypotension from dural cerebrospinal fluid leak. Ophthalmology 1994;101(2):244–51.

89. Pleasure SJ, Abosch A, Friedman J, et al. Spontaneous intracranial hypotension resulting in stupor caused by diencephalic compression. Neurology 1998;50(6): 1854–7.

90. Evan RW, Mokri B. Spontaneous intracranial hypotension resulting in coma. Headache 2002;42(2):159–60.

91. Pakiam AS, Lee C, Lang AE. Intracranial hypotension with parkinsonism, ataxia, and bulbar weakness. Arch Neurol 1999;56(7):869–72.

92. Hong M, Shah GV, Adams KM, et al. Spontaneous intracranial hypotension causing reversible frontotemporal dementia. Neurology 2002;58(8):1285–7.

93. Beck CE, Rizk NW, Kiger LT, et al. Intracranial hypotension presenting with severe encephalopathy. Case report. J Neurosurg 1998;89(3):470–3.

94. Nowak DA, Rodiek SO, Zinner J, et al. Broadening the clinical spectrum: unusual presentation of spontaneous cerebrospinal fluid hypovolemia. Case report. J Neurosurg 2003;98(4):903–7.

95. Mokri B, Ahlskog JE, Luetmer PH. Chorea as a manifestation of spontaneous CSF leak. Neurology 2006;67(8):1490–1.

96. Mokri B, Hunter SF, Atkinson JL, et al. Orthostatic headaches caused by CSF leak but with normal CSF pressures. Neurology 1998;51(3):786–90.

97. Mokri B, Parisi JE, Scheithauer BW, et al. Meningeal biopsy in intracranial hypotension: meningeal enhancement on MRI. Neurology 1995;45(10):1801–7.

Headaches and Brain Tumors

Sarah Kirby, MD, FRCPC, R. Allan Purdy, MD, FRCPC*

KEYWORDS

- Diagnosis • Brain tumor • Headache • Uncommon causes • Investigation
- Treatment

KEY POINTS

- Headache is a major symptom of brain tumors.
- When red flags are present, investigations are warranted, mainly neuroimaging.
- Even though brain tumors can present with what look like primary headaches, there usually are atypical features to the history to suggest a need to search for a secondary cause.
- Some less common headache disorders, such as trigeminal autonomic cephalalgias (TACs), can be associated with a variety of brain tumors, suggesting that most TACs should be investigated.

INTRODUCTION

Not much has changed since the authors' last review of this subject.[1] Brain tumors and headache are common companions and it is important to consider cerebral neoplasms in any patient who has only headache as a symptom and no other significant neurologic signs or symptoms. What may have changed is the increasing use of neuroimaging to make diagnoses in headache disorders, in particular chronic headache disorders.[2]

Many patients with headache and chronic daily headache have serious secondary disorders and these need investigation. Also, those patients with TACs, because of their relative rarity and frequent association with other pathologies, probably need to be investigated.

HEADACHES AND BRAIN TUMORS

Headache can be a cardinal symptom of serious disease, including primary cerebral neoplasms or metastatic disease. Headache is present in 48% to 71% of brain tumor

Disclosure Statement: The authors have no disclosures to make relevant to this publication.
Division of Neurology, Department of Medicine, QEII Health Sciences Centre, Dalhousie University, 1796 Summer Street, Halifax, Nova Scotia B3H3A7, Canada
* Corresponding author.
E-mail address: Allan.Prudy@cdha.nshealth.ca

Neurol Clin 32 (2014) 423–432
http://dx.doi.org/10.1016/j.ncl.2013.11.006
0733-8619/14/$ – see front matter © 2014 Elsevier Inc. All rights reserved.

patients in studies of unselected brain tumors in adults.[3–5] Primary brain tumors and metastatic lesions are equally likely to cause headache. Patients over 75 years of age are less likely to present with headache.[6]

Headaches are more common in brain tumor patients with a prior history of headache and 83% of patients noted an alteration in the character of their headache.[5,7] Among patients with a history of longstanding headaches, 64% had headache with their brain tumor but only 38% of patients without a prior history of headache developed headache as a symptom of their brain tumor.[5]

The classic brain tumor headache has been described as severe, early morning, or nocturnal headache associated with nausea and vomiting, but studies show that most brain tumor headaches are nonspecific, intermittent, moderate to severe in intensity, and progressive. The pain is variably described as aching, pressure, tightness, and throbbing or shooting.[3–5,7] Only 17% of patients in Forsyth and Posner's[3] study had classic brain tumor headaches. Most brain tumor headaches do not meet criteria for primary headache disorders. Up to 15% of patients report migraine-type headaches but these usually have atypical features. Tension-type headaches are reported in 29% to 39% of patients.[3,5,7]

The frequency of headaches depends on the location of the tumor. More than 90% of patients with intraventricular and midline tumors had headache. With infratentorial tumors, 70% to 84% of patients had headaches versus 55% to 60% of patients with supratentorial tumors.[8,9] Factors that may increase the risk of headache include raised intracranial pressure, degree of midline shift, and increasing edema.[3–5]

Tumor pathology also may affect the likelihood of headache. Valentinis and colleagues[5] found that headaches were more common in patients with glioblastomas and secreting pituitary adenomas. Slow-growing tumors may be less likely to cause headache because there is more time for the pain-sensitive structures to adapt than with a fast-growing tumor and usually there is less associated cerebral edema.

In patients with new undifferentiated headache, without known malignancy, the risk of a brain tumor is low (0.15%). If patients have a headache that meets criteria for a primary headache disorder, the risk is even lower (0.045%).[10]

DIAGNOSING SERIOUS HEADACHES, INCLUDING THOSE ASSOCIATED WITH BRAIN TUMORS

Red flags are as useful today as they always have been in neurologic diagnosis,[11] so it bears repeating that any patient who has the following red flags needs evaluation for serious or life-threatening causes of headache, including a brain tumor:

- Acute new, usually severe, headache or headache that has changed from prior headaches
- Headache on exertion or onset at night or early morning
- Headache that is progressive in nature
- Headache associated with fever or other systemic symptoms
- Headache with meningismus
- Headache with new neurologic signs
- Precipitation of head pain with the Valsalva maneuver (by bending down, coughing, sneezing, or straining)
- New headache onset in an adult, especially one who is over 50 years of age
- New headache in the elderly or children
- New or changed headache in a cancer patient

No matter what the ultimate cause of a patient's headache, it is vital to consider a longer differential diagnosis than primary headache disorder or neoplasm. It is best to consider a list of serious causes in the approach to patients, including

- Space-occupying lesion (tumor, abscess, hematoma, and so forth)
- Systemic infection, meningitis, encephalitis
- Stroke (infarction, intracerebral hemorrhage, and cerebral venous occlusion)
- Subarachnoid hemorrhage
- Systemic disorders (thyroid disease, posterior reversible encephalopathy syndrome [PRES], hypertension, pheochromocytoma, and so forth)
- Temporal arteritis
- Traumatic head injuries
- Serious ophthalmologic and otolaryngologic causes of headache

If consideration of red flags and serious causes is paired with a complete neurologic examination, most causes of headache can be sorted out at the bedside. The practice of classical neurologic diagnosis, based on principles of localization, misses little, even before a neuroimaging procedure or other diagnostic test is ordered. Some element of the history or physical findings suggests that a particular headache patient harbors a structural cause for the headache. Anyone with abnormal vital signs or systemic symptoms, cognitive dysfunction, or any focal neurologic signs needs further assessment and investigation.

BRAIN TUMORS PRESENTING AS HEADACHE

Adults with known malignancy, without any other neurologic symptoms or signs, who present with new or changed headache, frequently have intracranial metastases; 32% to 54% of patients with cancer and new or changed headache were found to have intracranial metastases.[12,13] In children with new headache and systemic cancer, the risk of metastatic brain tumors was 12% and primary brain tumors 1%.[14]

Headache is a common symptom of intracranial hemorrhage (ICH). Although hemorrhage into a brain tumor is an infrequent cause of spontaneous ICH (<10%) in the general population, it accounted for 61% of ICH in a study of 208 cancer patients with ICH from Memorial Sloan-Kettering Cancer Center. Most hemorrhages (77%) were in solid tumors, especially melanoma, lung, breast, and renal cell; 21% were in primary brain tumors, especially glioblastoma multiforme and oligodendroglioma.[15]

Headache as the only symptom of a brain tumor at diagnosis is uncommon, reported in only 2% to 8% of patients.[5,7,16] Most patients have other signs and symptoms by the time of diagnosis and, in a study by Vazquez-Barquero and colleagues,[16] all brain tumor patients who presented with isolated headache had developed other symptoms within 10 weeks.

MECHANISMS OF HEADACHE IN BRAIN TUMORS

In 1940, Ray and Wolfe[17] performed a classic series of experiments on patients undergoing craniotomies, in which they mapped pain-sensitive structures of the head. They found that the venous sinuses, dural arteries, cerebral arteries at the base of the brain, and some of the dura at the base of the brain were sensitive to pain. They postulated 6 mechanisms of headache pain:

- Traction causing displacement of the veins draining the large venous sinuses
- Traction on the middle meningeal artery
- Traction on the major arteries at the base of the brain

- Direct pressure on cranial nerves with pain afferent fibers from the head
- Distension and dilation of the extracranial and intracranial arteries
- Inflammation in or around the pain structures of the head.

Kunkle and colleagues[18] studied an additional 67 patients with brain tumors and concluded that distant and local traction on pain-sensitive structures, mass effect, and hydrocephalus caused most brain tumor headaches.

Brain tumor headache location does not predict tumor location. Wirth and Van Buren[19] applied electrical stimulation to the dura of patients having implanted epidural electrodes for treatment of movement disorders or evaluation of seizure disorders. They found that pain could be referred to all areas of the head and neck. The same area of stimulation could produce quite different areas of referred pain in different patients. Most patients had ipsilateral referral of pain, but, in 4 patients, unilateral stimulation produced bilateral or contralateral responses.

As might be predicted from these findings, the location of headache pain from brain tumors may be ipsilateral, contralateral, or bilateral. Skull-based tumors are more likely associated with frontal than occipital headache.[4,5] Raised intracranial pressure can cause headache. Plateau waves are acute elevations in intracranial pressure triggered by a vasodilatory cascade with loss of the autoregulatory response and can cause sudden intense headaches associated with dizziness and alterations in consciousness and motor control.[20]

UNCOMMON HEADACHES IN BRAIN TUMOR PATIENTS

Paroxysmal headaches are reported with brain tumors. The classic presentation of a colloid cyst is severe paroxysmal headache relieved by changes in position.[21] More recent series suggest, however, that colloid cysts are more likely to present as generalized intermittent headache, often without a positional component.[22] There may be associated papilledema, ataxia, decreased vision, and urinary incontinence. These tumors are important to diagnose because these patients can present with abrupt deterioration due to blockage of the foramen of Munro. In a case series of 78 patients with newly diagnosed colloid cysts by de Witt Hamer and colleagues,[23] there was a 12% mortality rate.

Craniopharyngiomas, dermoid, and epidermoid tumors have cysts that may rupture, spilling their contents into the cerebrospinal fluid. These contents are extremely irritating and may cause headache due to chemical meningitis.[24–26]

Pituitary tumors are associated with headache in 40% to 70% of patients.[27–29] The mechanism of headache seems variable—some mechanisms seem related to hormonal secretions, especially prolactin and growth hormone, and others to dural stretch and cavernous sinus invasion.[30] What is particularly unusual is the frequent association of TACs and pituitary tumors. Levy and colleagues[30] reported that in 84 patients with pituitary tumors and headache, there were 4 cases of short-lasting unilateral neuralgiform headache attacks with conjunctival injection and tearing (SUNCT), 3 cases of cluster headache, and 1 case of hemicrania continua. In a review of published symptomatic TAC cases, 29% of cluster cases, 67% of paroxysmal hemicranias cases, and 70% of SUNCT patients had pituitary tumors. Other tumors were found in the remaining patients with SUNCT or paroxysmal hemicrania.[31]

Although some patients had atypical features, others did not and many responded to the usual therapies. Despite the frequent association, the approximately 10% incidence of asymptomatic pituitary adenomas in the general population suggests that at least some are incidental.

Pituitary apoplexy is caused by hemorrhage or infarction of a pituitary tumor. Patients present with sudden onset of severe headache associated with visual loss, eye movement abnormalities, facial numbness, somnolence, and pituitary insufficiency.[32,33] If not recognized, patients may be left with permanent visual loss or diplopia and, rarely, patients die of pituitary insufficiency.[34]

Skull-based metastases may also cause headache. Greenberg and colleagues[35] described 5 clinical syndromes:

- Orbital: unilateral frontal headache, diplopia, ophthalmic division trigeminal sensory loss, and proptosis
- Parasellar: unilateral frontal headache, diplopia, and ophthalmic division trigeminal sensory loss
- Middle fossa: dull aching in the cheek, jaw, or forehead; occasional trigeminal neuralgia-type pain; and loss of sensation or numbness in the maxillary or mandibular divisions of the trigeminal nerve
- Jugular foramen: hoarseness and dysphagia; paralysis of the ninth, tenth, and eleventh cranial nerves; and unilateral dull retroauricular pain
- Occipital condyle: severe unilateral occipital pain aggravated by neck flexion and unilateral tongue paralysis. A more recent case series of this syndrome was published by Capobianco and colleagues[36] in 2002

HEADACHE ASSOCIATED WITH TREATMENT OF BRAIN TUMORS

Brain tumor patients are susceptible to headaches from the treatment of their brain tumors. Craniotomies can cause postsurgical headache. Rocha-Filho and colleagues[37] found that 91% of patients having surgery for intracranial aneurysms had headache postcraniotomy. Immediate postcraniotomy headache was reported in 30% of patients[38]; 58% of patients had craniofacial pain and functional jaw limitations 4 to 6 months after craniotomy.[39] Headaches are more frequent in patients having subocciptial craniotomies; 64% to 93% of patients with acoustic neuromas treated with surgery reported headache 3 months postoperatively, and 50% to 66% still had headache 3 years later.[40,41] The retrosigmoid approach is associated with a higher risk of postoperative pain.[42] Although dopamine agonists may shrink prolactin-secreting adenomas and normalize prolactin levels, some patients have headache from the dopamine agonists.[43] Rebound headaches can occur in patients treated with octreotide for growth hormone–secreting pituitary adenomas.[44]

Radiation therapy is a mainstay of treatment of both primary and metastatic brain tumors. It can cause headache immediately during therapy or even years later. Acute radiation encephalopathy associated with headache and worsening of other symptoms may occur at the initiation of radiotherapy. A subacute demyelinating radiation encephalopathy can occur 1 to 6 months postradiation, again associated with headache and deteriorating neurologic function.[45]

In malignant glioma patients treated with combined temozolomide chemotherapy and radiation, increased contrast enhancement and cerebral edema on both CT and MRI scans may be seen immediately after treatment. Edema may cause headaches and worsening symptoms but can be asymptomatic. Edema cannot be distinguished reliably from true tumor growth on imaging but probably reflects a good response to therapy because these patients have better survival rates than those who do not show pseudoprogression.[46]

Late complications of radiation therapy occurring months to many years after therapy include cerebral radiation necrosis, which presents with headache and focal neurologic symptoms. Another late complication is stroke-like migraine attacks after radiation therapy (SMART) syndrome. Patients with SMART syndrome have prolonged and usually reversible episodes of migraine-type headache, focal neurologic deficits, and sometimes seizures lasting hours to weeks. On MRI, there may be striking ribbon-like gadolinium enhancement of the cortex of the involved hemisphere during the episode.[47,48]

Chemotherapy drugs and medications used to treat side effects of chemotherapy can cause headache. Temozolomide, an alkylating agent used to treat malignant gliomas, causes headache in 25% of patients.[49] Agents to control nausea, such as the selective serotonin type-3 receptor antagonist, ondansetron, may cause headache in some patients.[50] Corticosteroids are often used to control cerebral edema, and their withdrawal can precipitate headache either from relapse of the edema or as a side effect of the steroid. Bevacizumab, a monoclonal antibody that binds to vascular endothelial growth factor, is used as second-line treatment of malignant gliomas and has been reported to cause headaches and, rarely, PRES.[51]

INVESTIGATION OF HEADACHE PATIENTS WHO HAVE SUSPECTED TUMOR

Patients presenting with suspected brain tumors need neuroimaging. A normal examination is reassuring and patients with red flags need to be investigated.[52] Chronic daily headache requires investigation, and, as Evans[2] points out, causes of these headache include neoplasms, among other serious secondary headache disorders. Although the yield of diagnostic testing is low, serious pathology can be easily overlooked without it.

The availability of CT head scans probably makes that imaging modality the first one used in patients with headache and suspected neoplasms. Unenhanced scans can miss lesions and, despite their expense, sometimes MRI is better in some patients especially if a posterior fossa or pituitary lesion is suspected.

TREATMENT OF HEADACHE PATIENTS WHO HAVE BRAIN TUMORS

The treatment of headache associated with brain tumor depends on type of tumor, patient functional status, and stage of the disease. Generally, treatment of the tumor improves the headache. Patients with brain metastases have a limited life expectancy and treatment is palliative. Acutely, corticosteroids, such as dexamethasone, often provide dramatic temporary relief of headache and other symptoms caused by cerebral edema, although steroid myopathies, sleep disturbance, mood changes, and other side effects may be troublesome.

Whole-brain radiotherapy is commonly used to try to control brain metastases. Recent prospective trials have suggested that improvement or stabilization of headache and lower requirements for corticosteroids were seen after whole-brain radiotherapy.[53,54]

For patients with stable systemic disease and few metastases, stereotactic radiosurgery or surgical resection may provide better local control and prolonged survival.[55–57] In most cases, chemotherapy is ineffective for brain metastases. Because survival is limited in these patients, usually 3 to 6 months, it is important to treat pain aggressively to maintain quality of life for as long as possible.

At presentation with a primary brain tumor, patients often have good symptom relief with corticosteroids to relieve cerebral edema while awaiting definitive treatment of the tumor. Analgesics may be required in addition. Treatment depends on the pathology of the tumor but usually includes surgery. Radiotherapy and chemotherapy, in addition to surgery, are the standard of care for high-grade gliomas. Valentinis and colleagues[5] reported that 98 of 116 patients with new or changed headache with their brain tumor had resolution or major improvement in their headaches postoperatively.

Not all patients improve. A small study of 13 long-term glioblastoma survivors prior to recurrence found that 10 of 13 reported headache and 3 of 10 ranked their headache as moderate to severe.[58] Studies investigating symptoms at recurrence of high-grade gliomas found that 36% to 52% of patients complain of headache.[59,60] Relapse of the headache often reflects relapse of the tumor. Most headaches respond to steroids but nonopioid or opioid analgesics may be required. Again, because survival is limited in these patients, good pain control is important to maintain quality of life.

Treatment of patients with potentially curable tumors or those with tumors with long survival rates can be more difficult. It is important to try and separate brain tumor–associated headaches from primary headache disorders. Patients with a history of primary headaches are more likely to have brain tumor–associated headaches.[3,5] If a headache meets criteria for a primary headache disorder, standard therapy for the primary headache is indicated. Even if there are atypical features, the headache may respond.

CONCLUDING REMARKS

Over time we have become impressed with the clinical, imaging, and treatment modalities available for brain tumor patients. Even when detected early, some tumors remain largely untreatable in the sense of cure, and some are amenable to therapy. Whether early discovery makes a difference or not in some currently untreatable tumors is uncertain. Headache remains a major symptom of brain tumor, however, so if early recognition allows better diagnosis and management, then that works in the best interests of patients. Brain tumors can present with symptoms similar to primary headache disorders, so astute clinicians and diagnosticians always need to consider cerebral tumors in headache patients. Most patients do not have brain tumors but some do and need to be investigated and treated.

REFERENCES

1. Purdy RA, Kirby S. Headaches and brain tumors. Neurol Clin North Am 2004;22: 39–53.
2. Evans R. Diagnostic testing for chronic daily headache. Curr Pain Headache Rep 2007;11(1):47–52.
3. Forsyth PA, Posner JB. Headaches in patients with brain tumors: a study of 111 patients. Neurology 1993;43(9):1678–83.
4. Pfund Z, Szapary L, Jaszberenyi O, et al. Headache in intracranial tumors. Cephalalgia 1999;19(9):787–90 [discussion: 765].
5. Valentinis L, Tuniz F, Valent F, et al. Headache attributed to intracranial tumours: a prospective cohort study. Cephalalgia 2010;30(4):389–98.
6. Lowry JK, Snyder JJ, Lowry PW. Brain tumors in the elderly: recent trends in a minnesota cohort study. Arch Neurol 1998;55(7):922–8.
7. Schankin CJ. Characteristics of brain tumour-associated headache. Cephalalgia 2007;27(8):904.
8. Childhood Brain Tumor Consortium. The epidemiology of headache among children with brain tumor. Headache in children with brain tumor. J Neurooncol 1991;10(1):31–46.
9. Wilne S. Presentation of childhood CNS tumours: a systematic review and meta-analysis. The Lancet Oncol 2007;8(8):685.

10. Kernick D, Stapley S, Goadsby PJ, et al. What happens to new-onset headache presented to primary care? A case-cohort study using electronic primary care records. Cephalalgia 2008;28(11):1188.
11. Purdy RA. Clinical evaluation of a patient presenting with headache. Med Clin North Am 2001;85(4):847–63, v.
12. Christiaans MH, Kelder JC, Arnoldus EP, et al. Prediction of intracranial metastases in cancer patients with headache. Cancer 2002;94(7):2063–8.
13. Argyriou AA, Chroni E, Polychronopoulos P, et al. Headache characteristics and brain metastases prediction in cancer patients. Eur J Cancer Care (Engl) 2006; 15(1):90–5.
14. Antunes NL. The spectrum of neurologic disease in children with systemic cancer. Pediatr Neurol 2001;25(3):227–35.
15. Navi BB, Reichman JS, Berlin D, et al. Intracerebral and subarachnoid hemorrhage in patients with cancer. Neurology 2010;74(6):494–501.
16. Vazquez-Barquero A, Ibanez FJ, Herrera S, et al. Isolated headache as the presenting clinical manifestation of intracranial tumors: a prospective study. Cephalalgia 1994;14(4):270–2.
17. Ray BS, Wolff HG. Experimental studies on headache: pain-sensitive structures of the head and their significance. Arch Surg 1940;41:813–56.
18. Kunkle EC, Ray BS, Wolff HG. Studies on headache: the mechanism and significance of the headache associated with brain tumor. Bull N Y Acad Med 1942; 18:400–22.
19. Wirth FP, Van Buren JM. Referral of pain from dural stimulation in man. J Neurosurg 1971;34(5):630–42.
20. Watling CJ, Cairncross JG. Acetazolamide therapy for symptomatic plateau waves in patients with brain tumors. Report of three cases. J Neurosurg 2002; 97(1):224–6.
21. Harris W. Paroxsymal and postural headaches from intraventricular cysts and tumors. Lancet 1944;2:654–5.
22. Desai KI, Nadkarni TD, Muzumdar DP, et al. Surgical management of colloid cyst of the third ventricle–a study of 105 cases. Surg Neurol 2002;57(5): 295–302 [discussion: 302–4].
23. de Witt Hamer PC, Verstegen MJ, De Haan RJ, et al. High risk of acute deterioration in patients harboring symptomatic colloid cysts of the third ventricle. J Neurosurg 2002;96(6):1041–5.
24. Satoh H, Uozumi T, Arita K, et al. Spontaneous rupture of craniopharyngioma cysts. A report of five cases and review of the literature. Surg Neurol 1993; 40(5):414–9.
25. Gormley WB, Tomecek FJ, Qureshi N, et al. Craniocerebral epidermoid and dermoid tumours: a review of 32 cases. Acta Neurochir (Wien) 1994;128(1–4): 115–21.
26. Stendel R, Pietila TA, Lehmann K, et al. Ruptured intracranial dermoid cysts. Surg Neurol 2002;57(6):391–8 [discussion: 398].
27. Levy MJ, Jager HR, Powell M, et al. Pituitary volume and headache: size is not everything. Arch Neurol 2004;61(5):721–5.
28. Chen L, White W, Spetzler R, et al. A prospective study of nonfunctioning pituitary adenomas: presentation, management, and clinical outcome. J Neurooncol 2011;102(1):129–38.
29. Schankin CJ, Reifferscheid AK, Krumbholz M, et al. Headache in patients with pituitary adenoma: clinical and paraclinical findings. Cephalalgia 2012;32(16): 1198–207.

30. Levy M. The association of pituitary tumors and headache. Curr Neurol Neurosci Rep 2011;11(2):164–70.
31. Cittadini E, Matharu M. Symptomatic trigeminal autonomic cephalalgias. Neurologist 2009;15(6):305–12.
32. Biousse V, Newman NJ, Oyesiku NM. Precipitating factors in pituitary apoplexy. J Neurol Neurosurg Psychiatr 2001;71(4):542–5.
33. Turgut M, Ozsunar Y, Başak S, et al. Pituitary apoplexy: an overview of 186 cases published during the last century. Acta Neurochir 2010;152(5):749–61.
34. Shields LB, Balko MG, Hunsaker JC. Sudden and unexpected death from pituitary tumor apoplexy. J Forensic Sci 2012;57(1):262–6.
35. Greenberg HS, Deck MD, Vikram B, et al. Metastasis to the base of the skull: clinical findings in 43 patients. Neurology 1981;31(5):530–7.
36. Capobianco DJ, Brazis PW, Rubino FA, et al. Occipital condyle syndrome. Headache 2002;42(2):142–6.
37. Rocha-Filho PA, Gherpelli JL, de Siqueira JT, et al. Post-craniotomy headache: a proposed revision of IHS diagnostic criteria. Cephalalgia 2010;30(5):560–6.
38. de Oliveira Ribeiro Mdo C, Pereira CU, Sallum AM, et al. Immediate post-craniotomy headache. Cephalalgia 2013;33(11):897–905.
39. Rocha-Filho PA. The long-term effect of craniotomy on temporalis muscle function. Oral Surg Oral Med Oral Pathol Oral Radiol Endod 2007;104(5): e17–21.
40. Ryzenman JM. Headache: a quality of life analysis in a cohort of 1,657 patients undergoing acoustic neuroma surgery, results from the acoustic neuroma association. Laryngoscope 2005;115(4):703.
41. Rimaaja T. Headaches after acoustic neuroma surgery. Cephalalgia 2007; 27(10):1128.
42. Ansari SF, Terry C, Cohen-Gadol AA. Surgery for vestibular schwannomas: a systematic review of complications by approach. Neurosurg Focus 2012; 33(3):E14.
43. Kars M, Pereira A, Smit J, et al. Long-term outcome of patients with macroprolactinomas initially treated with dopamine agonists. Eur J Intern Med 2009;20(4): 387–93.
44. Levy MJ, Matharu MS, Meeran K, et al. The clinical characteristics of headache in patients with pituitary tumours. Brain 2005;128(Pt 8):1921–30.
45. Schultheiss TE, Kun LE, Ang KK, et al. Radiation response of the central nervous system. Int J Radiat Oncol Biol Phys 1995;31(5):1093–112.
46. Brandsma D, Stalpers L, Taal W, et al. Clinical features, mechanisms, and management of pseudoprogression in malignant gliomas. Lancet Oncol 2008;9(5): 453–61.
47. Shuper A, Packer RJ, Vezina LG, et al. 'Complicated migraine-like episodes' in children following cranial irradiation and chemotherapy. Neurology 1995;45(10): 1837–40.
48. Kerklaan JP, Lycklama á Nijeholt GJ, Wiggenraad RG, et al. SMART syndrome: a late reversible complication after radiation therapy for brain tumours. J Neurol 2011;258(6):1098–104.
49. Yung WK, Albright RE, Olson J, et al. A phase II study of temozolomide vs. procarbazine in patients with glioblastoma multiforme at first relapse. Br J Cancer 2000;83(5):588–93.
50. Kalaycio M, Mendez Z, Pohlman B, et al. Continuous-infusion granisetron compared to ondansetron for the prevention of nausea and vomiting after high-dose chemotherapy. J Cancer Res Clin Oncol 1998;124(5):265–9.

51. Lou E, Turner S, Sumrall A, et al. Bevacizumab-induced reversible posterior leukoencephalopathy syndrome and successful retreatment in a patient with glioblastoma. J Clin Oncol 2011;29(28):e739–42.

52. De Luca GC, Bartleson JD. When and how to investigate the patient with headache. Semin Neurol 2010;30(2):131–44.

53. Steinmann D, Paelecke-Habermann Y, Geinitz H, et al. Prospective evaluation of quality of life effects in patients undergoing palliative radiotherapy for brain metastases. BMC Cancer 2012;12:283.

54. Wong J, Hird A, Zhang L, et al. Symptoms and quality of life in cancer patients with brain metastases following palliative radiotherapy. Int J Radiat Oncol Biol Phys 2009;75(4):1125–31.

55. Patchell RA, Tibbs PA, Walsh JW, et al. A randomized trial of surgery in the treatment of single metastases to the brain. N Engl J Med 1990;322(8):494–500.

56. Kondziolka D, Patel A, Lunsford LD, et al. Stereotactic radiosurgery plus whole brain radiotherapy versus radiotherapy alone for patients with multiple brain metastases. Int J Radiat Oncol Biol Phys 1999;45(2):427–34.

57. Sanghavi SN, Miranpuri SS, Chappell R, et al. Radiosurgery for patients with brain metastases: a multi-institutional analysis, stratified by the RTOG recursive partitioning analysis method. Int J Radiat Oncol Biol Phys 2001;51(2):426–34.

58. Schmidinger M, Linzmayer L, Becherer A, et al. Psychometric- and quality-of-life assessment in long-term glioblastoma survivors. J Neurooncol 2003;63(1): 55–61.

59. Pace A, Di Lorenzo C, Guariglia L, et al. End of life issues in brain tumor patients. J Neurooncol 2009;91(1):39.

60. Osoba D, Brada M, Prados MD, et al. Effect of disease burden on health-related quality of life in patients with malignant gliomas. Neuro-Oncol 2000;2(4):221–8.

Cough, Exercise, and Sex Headaches

F. Michael Cutrer, MD[a],*, Justin DeLange, DO[b]

KEYWORDS

- Cough • Sexual • Exercise • Headache • Neuroimaging • Benign • Structural
- Vascular

KEY POINTS

- Cough, exercise, and sex headaches are entities that are rare (or underrecognized) distinct but related syndromes, triggered in the context of rapid rises in intra-abdominal pressure.
- All 3 syndromes may occur as a manifestation of a possible underlying, symptomatic etiology, and additional diagnostics should typically be pursued to rule out serious causes.
- Cough headaches may be more common in certain subgroups or settings (ie, lung disease, pulmonary clinic).
- Exercise-related headache may be more common than previously thought, based on recent epidemiologic data.
- Different pain characteristics can be seen in sexual headaches; however, there is no evidence that different pain types are distinct from a pathophysiologic standpoint.
- Each of these headache syndromes is reported to be responsive to indomethacin.

INTRODUCTION

Headaches can be initiated in some individuals by exertional activities that result in rapid increases in intra-abdominal pressure. Three broad categories may be applied to such headaches: cough headache, exercise-induced headache, and sexual headache. Descriptions of these headaches have been in the medical literature since the 1930s.[1] The term primary exercise headache,[2] formerly exertional headache, encompasses headaches related to sustained, nonsexual effort, such as sports or work-related exercise or running. Primary cough headache is distinct in that it is triggered by a single or very short series of Valsalva maneuvers such as sneezing, coughing,

[a] Headache Section, Department of Neurology, Mayo Medical School, Mayo Clinic, 200 First Street Southwest, Rochester, MN 55905, USA; [b] Department of Neurology, Mayo Clinic, 200 First Street Southwest, Rochester, MN 55905, USA
* Corresponding author.
E-mail address: cutrer.michael@mayo.edu

Neurol Clin 32 (2014) 433–450
http://dx.doi.org/10.1016/j.ncl.2013.11.012
0733-8619/14/$ – see front matter © 2014 Elsevier Inc. All rights reserved.

or straining at stool. Primary headaches associated with sexual activity may arise during the build-up toward, at the moment of or during the minutes or hours after sexual orgasm resulting from intercourse or masturbation. The lifetime prevalence for cough headache, exercise headache (nonsexual), and sex-related headache has been reported by Rasmussen and Olesen[3] to be 1% each. Cough headaches[4] exercise headaches, and sex-triggered headaches may be either secondary (symptomatic of structural cranial or systemic disease) or primary (benign) disorders. In one series of 97 patients evaluated for cough, exertional, or sexual headache, 45% were found to have an underlying intracranial abnormality while 55% fulfilled International Headache Society (IHS) criteria for primary (benign) cough, exercise, or sex headache (**Box 1**).[2,5]

Before the reports of Symonds in 1956 and Rooke a decade later, cough and exertional headaches were always considered ominous symptoms, and there was no clear recognition that benign types of these headaches existed. In 1968, Rooke[6] noted that "in every patient with this complaint, an intracranial lesion of potentially serious nature,

---

Box 1
International Headache Society diagnostic criteria for primary cough, exertional, and sex headaches

Primary cough headache

A. At least 2 headache episodes fulfilling criteria B–D

B. Brought on by and occurring only in association with coughing, straining, and/or other Valsalva maneuver

C. Sudden onset

D. Lasting between 1 second and 2 hours

E. Not better accounted for by another International Classification of Headache Disorders 3rd edition (ICHD-3) diagnosis (secondary etiology must be ruled out)

Primary exercise headache

A. At least 2 headache episodes fulfilling criteria B and C

B. Brought on by and occurring only during or after strenuous physical exercise

C. Lasting less than 48 hours

D. Not better accounted for by another ICHD-3 diagnosis (secondary etiology must be ruled out)

Primary headache associated with sexual activity

A. At least 2 episodes of pain in the head and/or neck fulfilling criteria B–D

B. Brought on by and occurring only during sexual activity

C. Either or both of the following:

    1. Increasing in intensity with increasing sexual excitement

    2. Abrupt explosive intensity just before or with orgasm

D. Lasting from 1 minute to 24 hours with severe intensity and/or up to 72 hours with mild intensity

E. Not better accounted for by another ICHD-3 diagnosis (secondary etiology must be ruled out)

From Headache Classification Committee of the International Headache Society (IHS). The International Classification of Headache Disorders, 3rd edition (beta version). Cephalgia 2013;33(9):629–808; with permission.

such as brain tumor, aneurysm or vascular anomaly, has been suspected; and even when no such lesion could be identified, an uneasy uncertainty usually has remained." Symonds,[7] in his landmark article entitled "Cough Headache," clearly described cases of both secondary and primary cough headache. He presented patients with headache provoked by coughing, and noted that in these same patients sneezing, straining at stool, laughing, or stooping could also provoke the headache. In addition, Symonds outlined the clinical course of benign cough headache and suggested a pathophysiologic mechanism for the disorder. In 1968, Rooke[6] reviewed 93 patients with benign exertional headache. He did not separate cough headache from headaches caused by running. However, his data underscored Symonds' concept that cough headache could be benign. In the following decades it has become clear that cough, exercise, and sex headaches may represent either secondary or primary disorders.

COUGH HEADACHE
Clinical Manifestations of Cough Headache

Benign cough headache is typically bilateral, of sudden onset, and reaches its peak almost immediately, with improvement in pain over several seconds to a few minutes.[2] In fact, a recent study by Chen and colleagues[8] indicated that primary cough headache may last up to 2 hours. In their series, they found that 10.8% of patients with primary cough headache had headache duration longer than 30 minutes. It is precipitated rather than aggravated by coughing, and can be prevented by avoiding coughing. Cough headache may be encountered more commonly in a pulmonary clinic than in a headache subspecialty clinic.[9] Furthermore, there is a correlation between the frequency of the cough and the severity of the headache. Ozge and colleagues[9] also found that there was a 0.4-fold increase in the incidence of cough headache when cough frequency increased. The IHS criteria specify that structural lesions must be ruled out by neuroimaging before the diagnosis of benign cough headache can be made. It is not associated with nausea, vomiting, conjunctival injection, lacrimation, nasal congestion, or rhinorrhea.[4]

Because of their historical importance, Symonds' cases are reviewed here.[7] Eighteen of the 21 cases of benign cough headache reported were men. The age range was 37 to 77 years, with the average age being 55. Symonds' patients generally complained of severe bilateral head pain, lasting 2 to 10 minutes. Two patients had severe pain for a few minutes followed by a dull ache that lasted 1 to 2 hours. The quality of the pain was usually bursting. Most patients had pain at the vertex spreading to both frontal regions. As noted previously, other maneuvers besides cough could trigger the pain, but physical exercise was not mentioned as a precipitant. Two patients could trigger headache by quick rotation of the head. Two patients could cough without pain while lying down. Two patients noted that when they awoke in the morning they could cough without pain, but that the liability appeared after they assumed the vertical posture. One patient noted decreased pain severity if he coughed with his neck extended. Two patients had relief of cough headaches after lumbar puncture; one had relief for a few weeks and then had complete relief after air encephalography, and the second had complete relief after lumbar puncture when seen 6 months later. Two patients recovered after extraction of an infected tooth. Nine patients had eventual recovery, 6 had significant spontaneous improvement over a period of 18 months to 12 years, and the remaining 6 either had the disorder continue without change or died of an unrelated disease. Five patients had a history of migraine.

Rooke[6] considered cough headache to be a form of exertional headache, and reviewed the clinical features of 93 patients with benign exertional headache. The male to female ratio was 4:1, and exertional headache was twice as common in those older than 40 in comparison with those aged 10 to 40 years. Rooke outlined the generally favorable course of benign exertional headache. Seven of 31 patients noted a respiratory infection before their exertional headaches began, and 4 patients had unequivocal relief after dental extractions. One patient had complete headache relief after pneumoencephalography.

Pascual and colleagues[5] studied 28 patients with benign cough headache in detail. The mean age of the patients was 60 years (range 22–80 years), and 64% were female (which is interesting, as the literature points mainly to a male preponderance). The predominant location was either hemicranial (50% of cases) or bilateral (39%). The pain was variable and was described as a mixture of electric, pressing, and explosive quality in most patients. The pain usually lasted seconds in 78% of patients in this series. Furthermore, 100% of patients had cough as a trigger, while other triggers included sudden postural movements (56%), weightlifting (39%), laughing (33%), and defecating (22%). The disorder persisted for 1 month to 3.5 years. In this cohort, 7 patients were taking an angiotensin-converting enzyme inhibitor for hypertension. When this medication was stopped, symptoms of headache were improved in these patients.

Raskin[10,11] has reviewed the clinical features of benign cough headache. Many patients note headache onset during lower respiratory tract infections accompanied by cough, or during vigorous weightlifting programs. The headache arises moments after the cough, reaches its peak almost immediately, and then subsides over several seconds to a few minutes. Sometimes the pain remains at the peak for several seconds before receding. Most patients are pain-free between attacks, but some have a dull headache following the triggered attack that may persist for hours. Raskin warns that these patients often complain of continuous headaches, thus emphasizing the need to directly ask about triggering by cough. Nausea and other migrainous features are uncommon, and although the headache is usually bilateral, it can occasionally be unilateral.

Over the years some rare clinical characteristics have been reported. Bruyn[12] described a patient who could trigger headache by coughing or yawning. A case of cough headache presenting as unilateral toothache completely responsive to indomethacin has been reported.[13] This patient's pain was in the right maxillary region and radiated to the ipsilateral temple, ear, and occiput. Unilateral cough headache with circannual periodicity has been reported.[14] This patient's cough headaches were often induced by exertion as well. Unilateral benign cough headache coexisting with chronic paroxysmal hemicrania has been reported.[15]

Etiology of Cough Headache

The etiology of benign cough headache is not completely clear. It seems intuitive that it is associated with an increase in intracranial pressure (ICP), as coughing increases ICP. What causes the pain itself is unknown. Symonds[7] observed that in a normal person, coughing does not cause headache despite the fact that coughing should displace the brain toward the foramen magnum, causing stretching of pain-sensitive structures within the posterior fossa. He postulated that the degree and direction of traction was inadequate to cause headache in the normal person. Symonds later hypothesized that in benign cough headache "the pain is due to stretching of a pain-sensitive structure within the posterior fossa, which may be due to an adhesive arachnoiditis."[7]

Williams[16] measured cerebrospinal fluid (CSF) pressures from the lumbar region and the cisterna magna in 16 patients during coughing in the sitting position. All patients had "disease in the cervical region" requiring myelography. None of these patients had a complete blockage of the spinal subarachnoid space. During a cough, there was a phase during which the lumbar pressure exceeded the cisternal pressure, followed by a phase during which the cisternal pressure exceeded the lumbar pressure. Thus on coughing, the intrathoracic and intra-abdominal pressure was felt to be transmitted through the valveless veins around the vertebrae to the epidural veins, which then distended with blood.[17] Once distended, these veins compressed the spinal dura, causing a pressure wave that passed into the head and then rapidly downward again.[17] Williams commented that the upward passage of fluid was relatively easy, but that the downward rebound from the head toward the spine might cause tissue to crowd in the foramen magnum. This situation would create a pressure difference between the head and spine, which he termed the "craniospinal pressure dissociation."[16] He postulated that in Chiari I malformations, the ebb and flow of fluid through the foramen magnum could progressively impact the tonsils, leading to pain. Williams[17] subsequently investigated the etiology of cough headache in 2 patients with Chiari I malformations, in whom he verified the presence of a craniospinal pressure dissociation preoperatively. Decompression of the cerebellar tonsils relieved the cough headache and eliminated the craniospinal pressure dissociation. Nightingale and Williams[18] later described a further 4 similar patients who were successfully treated with surgical decompression.

By contrast, Sansur and colleagues[19] looked at the intrathecal pressures of 11 patients with Chiari I malformations and cough headache, and compared these values with those of healthy controls and patients with Chiari I malformation without headache. Preoperatively, It was noted that patients with cough headache had the highest intrathecal pressure during coughing, different from patients without headache and healthy volunteers. Specifically, in patients with Chiari I malformation but no cough headache, the peak cough-induced intrathecal pressure was not different from normal values. Moreover, baseline intrathecal pressures were also higher in the group with cough headache. Surgery was then performed on patients with Chiari I malformation, following which postoperative testing was done and compared with healthy controls, and between headache and nonheadache groups. Peak and baseline intrathecal pressures were found to have normalized in all surgical groups (Chiari I with cough headache, Chiari I without cough headache), and the presence of cough headache resolved or partially resolved. These investigators also refuted any craniocervical pressure dissociation and stated that the headache arises because obstruction, represented by increased intrathecal pressure, produces elevated ICPs and distention of the dura mater during coughing.

However, patients with benign cough headache do not have tonsillar herniation, so Raskin[10] has hypothesized that the pain in these circumstances is due to heightened sensitivity of yet unidentified receptors. Raskin successfully treated 4 patients with cough headache with repetitive intravenous dihydroergotamine, and suggested that unstable serotonergic neurotransmission might be important in the etiology of cough headache.[10] One case of cough headache has occurred after implantation of an electrode in the periaqueductal gray (PAG).[20] The phenotypic cough headache developed immediately after PAG-electrode implantation and was relieved by indomethacin. The patient used indomethacin for 4 months, and remained headache free after stopping the medication. She remained headache free at 5-year follow-up. After noting that benign cough headache could be provoked by a sudden increase in ICP and could remit after the sudden decrement in ICP that attended lumbar puncture, Raskin[11] later hypothesized that the nature of the receptors sensitive to ICP alterations was probably the key to understanding benign cough headache.

Wang and colleagues[21] postulated that benign cough headache was due to CSF hypervolemia, leading to an increased craniospinal pressure dissociation during coughing, thus explaining the response to acetazolamide, indomethacin, and lumbar puncture. The same group has reported in abstract form the association of benign cough headache with morphometric magnetic resonance imaging (MRI) evidence of posterior cranial fossa overcrowding.[22] Based on midline sagittal MRI, several parameters indicating posterior fossa crowding were measured in 15 patients with benign cough headache and 15 age-matched and sex-matched controls. Compared with the control group, patients with benign cough headache had a significantly higher mean brain tissue/posterior cranial fossa ratio, a shorter clivus length, and a shorter distance from the clivus to the mid-pons. There was also a significantly higher frequency of CSF space obliteration in the posterior cranial fossa in the patients with benign cough headache. The investigators suggested that posterior fossa overcrowding might be a contributing factor in the pathogenesis of benign cough headache.

The etiology of benign cough headache can be best summed up by Symonds himself, who in 1970 wrote "as far as I am aware its origin remains a mystery."[23]

Differential Diagnosis for Cough Headache

Before a diagnosis of benign cough headache can be made, intracranial masses and, specifically, posterior fossa lesions must be ruled out.[3,24] **Box 2** lists some secondary causes of cough headache. Pascual and colleagues[5] found clinical differences between patients with benign and symptomatic cough headache. Symptomatic cough headache started earlier in life (age 44 years), was mainly felt in the occipital area, had a longer attack duration (more than 50% cases lasted at least 1 minute), was associated with posterior fossa symptoms or signs in 33 of 40 patients, may have been triggered by other Valsalva (not by coughing) in one-third of all cases, and did

---

Box 2
Some secondary causes of cough headache

1. Chiari I malformation
2. Cerebrospinal fluid (CSF) volume depletion (low CSF pressure headache or spontaneous intracranial hypotension)
3. Middle cranial fossa or posterior fossa meningiomas
4. Medulloblastoma
5. Pinealoma
6. Chromophobe adenoma
7. Midbrain cyst
8. Basilar impression
9. Platybasia
10. Subdural hematoma
11. Brain tumor not otherwise specified
12. Reversible cerebral vasoconstriction syndrome
13. Cerebral aneurysms

Data from Refs.[2,4,7,24,31]

not respond to indomethacin. Chiari I malformation was the main cause of symptomatic cough headache in this study, in 32 patients (80% of cases). Similar findings were also seen in a previous study where 17 patients with symptomatic cough headache had a Chiari I malformation with occipital location of headache, longer duration, and Valsalva (not cough) trigger, and may have been accompanied by posterior fossa symptoms.[25] Indomethacin response should not be used to differentiate benign from symptomatic cough headache, as a patient with a Chiari I malformation–associated cough headache who responded completely to indomethacin has been reported.[26]

Unilateral cough headache has been reported with carotid stenosis,[27,28] but this has not been encountered by the authors. In the case reported by Britton and Guiloff,[27] the patient initially had right-sided cough-induced headaches without focal neurologic deficits. Two years later he developed episodic left-hand sensory symptoms. Later that same year he developed weakness in the left hand and numbness of the left face. He was admitted to hospital and found to have pyramidal weakness of the left hand. Computed tomography (CT) of the head was normal, and a myelogram showed no abnormality of the cord or foramen magnum. Twenty-four hours later he developed a continuous right-sided headache, "similar to the cough headache," and the next day developed a severe left hemiparesis. CT showed a large right anterior cerebral artery/middle cerebral artery infarct. A cerebral angiogram showed stenosis of the right internal carotid artery (ICA) close to its origin, and the possibility of dissection was raised. Echocardiography was normal. An angiogram 5 weeks later revealed an occluded right ICA. The patient was left with hemiparesis, but the cough headache had not recurred at the time of the case report. The investigators admitted that the relation of the cough headache to the abnormality of the right ICA was uncertain. Understandably, they recommended studying the carotid arteries in patients with cough headache when the headache is associated with focal neurologic symptoms or signs and no intracranial or foramen magnum lesion can be found.[27] The patient described by Rivera and colleagues[28] initially had right-sided cough headache alone. Four months later the cough headache was associated with focal neurologic symptoms (right blunted vision, weakness of the left arm, facial paresis, dysarthria, abnormal spontaneous movements of the left arm). The focal symptoms occurred after coughing and also with episodes of hypotension during dialysis, and lasted 10 to 15 minutes. He was admitted to the hospital and found to have bilateral carotid bruits with an otherwise normal neurologic examination. CT of the head was normal, and carotid ultrasonography showed significant left common carotid stenosis. The patient was treated with antiplatelet agents and codeine with "transient improvement," and died 18 months after his cough headache started.[28] Whether the cough headache in this case was actually caused by the carotid stenosis is unclear.

Cough headache secondary to an unruptured cerebral aneurysm has been reported.[29] The patient was a 42-year-old woman who for 24 days complained of a right temporal, severe pain induced by coughing or bending forward. The pain lasted 1 to 5 minutes, followed by a dull ache lasting 1 hour. Neurologic examination was normal 2 weeks after the onset of symptoms, and indomethacin failed to give her relief. Twenty-four days after headache onset, she complained of a continuous right-sided head pain worsened by cough, strain, or bending forward. On examination she was found to have right-sided ptosis, and the next day developed more complete third nerve palsy. CSF showed 16 red blood cells per mm^3 and 11 white blood cells per mm^3, and cerebral angiography revealed an 8-mm right-sided aneurysm at the junction of the posterior communicating artery and the internal carotid artery. She was free of cough headache postoperatively at 1-year follow-up.[26] Rooke,[6] however, reported that none of the 14 patients with unruptured aneurysms that he studied complained of exertional headache. A patient with a large venous angioma of the posterior fossa presenting with cough headache has been reported.[30] However, close inspection of this case reveals that the headache was exacerbated, not elicited, by coughing, and thus would not readily be confused with benign cough headache.

Patients with CSF volume depletion (low-pressure headache) can present with intermittent, transient, severe headaches provoked by Valsalva-type maneuvers in the absence of orthostatic headache.[31] One case of cough headache caused by pneumocephalus and pneumococcal meningitis has also been described in the literature.[32] Migraine, cluster headache, and headache associated with idiopathic intracranial hypertension can be aggravated, but not elicited, by cough.[3,33]

Pascual and colleagues[5] found differences between patients with benign cough headache, benign exercise headache, and sexual headache, lending credence to their separate classification. Cough headache was triggered by cough or Valsalva maneuvers, whereas exercise headache was triggered only by sustained physical exercise. Benign cough headache affected a much older population than that affected by benign exercise headache or benign sexual headache. The average age of patients afflicted with benign cough headache was 60 years, whereas the age of patients with benign exercise headache and benign sexual headache was some 20 years younger. Benign cough headache was shorter than benign exercise headache, and treatment responses were somewhat different. Benign cough headache was typically electric, exploding, or pressure, whereas benign exercise headache was described as pulsating.

Diagnostic Evaluation for Cough Headache

Given the differential diagnosis already outlined, every patient with cough headache should have an MRI of the brain to rule out a posterior fossa lesion. The MRI should be done with gadolinium to look for pachymeningeal enhancement, given that CSF volume depletion (low-pressure headache or spontaneous intracranial hypotension) can present as cough headache alone with no orthostatic component.[31] Whether a patient with an unruptured aneurysm can present with cough headache is not clear, but it seems reasonable to obtain a magnetic resonance angiogram (MRA) of the intracranial circulation in most cases. The authors do not typically perform carotid ultrasonography or MRA of the extracranial circulation in the evaluation of cough headache, unless the patient furnishes a history consistent with transient ischemic attacks.

Management of Cough Headache

Any chest disease that may be causing the cough should be identified and treated.[34] Because of the typical short duration of benign cough headache, preventive rather than abortive treatment is used. Mathew[35] established the efficacy of indomethacin at a dose of 150 mg/d in a double-blind study involving 2 patients with benign cough headache. Of 16 patients treated with indomethacin, Raskin[36] reported that 10 responded completely, 4 had moderate improvement, and 2 had no response. The effective dosage ranged from 50 to 200 mg, with an average of 78 mg. The duration of treatment was 6 months to 4 years.[36] Raskin[10] has noted that indomethacin rarely fails, but that the dosage sometimes must approach 250 mg daily. The authors have had success in using indomethacin in the range of 25 to 150 mg per day, and usually combine this with a proton-pump inhibitor in those patients who require long-term treatment. Indomethacin decreases ICP,[37] which may be why it is effective in this condition in comparison with other nonsteroidal anti-inflammatories. Because some patients lose the liability to benign cough headache over time, treatment should be withdrawn periodically.

Acetazolamide[21] and methysergide[38,39] have been reported to be effective in open-label trials. In the study by Wang and colleagues,[21] 4 of 5 patients with indomethacin-responsive benign cough headache responded favorably to acetazolamide at maximum doses of 1125 to 2000 mg/d. Two of these patients responded completely to acetazolamide. The patients were allowed to adjust the maintenance dose to treatment effectiveness or side effects, and the mean maintenance dose was 656 mg. One patient withdrew from the study because of intolerable distal limb numbness. The methysergide-responsive patient described by Calandre and colleagues[38] had unilateral, throbbing, cough-induced headaches lasting 30 minutes to a "few hours." This patient only had headache with coughing, straining, and stooping, and responded completely to methysergide at an unknown dose after failing nicardipine and propranolol and after partially responding to amitriptyline. The methysergide-responsive patient described by Bahra and Goadsby[39] had unilateral cough-induced headaches lasting 15 to 30 minutes. She required 2 mg daily and then lower doses for 9 weeks in total, and was then headache free after cessation.

Several investigators have written of the occasional efficacy of lumbar puncture.[6,7,36] Raskin[36] noted the effectiveness of a 40-mL lumbar puncture in 6 of 14 patients. Three had immediate relief after the procedure, and in the other 3 relief came over 2 days. One of the responders redeveloped cough headache 6 weeks after initial lumbar puncture, but responded completely to repeat spinal tap. Six of the 8 patients who failed lumbar puncture responded to indomethacin.

Raskin[10] has written of the effectiveness of naproxen, ergonovine, intravenous dihydroergotamine, and phenelzine, but found propranolol to be ineffective. Mateo and Pascual[15] found naproxen to be partially effective in 1 case. Of the 6 patients with cough headache and normal MRI described by Calandre and colleagues,[38] 1 found propranolol effective while 2 found it ineffective. Aside from Raskin's observations,[10] there is one other report of the efficacy of intravenous dihydroergotamine in treating cough headache.[40] Furthermore, small case series have also described the benefit of topiramate and intravenous metoclopramide for treatment.[41,42]

EXERCISE HEADACHE
Clinical Features of Primary Exercise Headache

Exercise headaches,[2] formerly known as exertional headaches, are generally described as bilateral in onset, often with a throbbing pulsatile quality.[43] However, pulsatile quality is no longer required for diagnosis of the primary (benign) form.[44] The headaches lasts from minutes[43] up to 48 hours, occur particularly at high altitude or in hot weather,[2] arise from sustained physical exercise, and may be prevented by avoidance of excessive physical exertion.[5] Although not usually associated with nausea or vomiting,[6] migraine has often been associated with exercise headache.[45,46] Previously the defining features arose from a small number of cases.[6,25,47–49] However, recent studies have further refined the definition and clinical characteristics, and have added further evidence to this often missed entity.[5,43,46] In contrast to a previous population-based study that estimated the prevalence of exercise headache at 1%,[3] recent epidemiologic studies suggest that this entity may be more common than previously thought. The Vågå study from Norway included 1646 survey respondents and found a prevalence of 12.3%,[43] and a recent study by Chen and colleagues[46] found a prevalence of 10.2% in an adolescent population when modified IHS criteria were applied. It may also be more prevalent in athletes who engage in intense exercise, as found by van der Ende-Kastelijn and colleagues.[50] In their 2012 study, based on an online survey of 4000 cyclists, 1045 (26%) met IHS criteria for primary exertional headache.

Etiology: Symptomatic Versus Primary Exercise Headaches

Exercise may trigger both benign primary headaches and secondary headaches symptomatic of intracranial disease. The relative frequency of primary versus secondary headaches differs from one case series to another; however, as neuroimaging techniques have improved, the proportion of symptomatic headaches relative to benign primary headaches has increased. The large case series of patients reported on and followed by Rooke[6] in the 1960s found that of the 103 patients initially presenting with exertional headaches (including those triggered by coughing) and normal neurologic examinations, 10 had developed an intracranial lesion after 3 years of follow-up. Of the remaining 93 patients, 11 had complete relief of their headaches at 1 year, 30 had complete relief within 5 years, and after 10 years 73 were significantly improved or were headache free. More than 2 decades later, in a large literature review of 219 nonconsecutive patients that included cough headache as well as exertional headache, Sands and colleagues[51] determined that in 48 patients the headaches were symptomatic of a structural lesion, whereas the remaining 171 represented a benign primary headache disorder.

A less comforting distribution of primary versus secondary headaches was also reported by Pascual and colleagues[25] in a previous series of patients with exertional headache. In this series, 12 of 28 (43%) cases were found to have intracranial abnormality. Of the 12 patients with symptomatic headaches, 10 were found on CT or lumbar puncture to have had a subarachnoid hemorrhage. These patients described their headache as a single episode of severe, sudden-onset, bilateral explosive head pain that occurred with exertion and persisted for 1 to 30 days. The headaches were associated with vomiting as well as nausea and in 4 instances, with diplopia. Of the 2 remaining symptomatic headaches, one was due to pansinusitis and cleared with antibiotic treatment, and the other was due to multiple brain metastases from breast carcinoma and was associated with papilledema and bilateral sixth nerve palsy. By contrast, the 16 patients from this series diagnosed with benign exertional headaches[25] had pain that always began during the exertion, could be either bilateral or unilateral, was throbbing but nonexplosive in quality, and of moderate to severe intensity. The benign exertional headaches persisted from minutes up to 2 days. Although sometimes accompanied by nausea and photophobia, the benign headaches were not associated with vomiting, neck stiffness, or focal neurologic symptoms. The underlying abnormalities most often associated with exertional headaches include supratentorial and posterior fossa space-occupying lesions (both metastatic and primary), sites of traumatic injury, vascular abnormalities such as aneurysm, arterial dissection, reversible cerebral vasoconstriction syndrome (RCVS),[2] arteriovenous malformation, and intracranial hemorrhage. A more recent study by Pascual and colleagues[5] looked at 11 patients with exertional headache, of whom 9 (82%) were diagnosed as primary and 2 (18%) as having a symptomatic cause, which in these 2 patients was subarachnoid hemorrhage. Other types of paroxysmal headaches that may be triggered by exertion include pheochromocytoma-related headaches[52]; headaches resulting from intermittent obstruction of CSF flow, such those arising from third ventricular colloid cysts or lateral ventricular tumors[51] and in patients with risk factors for coronary disease; and cardiogenic headaches. It should also be remembered that exercise can be a trigger in some migraine patients for their typical migrainous headaches.

Pathophysiology of Exercise Headache

The pathophysiology of exercise headaches is poorly understood. Most theories invoke, quite logically, the transmission of increases in intra-abdominothoracic pressure into the cranium via the venous system with distension of or traction on pain-sensitive vascular or meningeal structures.[1] Furthermore, a recent study by Doepp and colleagues[53] postulated that transient cerebral venous congestion might play a causative role in exercise headache and that internal jugular vein valve incompetence could be an underlying risk factor. In their study, 20 patients with exertional (exercise) headache and 40 age-matched controls underwent bilateral internal jugular venous duplex ultrasonography to evaluate for internal jugular vein valve incompetence (IJVVI). Fourteen of 20 patients with exertional headache (70%) and 8 of 40 controls (20%) demonstrated IJVVI. This difference between the 2 groups was found to be statistically significant. In addition, in the exertional group IJVVI was also more likely to be bilateral or ipsilateral to the dominant venous outflow. This finding may explain how certain individuals become vulnerable to repeated activations of the trigeminocervical pain system, possibly because of a propensity for engorged venous sinuses. However, Doepp and colleagues[53] also pointed out that exertional headache may spontaneously remit, and IJVVI does not. Furthermore, not every patient with IJVVI has exertional headaches. Therefore, other mechanisms should be explored. Possibilities might include factors that cause lowered activation thresholds in primary or second-order nociceptive trigeminocervical neurons, alterations in central nociceptive processing, or other factors that result in inordinately large fluctuations in ICP. It has also been suggested, based on transcranial Doppler studies, that exertional and sexual headache may be the result of impaired autoregulation of cerebrovascular smooth muscle. The dysregulation might render resistance vessels unable to adequately respond to increased blood pressure during exercise, resulting in abnormal vasodilation, vessel-wall edema, or increased cephalic blood volume.[48] Cardiac cephalalgia is another entity that should also be considered, often presenting as a headache aggravated by exercise.[54]

Evaluation of Exercise Headache

The evaluation of exercise headaches should include MRI and vessel imaging such as MRA or CT angiography to rule out structural cause or vascular abnormality. The need for such investigations increases when the headaches are prolonged beyond a few hours, are accompanied by focal neurologic symptoms and vomiting, or appear de novo after the age of 40 years. Obviously any symptoms suggestive of subarachnoid hemorrhage including rapid onset, alteration in consciousness, or meningeal symptoms also argue for emergent evaluation.

Treatment of Exercise Headaches

Once structural or vascular causes have been eliminated, treatment should begin. Treatment of exercise headaches is usually prophylactic because the brief duration of most of these headaches makes it unlikely that oral abortive therapies will have much therapeutic effect. When exertion is predictable, use as needed of several agents, minutes to an hour before exertion, may be effective. Indomethacin is the de facto drug of choice for primary exercise headaches.[35,55] The therapeutic dose may range from 25 to 150 mg per day, although higher doses up to 250 mg may be necessary. The mechanism of indomethacin's effect in these syndromes is not well understood, although its effect on CSF pressure has been suggested.[37] β-Blockers such as nadolol or propranolol may be another alternative at doses of

1 to 2 mg/kg daily.[5] Other therapies such as naproxen, phenelzine, and ergonovine have also been reported to be effective in some patients.[10]

Exercise Headache Versus Sexual Headache

The exact relationship between exercise headache and sexual headache is unclear. In one series, about 40% of patients experiencing sexual headache also reported headaches with other nonsexual exertion.[48] Pascual[5] noted that sexual headaches share several characteristics with exercise headache. Lance,[56] on the other hand, reported that the activation of head pain in at least some of his patients with coital headache seemed to be more related to the degree of sexual excitement and the selective contraction of neck and facial muscles than to exertion per se.

SEX HEADACHE
Simplification to the Classification of Sexual Headaches

In the original 1988 IHS criteria, 3 characteristic headache types were associated with sexual activity.[57] Type 1 consists of a bilateral, usually occipital pressure-like headache that gradually increases with mounting sexual excitement. Type 2 has an explosive, throbbing quality and appears just before or at the moment of orgasm. Like type 1, they often arise occipitally but may generalize rapidly. The third type of coital headache is holocephalic, positional, occurs after coitus,[2] and has many clinical features consistent with low-CSF pressure headache. In the 2004 IHS criteria, this third type of coital headache was moved and placed into the category of low-CSF pressure headache, and is therefore no longer considered a sex headache.[58] The most recent IHS criteria now include both type 1 and type 2 as one entity, no longer subdivided into orgasmic and preorgasmic subtypes.[44]

Etiology and Differential Diagnosis of Sexual Headaches

Symptomatic sexual headache

Although sexual headaches may be manifestations of a benign primary headache disorder, they may also be symptomatic of an underlying pathologic process. The differential diagnosis for sexual headache includes: RCVS,[59] arterial dissection,[57] subarachnoid hemorrhage (SAH) caused by aneurysmal rupture or arteriovenous malformation (AVM),[60] nonhemorrhagic strokes, meningitis,[61] encephalitis,[61] hemorrhage into a cerebral tumor,[61] and pheochromocytoma.[62] Given that myocardial ischemia may occur during sexual intercourse,[63] referred cardiac pain should be considered as a potential cause of sexual headache in individuals with risk factors for coronary artery disease. The use of several drugs has also been linked in case reports to sexual headaches associated with neurologic symptoms. These agents include amiodarone,[64] birth control pills,[61] pseudoephedrine,[56] and cannabis.[65] Several other nonneurologic disorders have been suggested as possible causes for sexual headache, including glaucoma, myxedema, anemia, chronic obstructive pulmonary disease, sinusitis, hypoglycemia, Cushing disease,[51] and occlusion of the abdominal aorta.[66]

Of the 3 types of sexual headache, the type 2 explosive headache is the most common and the only one that is associated with stroke.[25,49,56,67] That the explosive type 2 sexual headaches, with their sudden onset and rapid ascent to maximal severity, are linked with cerebral infarction is not surprising given that they are qualitatively similar to the classic headaches of SAH. Sexual intercourse has been reported as the precipitating cause of SAH in 3.8% to 12% of those patients whose bleeding was due to aneurysmal rupture.[68,69]

In one small series of 18 consecutive cases of sexual headache,[5] 2 cases of symptomatic headache were identified. One patient was found to have hydrocephalus caused by aqueductal stenosis and the other patient was found to have a cervical AVM. Another more recent study by Yeh and colleagues[59] looked at 30 patients with headache triggered by sexual activity. Each patient with headache received MRI of the brain and MRA (if they did not have SAH). Twenty patients (67%) in this study had secondary causes for their headaches. Eighteen of these patients were diagnosed as having RCVS while 1 patient had SAH and 1 had basilar dissection. Though uncommon, pheochromocytoma should also be ruled out.[62] Lance[56] points out that many clinical features of type 2 sexual headache are shared with pheochromocytoma headache, including abrupt onset, extreme severity, throbbing quality, and occipital or generalized location. In addition, the abrupt, extreme increases in blood pressure seen during pheochromocytoma[70] have also been recorded in subjects whose blood pressure was measured during sexual orgasm.[71] It should also be noted, however, that the same clinical features linked to pheochromocytoma headaches may also suggest SAH.

Primary sexual headache

The IHS classification defines primary headache associated with sexual activity as headaches precipitated by sexual excitement (masturbation or coitus), occurring either with increasing sexual intensity, or abruptly with orgasm, which occur in the absence of any intracranial disorder (see **Box 1**). Although not necessary for diagnosis, the pain is often described as pulsating,[5] may last from 1 minute to 72 hours,[2] and is typically bilateral and diffuse or occipital.[72] A male preponderance is typically demonstrated in the literature.[5,25,72] The typical age of onset has been described from the second to the fourth decade,[4,57,72] although some recent cases have elucidated onset in adolescents.[73,74] Sexual headaches are unpredictable and are not necessarily precipitated with every sexual encounter.[56,67] Type 1 (dull tension type) and type 3 (low CSF pressure) sexual headaches combined account for less than one-third of the benign coital headaches reported in the literature. The explosive type 2 headaches are both the most common and the most worrisome. In Pascual and colleagues'[25] small series of patients with sexual headaches from the mid-1990s, 13 of 14 were found to have type 2 benign sexual headache. In all 13 cases the headache began explosively with orgasm and rapidly reached severe intensity. In 10 of 13 patients, the headache was bilateral. In 12 of 13, the headache was throbbing. On average, the coital headaches persisted about 30 minutes (range 1–180 minutes) and the frequency of the headaches was related to that of orgasm. Four of 13 patients also had exertional headaches.

Primary sexual headache has been associated with migraine headache,[75] and previously had been suggested by some to be a variant of migraine.[61,67] For example, Martinez and colleagues[62] suggest that coital headaches associated with neurologic symptoms that occur in patients with a history of migraine should be considered a complicated form of migraine caused by hemodynamic changes occurring during orgasm. Moreover, a case-control study published in 2007 by Biehl and colleagues[75] examined 100 migraineurs and 100 controls for sexual headache. A questionnaire and personal interview were used to make all appropriate diagnoses. In the control group there were no patients with sexual headache, whereas 5 patients (5.2%) in the migraine group had sexual headache. This study showed that the association between migraine and headache associated with sexual activity is bilateral. In general, the prognosis for coital headache is reasonable, even for those cases associated with neurologic symptoms.[43,62,71] However, persistent neurologic deficits following coital headaches have also been reported.[65]

Pathophysiology of Sexual Headaches

The pathophysiologic mechanisms proposed for sexual headaches are largely speculative. Historically, Lance[56] suggested that type 1 sexual headache arises from excessive contraction of neck and jaw muscles during sexual activity, and that it might be avoided by conscious relaxation of these muscles during intercourse. Explosive (type 2) headaches have been attributed to rapid increases in blood pressure and heart rate that occur during orgasm.[56] However, the symptoms and characteristics of both types often overlap[59,76] and, at least at this point in time, there is no evidence that type 1 and type 2 are distinct from a pathophysiologic standpoint.[72]

Evaluation of Sexual Headaches

It has been pointed out that unlike primary sexual headache, SAH-related headache is associated with neck stiffness, focal neurologic symptoms, and loss of consciousness, and is in general more protracted.[49] Despite these potentially discriminating factors, when confronted with a patient experiencing coital headaches, prudence suggests evaluation for vascular abnormality or SAH with neuroimaging, CT, and lumbar puncture if within hours of the onset, and MRI with gadolinium and MRA with or without lumbar puncture if days or weeks have elapsed. This protocol is especially important when the headaches are of the explosive type 2. In fact, to meet the IHS criteria for the diagnosis of primary headache associated with sexual activity, structural causes must be excluded. When suggestive accompanying symptoms such as prominent flushing and tachycardia are present, urine testing for evidence of pheochromocytoma (metanephrines and vanillylmandelic acid) is also probably warranted.

Treatment of Sexual Headaches

Once underlying pathologic factors have been excluded, treatment should be offered. In one case series, the advice to engage in sexual intercourse more frequently but less strenuously resulted in an apparent reduction in headaches.[77] In a recent case series, 9 of 10 patients with sexual headache were satisfied with indomethacin for the prevention of sexual headache. Furthermore, 10 of 13 patients who underwent prophylaxis with β-blockers for sexual headache showed similar satisfaction.[76] Indomethacin can be used in doses from 25 to 200 mg/d for preventive or acute purposes.[11,76] Other therapies reported to be effective for the treatment of sexual headache include propranolol (40–200 mg/d),[51,77] Bellergal,[77] and triptans.[78,79]

SUMMARY

Cough, exercise, and sex headaches are 3 relatively uncommon, distinct but related syndromes, all of which are triggered in the context of rapid rises in intra-abdominal pressure. Cough headache occurs after a single or brief series of such rises, whereas exercise and sexual headache typically arise after more prolonged provocations. All 3 syndromes may occur as the manifestation of an underlying, potentially serious cause, and appropriate management involves the elimination of intracranial structural or vascular abnormalities. The pathophysiology of the 3 syndromes remains poorly understood. These headache syndromes share several clinical features, including relatively brief duration and a response to indomethacin.

REFERENCES

1. Tinel J. La céphalée à l'effort - syndrome de distension douloureuse des veines intracrâniennes. Médecine (Paris) 1932;13:113–8.

2. Headache Classification Committee of the International Headache Society (IHS). The international classification of headache disorders, 3rd edition (beta version). Cephalalgia 2013;33:629–808.

3. Rasmussen BK, Olesen J. Symptomatic and nonsymptomatic headaches in a general population. Neurology 1992;42:1225–31.

4. Ekbom K. Cough headache. In: Rose FC, editor. Headache. Handbook of clinical neurology, vol. 4 (48). Amsterdam: Elsevier Science Publishers; 1986. p. 367–71.

5. Pascual J, Gonzalez-Mandly A, Martin R, et al. Headaches precipitated by cough, prolonged exercise or sexual activity: a prospective etiological and clinical study. J Headache Pain 2008;9:259–66.

6. Rooke ED. Benign exertional headache. Med Clin North Am 1968;52:801–8.

7. Symonds C. Cough headache. Brain 1956;79:557–68.

8. Chen PK, Fuh JL, Wang SJ. Cough headache: a study of 83 consecutive patients. Cephalalgia 2009;29(10):1079–85.

9. Ozge C, Ozge A, Nass Duce M, et al. Cough headache: frequency, characteristics and the relationship with the characteristics of cough. Eur J Pain 2005; 9(4):383–8.

10. Raskin NH. The indomethacin-responsive syndromes. In: Raskin NH, editor. Headache. 2nd edition. New York: Churchill Livingstone; 1988. p. 255–68.

11. Raskin NH. Short-lived head pains. Neurol Clin 1997;15:143–52.

12. Bruyn GW. Cough headache. In: Vinken PJ, Bruyn GW, editors. Headache and cranial neuralgias. Handbook of clinical neurology, vol. 5. Amsterdam: North-Holland Publishing Company; 1968. p. 185–7.

13. Moncada E, Graff-Radford SB. Cough headache presenting as a toothache: a case report. Headache 1993;33:240–3.

14. Perini F, Toso V. Benign cough "cluster" headache. Cephalalgia 1998;18:493–4.

15. Mateo I, Pascual J. Coexistence of chronic paroxysmal hemicrania and benign cough headache. Headache 1999;39:437–8.

16. Williams B. Cerebrospinal fluid pressure changes in response to coughing. Brain 1976;99:331–46.

17. Williams B. Cough headache due to craniospinal pressure dissociation. Arch Neurol 1980;37:226–30.

18. Nightingale S, Williams B. Hindbrain hernia headache. Lancet 1987;1:731–4.

19. Sansur CA, Heiss JD, DeVroom HL, et al. Pathophysiology of headache associated with cough in patients with Chiari I malformation. J Neurosurg 2003;98(3): 453–8.

20. Raskin NH, Hosobuchi Y, Lamb S. Headache may arise from perturbation of brain. Headache 1987;27:416–20.

21. Wang SJ, Fuh JL, Lu SR. Benign cough headache is responsive to acetazolamide. Neurology 2000;55:149–50.

22. Chen YY, Lirng JF, Fuh JL, et al. Benign cough headache is associated with posterior cranial fossa overcrowding: a morphometric MRI study. Neurology 2003; 60:A157.

23. Symonds C. Cough headache. In: Studies in neurology. London: Oxford University Press; 1970. p. 216–26.

24. Eross EJ, Swanson JW, Krauss WE, et al. A rare cause of cough headache in an adult. Headache 2002;42:382.

25. Pascual J, Iglesias F, Oterino A, et al. Cough, exertional, and sexual headaches: an analysis of 72 benign and symptomatic cases. Neurology 1996;46(6):1520–4.

26. Ertsey C, Jelencsik I. Cough headache associated with Chiari type-I malformation: responsiveness to indomethacin. Cephalalgia 2000;20:518–20.

27. Britton TC, Guiloff RJ. Carotid artery disease presenting as cough headache. Lancet 1988;1:1406–7.

28. Rivera M, del Real MA, Teruel JL, et al. Carotid artery disease presenting as cough headache in a patient on haemodialysis. Postgrad Med J 1991;67:702.

29. Smith WS, Messing RO. Cerebral aneurysm presenting as cough headache. Headache 1993;33:203–4.

30. Senegor M, Dohrmann GJ, Wollmann RL. Venous angiomas of the posterior fossa should be considered as anomalous venous drainage. Surg Neurol 1983;19:26–32.

31. Mokri B. Spontaneous CSF leaks mimicking benign exertional headaches. Cephalalgia 2002;22:780–3.

32. Jacome DE, Stamm MA. Malignant cough headache. Headache 2004;44(3): 259–61.

33. Wall M, Silberstein SD, Aiken RD. Headache associated with abnormalities in intracranial structure or function: high cerebrospinal fluid pressure headache and brain tumor. In: Silberstein SD, Lipton RB, Dalessio DJ, editors. Wolff's headache and other head pain. Oxford (United Kingdom): Oxford University Press; 2001. p. 393–416.

34. Edmeads J. The worst headache ever: 2. Innocuous causes. Postgrad Med 1989;86:107–10.

35. Mathew NT. Indomethacin responsive headache syndromes. Headache 1981; 21:147–50.

36. Raskin NH. The cough headache syndrome: treatment. Neurology 1995;45: 1784.

37. Slavik RS, Rhoney DH. Indomethacin: a review of its cerebral blood flow effects and potential use for controlling intracranial pressure in traumatic brain injury patients. Neurol Res 1999;21:491–9.

38. Calandre L, Hernandez-Lain A, Lopez-Valdes E. Benign Valsalva's maneuver-related headache: an MRI study of six cases. Headache 1996;36:251–3.

39. Bahra A, Goadsby PJ. Cough headache responsive to methysergide. Cephalalgia 1998;18:495–6.

40. Hazelrigg RL. IV DHE-45 relieves exertional cephalgia. Headache 1986;26:52.

41. Medrano V, Mallada J, Sempere AP, et al. Primary cough headache responsive to topiramate. Cephalalgia 2005;25(8):627–8.

42. Gupta VK. Metoclopramide aborts cough-induced headache and ameliorates cough—a pilot study. Int J Clin Pract 2007;61(2):345–8.

43. Sjaastad O, Bakketeig LS. Exertional headache I. Vågå study of headache epidemiology. Cephalalgia 2002;22:784–90.

44. Levin M. The international classification of headache disorders, 3rd edition (ICHD-III)-changes and challenges. Headache 2013;53(8):1383–95.

45. Sjaastad O, Bakketeig LS. Exertional headache-II. Clinical features Vågå study of headache epidemiology. Cephalalgia 2003;23:803–7.

46. Chen SP, Fuh JK, Lu SR, et al. Exertional headache—a survey of 1963 adolescents. Cephalalgia 2009;29(4):401–7.

47. Diamond S. Prolonged exertional headache: its clinical characteristics and response to indomethacin. Headache 1982;22:96–8.

48. Heckmann JG, Hilz MJ, Muck-Weymann M, et al. Benign exertional headache/benign sexual headache: a disorder of myogenic cerebrovascular autoregulation? Headache 1997;37(9):597–8.

49. Silbert PL, Edis RH, Stewart-Synne EG, et al. Benign vascular sexual headache and exertional headache. J Neurol Neurosurg Psychiatry 1991;54:417–21.

50. van der Ende-Kastelijn K, Oerlemans W, Goedegebuure S. An online survey of exercise-related headaches among cyclists. Headache 2012;52(10):1566–73.
51. Sands GH, Newman L, Lipton R. Cough, exertional, and other miscellaneous headaches. Med Clin North Am 1991;75(3):733–47.
52. Paulson GW, Zipf RE, Beekman JF. Pheochromocytoma causing exercise-related headache and pulmonary edema. Ann Neurol 1979;5:96–9.
53. Doepp F, Valdueza JM, Schreiber SJ. Incompetence of internal jugular valve in patients with primary exertional headache: a risk factor? Cephalalgia 2007;28:182–5.
54. Lance JW, Lambros J. Unilateral exertional headache as a symptom of cardiac ischemia. Headache 1998;38:315–6.
55. Diamond S, Medina JL. Benign exertional headache: successful treatment with indomethacin. Headache 1979;19:249.
56. Lance JW. Headaches related to sexual activity. J Neurol Neurosurg Psychiatry 1976;39:1226–30.
57. Allena M, Rossi P, Tassorelli C, et al. Focus on therapy of the chapter IV headaches: primary cough headache, primary exertional headache, and primary headache associated with sexual activity. J Headache Pain 2010;11:525–30.
58. Headache Classification Subcommittee of the International Headache Society. The international classification of headache disorders, 2nd edition. Cephalalgia 2004;24(Suppl 1):9–160.
59. Yeh YC, Fuh JL, Chen SP, et al. Clinical features, imaging findings and outcomes of headache associated with sexual activity. Cephalalgia 2010;30:1329–35.
60. Malignant coital headache. Headache 2002;42(3):230.
61. Porter M, Jankovic J. Benign coital cephalalgia: differential diagnosis and treatment. Arch Neurol 1981;38:710–2.
62. Martinez JM, Roig C, Arboix A. Complicated coital cephalalgia, Three cases with benign evolution. Cephalalgia 1988;8:265–8.
63. Servoss SJ, Januzzi JL, Muller JE. Triggers of acute coronary syndromes. Prog Cardiovasc Dis 2002;44(5):369–80.
64. Biran I, Steiner I. Coital headaches induced by amiodarone. Neurology 2002; 58(3):501–2.
65. Alvaro LC, Iriondo I, Villaverde FJ. Sexual headache and stroke in a heavy cannabis smoker. Cephalalgia 2002;42(3):224–6.
66. Staunton HP, Moore J. Coital cephalgia and ischaemic muscular work of the lower limbs. J Neurol Neurosurg Psychiatry 1978;41:930–3.
67. Johns DR. Benign sexual headache within a family. Arch Neurol 1986;43: 1158–60.
68. Lundberg PO, Osterman PO. The benign and malignant forms of orgasmic cephalgia. Headache 1971;13:164–5.
69. Locksley HB. Natural history of subarachnoid hemorrhage, intracranial aneurysms and arteriovenous malformations based on 6368 cases in the cooperative study. J Neurosurg 1966;25:219–39.
70. Lance JW, Hinterberger H. Symptoms of pheochromocytoma with particular reference to headache correlated with catecholamine production. Arch Neurol 1976;31:281–8.
71. Littler WA, Honour AJ, Sleight P. Direct arterial pressure, heart rate and electrocardiogram during human coitus. J Reprod Fertil 1974;40:321–31.
72. Frese A, Eikermann A, Frese K, et al. Headache associated with sexual activity: demography, clinical features, and comorbidity. Neurology 2003;61:796–800.
73. Gelfand AA, Goadsby PJ. Primary sex headache in adolescents. Pediatrics 2012;130(2):e439–41.

74. Evers S, Peikert A, Frese A. Sexual headache in young adolescence: a case report. Headache 2009;49:1234–5.
75. Biehl K, Evers S, Frese A. Comorbidity of migraine and headache associated with sexual activity. Cephalalgia 2007;27:1271–3.
76. Frese A, Rahmann A, Gregor N, et al. Headache associated with sexual activity: prognosis and treatment options. Cephalalgia 2007;27:1265–70.
77. Paulson GW, Klawans HL. Benign orgasmic cephalgia. Headache 1974;13: 181–7.
78. Evans RW, Pascual J. Orgasmic headaches: clinical features, diagnosis, and management. Headache 2000;40:491–4.
79. Frese A, Gantenbein A, Marziniak M, et al. Triptans in orgasmic headache. Cephalalgia 2006;26(12):1458–61.

Metabolic Headaches

Ana Marissa Lagman-Bartolome, MD[a],
Jonathan Gladstone, MD, FRCPC[b],*

KEYWORDS

- Homeostasis • Hypoxia • Dialysis • Hypertension • Hypothyroidism • Fasting
- Cardiac cephalalgia

KEY POINTS

- Clinicians caring for patients with headache need to be aware that there are numerous secondary causes of headache related to a wide range of disorders of homeostasis, and these headaches can mimic the phenotype of common primary headache disorders (ie, migraine, tension-type headache, and primary exertional headache).
- Failure to recognize a secondary cause of headache attributed to a disorder of homeostasis can lead to significant morbidity due to an unrecognized (and untreated) underlying medical condition (ie, hypothyroidism, hypertension, and sleep apnea).
- Failure to recognize a secondary cause of headache attributed to a disorder of homeostasis can lead to significant morbidity or mortality due to inappropriate treatment of a presumed primary headache disorder (ie, therapeutic trial of a triptan for presumed migraine in a patient with actual cardiac cephalgia).

INTRODUCTION

Headaches attributed to disorders of homeostasis were referred to as "headaches associated with metabolic or systemic diseases" in the first edition of the International Headache Society *International Classification of Headache Disorders (ICHD)-1*.[1] The recent third edition the *ICHD-3 (beta version)*, states that if a headache occurs for the first time in close temporal relation to a disorder of homeostasis, it is coded as a secondary headache attributed to that disorder.[2] *ICHD-3 beta* includes headaches attributed to (1) hypoxia and/or hypercapnia (high altitude, diving, and sleep apnea), (2) dialysis, (3) arterial hypertension (pheochromocytoma, hypertensive crisis without hypertensive encephalopathy, hypertensive encephalopathy, preeclampsia or eclampsia, and autonomic dysreflexia), (4) hypothyroidism, (5) fasting, (6) cardiac

Funding Sources: Dr A.M. Lagman-Bartolome: Canadian Headache Society.
Conflict of Interest: Nil.
[a] Division of Pediatric Neurology, Hospital for Sick Children, Women's College Hospital, University of Toronto, 555 University Avenue, Toronto, ON M5G1X8, Canada; [b] Gladstone Headache Clinic, 1333 Sheppard Avenue East, Suite 122, Toronto, ON M2J 1V1, Canada
* Corresponding author.
E-mail address: jon.gladstone@utoronto.ca

CASE VIGNETTE

A 72-year-old gentleman presented with a 3-week history of headaches. The headaches were intermittent, occurring approximately 2 to 3 days per week. The headaches were pulsating in quality, were moderate to severe in intensity, and lasted less than an hour. There was no associated nausea, vomiting, photophobia, or phonophobia. There were no trigeminal autonomic symptoms. There were no symptoms suggestive of polymyalgia rheumatica and there were no claudication symptoms. There was no prior history of headaches and no known past medical history. He was not on any medications. On further directed questioning regarding potential triggers for his headaches, it was noted that the headaches typically occurred when outside gardening. Further probing noted that gardening represented his most strenuous physical activity and, at times, he was aware that his heart seemed to be beating quickly and strongly while gardening. He attributed this to the physical exertion associated with gardening. Given the new onset of an exertion-related headache in a 72-year-old gentleman, an exercise stress test was ordered. During the treadmill stress test, the gentleman developed his typical pulsating headache and his ECG noted significant ventricular tachycardia. He was admitted urgently to hospital under cardiology; definitive treatment was initiated with an implantable cardioverter defibrillator, and headaches ceased.

cephalalgia, and (7) other disorder of homeostasis. Although there are varied mechanisms behind causation of these different subtypes of headache attributed to a disorder of homeostasis, there are general diagnostic criteria applicable in most cases, as seen in **Box 1**.

HEADACHE ATTRIBUTED TO HYPOXIA OR HYPERCAPNIA

This group of headache disorders is caused by hypoxia and/or hypercapnia and occurs in conditions of exposure to one or both of those conditions (**Box 2**). According to the *ICHD-2*, it is difficult to separate the effects of hypoxia and hypercapnia.[3] The *ICHD-2* criteria for headache secondary to hypoxia state that headache begins within 24 hours after acute onset of hypoxia with PaO_2 less than 70 mm Hg or in chronically hypoxic patients with PaO_2 persistently at or below these levels.[3] Diseases or situations that are related to acute or chronic hypoxia/hypercapnia may be associated with headache. In brief, any disease that induces a hypoxic state, such as pulmonary diseases (asthma or chronic obstructive pulmonary disease), cardiac disease

---

Box 1
Headache attributed to a disorder of homeostasis

A. Headache fulfilling criterion C.

B. A disorder of homeostasis known to be able to cause headache has been diagnosed.

C. Evidence of causation demonstrated by at least 2 of the following:

 1. Headache has developed in temporal relation to the onset of the disorder of homeostasis.

 2. Either or both of the following:

  a. Headache has significantly worsened in parallel with worsening of the disorder of homeostasis.

  b. Headache has significantly improved after resolution of the disorder of homeostasis.

 3. Headache has characteristics typical for the disorder of homeostasis.

D. Not better accounted for by another *ICHD-3* diagnosis.

Box 2
Headache attributed to hypoxia or hypercapnia

A. Any headache fulfilling criterion C.

B. Exposure to conditions of hypoxia and/or hypercapnia.

C. Evidence of causation demonstrated by at least 1 of the following:

1. Headache has developed in temporal relation to the exposure.

2. Either or both of the following:

a. Headache has significantly worsened in parallel with increasing exposure to hypoxia and/or hypercapnia.

b. Headache has significantly improved in parallel with improvement in hypoxia and/or hypercapnia.

D. Not better accounted for by another *ICHD-3* diagnosis.

(congestive heart failure), or hematologic disorders (with significant anemia), may be associated with headache.

The *ICHD-3 beta* outlines 4 specific situations associated with headaches attributed to hypoxia that are potentially manageable, including (1) high altitude, (2) airplane travel, (3) diving, and (4) sleep apnea. Each of these specific headache conditions is discussed in detail.

High-Altitude Headache

Headache attributed to high altitude is a headache that develops in temporal relation to an ascent above 2500 m that worsens during continued ascent and/or resolves within 24 hours after descent to below 2500 m (**Box 3**). Although the criteria suggest that the headaches are more often bilateral, unilateral headaches can occur, and this is seen more often in migraineurs who typically experience unilateral migraine attacks attributable to altitude.[4] High-altitude headache is the most frequent symptom of acute exposure to high altitude, with incidence as high as 73.3% to 86.7%.[5,6]

Box 3
Headache attributed to high altitude

A. Any headache fulfilling criterion C.

B. Ascent to altitude above 2500 m has taken place.

C. Evidence of causation demonstrated by at least 2 of the following:

1. Headache has developed in temporal relation to the ascent.

2. Either or both of the following:

a. Headache has significantly worsened in parallel with continuing ascent.

b. Headache has resolved within 24 hours after descent to below 2500 m.

3. Headache has at least 2 of the following 3 characteristics:

a. Bilateral location

b. Mild or moderate intensity

c. Aggravated by exertion, movement, straining, coughing, and/or bending

D. Not better accounted for by another *ICHD-3* diagnosis.

High-altitude headache is often associated with nausea, photophobia, vertigo, poor concentration, and, in severe cases, impaired judgment and signs that suggest brain edema. Risk factors include a history of migraine, low arterial oxygen saturation, high perceived degree of exertion, fluid intake less than 2 L in 24 hours, insomnia, high heart rate, and high Self-Rating Anxiety Scale score.[4,5]

The exact pathophysiologic process that causes high altitude headache is still unknown. Hypoxia elicits neurohumoral and hemodynamic responses that result in overperfusion of microvascular beds, increased hydrostatic capillary pressure, capillary leakage, and consequent edema.[7] Several neuroimaging studies have demonstrated mild increase in brain volume associated with an increased T2 relaxation time and apparent diffusion coefficient, which were consistently associated with the severity of neurologic symptoms. The investigators suggested that the brain edema is predominantly vasogenic (with movement of fluid and proteins out of the vascular compartment into extracellular brain areas) rather than a cytotoxic edema (due to cellular swelling). Mild extracellular vasogenic edema contributes to the generalized brain swelling observed at high altitude and may be of significance in headache attributed to altitude.[8] This was supported by findings that elderly people have fewer headaches than younger people after exposure to high altitude, probably due to a certain degree of brain atrophy.[9]

A recent study examined indices of brain white matter water mobility after 2 and 10 hours in normoxia (21% O_2) and hypoxia (12% O_2) using MRI whole-brain analysis (tract-based spatial statistics). The results of this study indicate that acute periods of hypoxemia cause a shift of water into the intracellular space within the cerebral white matter, which were found related to the intensity of high-altitude headache, whereas no evidence of brain edema (a volumetric enlargement) was identifiable.[10] Furthermore, efforts to demonstrate a specific genotype associated with a predisposition to develop this headache led to the suggestion that low ATP1A1 subunit of the ATPase gene mRNA expression may be of importance.[11]

Medical treatment of this disorder involves simple analgesics, such as paracetamol (acetaminophen) or ibuprofen and antiemetic agents as well as acetazolamide, at 125 mg to 250 mg twice daily, or steroids (eg, dexamethasone).[12,13] Randomized, placebo-controlled trials also showed a significant reduction in the risk of headache with the use of acetylsalicylic acid at a dose of 320 mg taken 3 times at 4-hour intervals, starting 1 hour before ascent,[14] or ibuprofen at a dose of 600 mg 3 times per day,[15,16] starting a few hours before ascent to altitudes between 3480 m and 4920 m. Other nonpharmacologic strategies include 2 days of acclimatization prior to engaging in strenuous exercise at high altitudes, slow ascent, liberal fluid intake, and avoidance of alcohol.[13]

Headache Attributed to Airplane Travel

Headache attributed to airplane travel, also called airplane headache, is a recent addition to the ICHD-3 beta (**Box 4**). This headache is often severe, usually unilateral and periocular, and without autonomic symptoms, occurring during and caused by airplane travel, and it remits after landing.[2] The largest case series of airplane headache showed the stereotypical nature of the attacks, which include the short duration of the pain (lasting less than 30 minutes in up to 95% of the cases), clear relationship with landing phase, male preponderance, and absence of accompanying signs and/or symptoms.[17] It occurs during landing in more than 85% of patients.[18] The pathophysiology of airplane headache remains unclear. This rare headache, felt on aircraft descent, is thought, however, due to the squeeze effect on the frontal sinus wall, when air trapped inside it contracts, producing a negative pressure, leading to

---

Box 4
Headache attributed to airplane travel

A. At least 2 episodes of headache fulfilling criterion C.

B. The patient is traveling by airplane.

C. Evidence of causation demonstrated by at least 2 of the following:

   1. Headache has developed exclusively during airplane travel.

   2. Either or both of the following:

      a. Headache has worsened in temporal relation to ascent after take-off and/or descent prior to landing of the airplane.

      b. Headache has spontaneously improved within 30 minutes after the ascent or descent of the airplane is completed.

   3. Headache is severe, with at least 2 of the following 3 characteristics:

      a. Unilateral location

      b. Orbitofrontal location (parietal spread may occur)

      c. Jabbing or stabbing quality (pulsation may also occur)

D. Not better accounted for by another *ICHD-3* diagnosis.

---

mucosal edema, transudation, and intense pain.[19] Another proposed theory states that this type of headache generally results from the temporary local inflammation caused by hypoxia or dryness in the sinus mucosa or sinus barotraumas.[20]

Prophylactic therapy for this type of headache includes simple analgesics; nonsteroidal antiinflammatory drugs (NSAIDs), like naproxen sodium (550 mg); antihistamines, like pseudoephedrine; and nasal decongestants administered 30 minutes to 1 hour prior to travel, were found effective.[18,19] Performing spontaneous maneuvers (ie, pressure on the pain area, Valsalva maneuver, relaxation methods, chewing, and extension of the earlobe) have been shown to decrease the pain intensity by 25%.[18]

Diving Headache

The best clinical example of headache attributed to hypercapnia is diving headache (**Box 5**). This headache disorder is caused by diving below 10 m and occurs during the dive, is often intensified on resurfacing, and occurs in the absence of decompression illness. It is usually accompanied by symptoms of CO_2 intoxication. It remits quickly with oxygen or, if this is not given, spontaneously within 3 days after the dive has ended.[2] There is some evidence that hypercapnia (arterial Pco_2 >50 mm Hg) is known to cause relaxation of cerebrovascular smooth muscle, leading to intracranial vasodilatation and increased intracranial pressure, leading to headache.[21] CO_2 may accumulate in a diver who intentionally holds his or her breath intermittently (skip breathing) in a mistaken attempt to conserve air or takes shallow breaths to minimize buoyancy variations in the narrow passages of a wreck or cave. Divers may also hypoventilate unintentionally when a tight wetsuit or buoyancy compensator jacket restricts chest wall expansion or when ventilation is inadequate in response to physical exertion. Strenuous exercise increases the rate of CO_2 production more than 10-fold, resulting in a transient elevation of Pco_2 to more than 60 mm Hg. Inadequate ventilation of compressed gases can lead to CO_2 accumulation, cerebral vasodilation, and headache.[21] Diving headache usually intensifies during the decompression phase of the dive or on resurfacing. A recent study, however, showed that the prevalence of

---

Box 5
Diving headache

A. Any headache fulfilling criterion C.

B. Both of the following:

   1. The patient is diving at a depth greater than 10 m.

   2. There is no evidence of decompression illness.

C. Evidence of causation demonstrated by at least 1 of the following:

   1. Headache has developed during the dive.

   2. Either or both of the following:

      a. Headache has worsened as the dive is continued.

      b. Either of the following:

         i. Headache has spontaneously resolved within 3 days of completion of the dive.

         ii. Headache has remitted within 1 hour after treatment with 100% oxygen.

   3. At least 1 of the following symptoms of CO_2 intoxication:

      a. Mental confusion

      b. Light-headedness

      c. Motor incoordination

      d. Dyspnea

      e. Facial flushing

D. Not better accounted for by another *ICHD-3* diagnosis.

---

headache among male divers and matched controls was not significant (16% vs 22%) and concluded that scuba diving is not associated with headache.[22]

It is well established that headache in divers, although uncommon (4.5%–23%) and relatively benign, can occasionally signify serious consequences of hyperbaric exposure, such as arterial gas embolism, decompression sickness, and otic or paranasal sinus barotrauma.[23–25] For patients in whom the headache is not obviously benign, the diagnostic evaluation should consider otic and paranasal sinus barotrauma, arterial gas embolism, decompression sickness, CO_2 retention, carbon monoxide toxicity, hyperbaric-triggered migraine, cervical and temporomandibular joint strain, supraorbital neuralgia, carotid artery dissection, and exertional and cold stimulus headache syndromes.[21]

Focal neurologic symptoms, even in the migraineur, should not be ignored but rather treated with 100% oxygen acutely, and patients should be referred without delay to a facility with a hyperbaric chamber.[23] A potential relationship between patent foramen ovale and migraine with aura was first described in scuba divers.[26] Therefore, it is prudent to screen for patent foramen ovale before assigning a diagnosis of diving headache.

Sleep Apnea Headache

Sleep apnea headache is a recurrent morning headache (**Box 6**), usually bilateral and with a duration of less than 4 hours, caused by sleep apnea diagnosed using polysomnography with apnea-hypopnea index (AHI) greater than or equal to 5. AHI is calculated by dividing the number of apneic events by the number of hours of sleep.[2] This headache disorder resolves with successful treatment of the sleep apnea.[27,28]

Box 6
Headache attributed to sleep apnea

A. Headache present on awakening after sleep and fulfilling criterion C.

B. Sleep apnea (AHI ≥5) has been diagnosed.

C. Evidence of causation demonstrated by at least 2 of the following:

    1. Headache has developed in temporal relation to the onset of sleep apnea.

    2. Either or both of the following:

        a. Headache has worsened in parallel with worsening of sleep apnea.

        b. Headache has significantly improved or remitted in parallel with improvement in or resolution of sleep apnea.

    3. Headache has at least 1 of the following 3 characteristics:

        a. Recurs on >15 days per month

        b. All of the following:

            i. Bilateral location

            ii. Pressing quality

            iii. Not accompanied by nausea, photophobia, or phonophobia

        c. Resolves within 4 hours

D. Not better accounted for by another *ICHD-3* diagnosis.

The relationship between headache and sleep disorders is complex. First, sleep disturbances may trigger migraine.[29] Second, snoring and other sleep disorders are risk factors for migraine progression.[30] Third, sleep apnea is a risk factor for cluster headache and morning headaches.[31,32] Although morning headache is significantly more frequent in patients with obstructive sleep apnea (OSA) (11.8% vs 4.6%) than those without OSA, headache present on awakening is a nonspecific symptom, which occurs in a variety of primary and secondary headache disorders, in sleep-related respiratory disorders other than sleep apnea (eg, pickwickian syndrome and chronic obstructive pulmonary disorder), and in other primary sleep disorders, such as periodic leg movements of sleep.[33] Prior studies have shown higher prevalence (27.2%–74%) of morning headaches among patients with OSA,[28,32,34,35] habitual snoring (23.5%),[32] and insomnia (48%).[35] Other predictors for sleep apnea headache include female gender, history of migraine, psychological distress, and obesity.[32,35]

The exact pathophysiology of sleep apnea headache remains debatable. Several possible mechanisms include hypoxia or oxygen desaturation, hypercapnia, or disturbance in sleep architecture (ie, shorter rapid-eye-movement sleep) as well as increase intracranial pressure.[28,32,34,35]

DIALYSIS HEADACHE

Dialysis headache is a type of secondary headache disorder with no specific characteristics occurring during and caused by hemodialysis (**Box 7**). It resolves spontaneously within 72 hours after the hemodialysis session has ended or headache episodes may stop altogether after a successful kidney transplantation and termination of hemodialysis.[2] This type of headache has been recognized for years as a known emerging symptom of hemodialysis treatment.[36] Dialysis headache occurs in 30% to 70% of patients receiving hemodialysis.[37–39] In a prospective study, however,

---

Box 7
Dialysis headache

A. At least 3 episodes of acute headache fulfilling criterion C.

B. The patient is on hemodialysis.

C. Evidence of causation demonstrated by at least 2 of the following:

    1. Each headache has developed during a session of hemodialysis.

    2. Either or both of the following:

        a. Each headache has worsened during the dialysis session.

        b. Each headache has resolved within 72 hours after the end of the dialysis session.

    3. Headache episodes cease altogether after successful kidney transplantation and termination of hemodialysis.

D. Not better accounted for by another *ICHD-3* diagnosis.

---

approximately one-third of patients with otherwise typical dialysis headache had similar headache in-between the dialysis sessions and the headaches occurred mainly in the second half of the hemodialysis (86%).[40] There is no consensus on pathophysiology of dialysis headache; however, it commonly occurs in association with hypotension and dialysis disequilibrium syndrome. This syndrome may begin as headache and then progress to obtundation and coma, with or without seizures. The most consistent triggers for dialysis headache found in several studies include arterial hypertension (38%), arterial hypotension (12%), and changes in weight during the hemodialysis sessions (6%).[39,41] Reduced serum osmolality and low magnesium and high sodium levels may be risk factors for developing dialysis headache.[38] Dialysis headache may be prevented by changing dialysis parameters.

There is no specific treatment of dialysis headache. Acute treatment is mainly symptomatic and complicated by the chronic renal insufficiency status. Analgesics and NSAIDs are often used during dialysis sessions. The use of preventative medication may be necessary to improve headache burden; however, evidence for this is limited. Angiotensin-converting enzyme inhibitors (ie, lisinopril and fosinopril) were given to one patient with good response in a case report.[42]

HEADACHE ATTRIBUTED TO HYPERTENSION

Headache attributed to hypertension is often bilateral and pulsating, caused by arterial hypertension, usually during an acute rise in systolic (to ≥180 mm Hg) and/or diastolic (to ≥120 mm Hg) blood pressure (**Box 8**). It remits after normalization of blood pressure.[2] Mild (140–159/90–99 mm Hg) or moderate (160–179/100–109 mm Hg) chronic arterial hypertension does not seem to cause headache. Ambulatory blood pressure monitoring in patients with mild and moderate hypertension has shown no convincing relationship between blood pressure fluctuations over a 24-hour period and presence or absence of headache.[43,44] Some investigators have reported a significant correlation between blood pressure levels and headache and reduced headache frequency with treatment of hypertension.[45–47] Whether moderate hypertension predisposes to headache at all remains controversial, but there is some evidence that it does.

Several studies documented association of headache with pheochromocytoma,[48–51] hypertensive encephalopathy,[52,53] and preeclampsia and eclampsia[54,55]

Box 8
Headache attributed to hypertension

A. Any headache fulfilling criterion C.

B. Hypertension defined as systolic pressure $\geq$180 mm Hg and/or diastolic pressure $\geq$120 mm Hg has been demonstrated.

C. Evidence of causation demonstrated by either or both of the following:

　1. Headache has developed in temporal relation to the onset of hypertension.

　2. Either or both of the following:

　　a. Headache has significantly worsened in parallel with worsening hypertension.

　　b. Headache has significantly improved in parallel with improvement in hypertension.

D. Not better accounted for by another *ICHD-3* diagnosis.

---

as well as autonomic dysreflexia.[56] The proposed mechanism for this type of headache is failure of the normal baroreceptor reflex.[46]

Headache Attributed to Pheochromocytoma

Headaches attributed to pheochromocytoma are usually severe and of short duration (less than 1 hour); headache attacks are accompanied by sweating, palpitations, pallor, and/or anxiety, caused by pheochromocytoma (**Box 9**).[2] This type of headache occurs as a paroxysmal headache in 51% to 80% of patients with pheochromocytoma.[48,49] It is often severe, frontal, or occipital and usually described as pulsating or constant in quality. An important feature of the headache is its short duration: less than 15 minutes

---

Box 9
Headache attributed to pheochromocytoma

A. Recurrent discrete short-lasting headache episodes fulfilling criterion C.

B. Pheochromocytoma has been demonstrated.

C. Evidence of causation demonstrated by at least 2 of the following:

　1. Headache episodes have commenced in temporal relation to development of the pheochromocytoma, or led to its discovery.

　2. Either or both of the following:

　　a. Individual headache episodes develop in temporal relation to abrupt rises in blood pressure.

　　b. Individual headache episodes remit in temporal relation to normalization of blood pressure.

　3. Headache is accompanied by at least 1 of the following:

　　a. Sweating

　　b. Palpitations

　　c. Anxiety

　　d. Pallor

　4. Headache episodes remit entirely after removal of the pheochromocytoma.

D. Not better accounted for by another *ICHD-3* diagnosis.

---

in 50% of patients and less than 1 hour in 70% of patients.[48] Associated features include apprehension and/or anxiety, often with a sense of impending death, tremor, visual disturbances, abdominal or chest pain, nausea, vomiting, facial flushing, and occasionally paresthesia.[48,50] A diagnosis of pheochromocytoma is established by the demonstration of increased excretion of catecholamines or catecholamine metabolites and can usually be secured by analysis of a single 24-hour urine sample collected when a patient is hypertensive or symptomatic.[48,50,51] The variable duration and intensity of the headache correlates with the pressor and cranial vasoconstrictor effects of the secreted amines.[50]

Headache Attributed to Hypertensive Crisis Without Hypertensive Encephalopathy

Headache attributed to hypertensive crisis without hypertensive encephalopathy is usually a bilateral and pulsating headache (**Box 10**), caused by a paroxysmal rise of arterial hypertension (systolic ≥180 mm Hg and/or diastolic ≥120 mm Hg). It remits after normalization of blood pressure.[2] A hypertensive crisis is defined as a paroxysmal rise in systolic (to ≥180 mm Hg) and/or diastolic (to ≥120 mm Hg) blood pressure. Paroxysmal hypertension may occur in association with failure of baroreceptor reflexes (after carotid endarterectomy or subsequent to irradiation of the neck) or in patients with enterochromaffin cell tumors.

Headache Attributed to Hypertensive Encephalopathy

Headache, usually bilateral and pulsating, is caused by persistent blood pressure elevation to 180/120 mm Hg or above and accompanied by symptoms of encephalopathy, such as confusion, lethargy, visual disturbances, or seizures (**Box 11**). It improves after normalization of blood pressure.[2] Hypertensive encephalopathy presents with persistent elevation of blood pressure to greater than or equal 180/120 mm Hg and at least 2 of the following: confusion, reduced level of consciousness, visual disturbances, including blindness, and seizures.[52,53] Headache is one of the

---

Box 10
Headache attributed to hypertensive crisis without hypertensive encephalopathy

A. Headache fulfilling criterion C.

B. Both of the following:

　1. A hypertensive crisis is occurring.

　2. There are no clinical features or other evidence of hypertensive encephalopathy.

C. Evidence of causation demonstrated by at least 2 of the following:

　1. Headache has developed during the hypertensive crisis.

　2. Either or both of the following:

　　a. Headache has significantly worsened in parallel with increasing hypertension.

　　b. Headache has significantly improved or resolved in parallel with improvement in or resolution of the hypertensive crisis.

　3. Headache has at least 1 of the following 3 characteristics:

　　a. Bilateral location

　　b. Pulsating quality

　　c. Precipitated by physical activity

D. Not better accounted for by another *ICHD-3* diagnosis.

> **Box 11**
> **Headache attributed to hypertensive encephalopathy**
>
> A. Headache fulfilling criterion C.
>
> B. Hypertensive encephalopathy has been diagnosed.
>
> C. Evidence of causation demonstrated by at least 2 of the following:
>
>   1. Headache has developed in temporal relation to the onset of the hypertensive encephalopathy.
>
>   2. Either or both of the following:
>
>   a. Headache has significantly worsened in parallel with worsening of the hypertensive encephalopathy.
>
>   b. Headache has significantly improved or resolved in parallel with improvement in or resolution of the hypertensive encephalopathy.
>
>   3. Headache has at least 2 of the following 3 characteristics:
>
>   a. Diffuse pain
>
>   b. Pulsating quality
>
>   c. Aggravated by physical activity
>
> D. Not better accounted for by another *ICHD-3* diagnosis.

most frequent signs (22%) at presentation in hypertensive urgencies.[52] It is thought to occur when compensatory cerebrovascular vasoconstriction can no longer prevent cerebral hyperperfusion as blood pressure rises.[57] As normal cerebral autoregulation of blood flow is overwhelmed, endothelial permeability increases and cerebral edema occurs.[52] On MRI, this is often most prominent in the parieto-occipital white matter.[58] Although hypertensive encephalopathy in patients with chronic arterial hypertension is usually accompanied by a diastolic blood pressure of greater than 120 mm Hg and by grade III or IV hypertensive retinopathy (Keith-Wagener-Barker classification), previously normotensive individuals may develop signs of encephalopathy with blood pressures as low as 160/100 mm Hg.[59]

Headache Attributed to Preeclampsia or Eclampsia

Headache attributed to preeclampsia or eclampsia is usually bilateral and pulsating headache, occurring in women during pregnancy or the immediate puerperium with preeclampsia or eclampsia (**Box 12**). It remits after resolution of the preeclampsia or eclampsia.[2] Preeclampsia and eclampsia seem to involve a strong maternal inflammatory response, with broad immunologic systemic activity.[54] Preeclampsia and eclampsia are multisystem disorders with various forms. Their diagnosis requires hypertension (>140/90 mm Hg) documented on 2 blood pressure readings at least 4 hours apart, or a rise in diastolic pressure of greater than or equal to 15 mm Hg or in systolic pressure of great than or equal to 30 mm Hg, coupled with urinary protein excretion greater than 0.3 g/24 h. In addition, tissue edema, thrombocytopenia, and abnormalities in liver function can occur.[54] A case-control study found that headache was significantly more frequent in patients with preeclampsia (63%) than in controls (25%) (odds ratio [OR] 4.95; 95% CI, 2.47–9.92).[60]

Headache Attributed to Autonomic Dysreflexia

Headache attributed to autonomic dysreflexia is a throbbing severe headache, with sudden onset, in patients with spinal cord injury (SCI) and autonomic dysreflexia

Box 12
Headache attributed to preeclampsia or eclampsia

A. Headache, in a woman who is pregnant or in the puerperium (up to 4 weeks postpartum), fulfilling criterion C.

B. Preeclampsia or eclampsia has been diagnosed.

C. Evidence of causation demonstrated by at least 2 of the following:

   1. Headache has developed in temporal relation to the onset of the preeclampsia or eclampsia.

   2. Either or both of the following:

      a. Headache has significantly worsened in parallel with worsening of the preeclampsia or eclampsia.

      b. Headache has significantly improved or resolved in parallel with improvement in or resolution of the preeclampsia or eclampsia.

   3. Headache has at least 2 of the following 3 characteristics:

      a. Bilateral location

      b. Pulsating quality

      c. Aggravated by physical activity

D. Not better accounted for by another *ICHD-3* diagnosis.

(**Box 13**).[2] The latter, which can be life threatening, manifests as a paroxysmal rise in blood pressure, among other symptoms and clinical signs.[56] This type of headache is a sudden-onset, severe headache accompanied by several other symptoms and clinical signs, including increased blood pressure, altered heart rate, and diaphoresis cranial to the level of SCI. Severe headaches occur in 56% to 85% of the patients with autonomic dysreflexia.[61,62] These are triggered by noxious or non-noxious stimuli, usually of visceral origin (bladder distension, urinary tract infection, bowel distension

Box 13
Headache attributed to autonomic dysreflexia

A. Headache of sudden onset, fulfilling criterion C.

B. Presence of SCI and autonomic dysreflexia documented by a paroxysmal rise above baseline in systolic pressure of $\geq$30 mm Hg and/or diastolic pressure $\geq$20 mm Hg.

C. Evidence of causation demonstrated by at least 2 of the following:

   1. Headache has developed in temporal relation to the rise in blood pressure.

   2. Either or both of the following:

      a. Headache has significantly worsened in parallel with increase in blood pressure.

      b. Headache has significantly improved in parallel with decrease in blood pressure.

   3. Headache has at least 2 of the following 4 characteristics:

      a. Severe intensity

      b. Pounding or throbbing (pulsating) quality

      c. Accompanied by diaphoresis cranial to the level of the SCI

      d. Triggered by bladder or bowel reflexes

D. Not better accounted for by another *ICHD-3* diagnosis.

or impaction, urologic procedures, gastric ulcer) but also of somatic origin (pressure ulcers, ingrown toenail, burns, trauma, and surgical or invasive diagnostic procedures).[62] The time to onset of autonomic dysreflexia after SCI is variable and has been reported from 4 days to 15 years.[61] The most important predictors of autonomic dysreflexia are the level and severity of SCI. Patients with complete SCI are at greater risk of development of autonomic dysreflexia and consequently more susceptible to develop headaches.[56] Little is known about mechanism of headache attributed to autonomic dysreflexia; however, it was suggested that this type of headache has a vasomotor nature and may result from passive dilation of cerebral vessels or increased circulating prostaglandin E2.[56] Given that autonomic dysreflexia can be a life-threatening condition, its prompt recognition and adequate management are critical. The primary treatment of this type of autonomic headache involves management of actual episode of autonomic dysreflexia, which includes close monitoring of blood pressure and heart rate as the following steps are followed: (1) patient is placed in a sitting position; (2) removal/loosening of clothing or constrictive devices; (3) scrutinizing for potential triggers (ie, bladder distension and bowel impaction); and (4) pharmacologic treatment with rapid-onset and short-duration antihypertensive agent (ie, nifedipine or nitrates) for elevated systolic blood pressure ≥ 150 mm Hg.[56]

HEADACHE ATTRIBUTED TO HYPOTHYROIDISM

Headache attributed to hypothyroidism is usually bilateral and nonpulsatile headache and remits after normalization of thyroid hormone levels (**Box 14**).[2,63] Approximately 30% of patients with hypothyroidism suffer from headache.[63] In migraineurs with subclinical hypothyroidism, treatment of borderline hypothyroidism is sometimes followed by dramatic improvement in the control of the headache.[64] The headache begins within 2 months after the onset of hypothyroidism and lasts less than 3 months after its effective treatment.[65] Its mechanism is unclear. There is a female preponderance and often a history of migraine in childhood.

Box 14
Headache attributed to hypothyroidism

A. Headache fulfilling criterion C.

B. Hypothyroidism has been demonstrated.

C. Evidence of causation demonstrated by at least 2 of the following:

   1. Headache has developed in temporal relation to the onset of hypothyroidism or led to its discovery.

   2. Either or both of the following:

      a. Headache has significantly worsened in parallel with worsening of the hypothyroidism.

      b. Headache has significantly improved or resolved in parallel with improvement in or resolution of the hypothyroidism.

   3. Headache has at least 1 of the following 3 characteristics:

      a. Bilateral location

      b. Nonpulsatile quality

      c. Constant over time

D. Not better accounted for by another *ICHD-3* diagnosis.

Hypothyroidism was noted as an important risk factor for new daily persistent headache in a clinic-based case-control study, when the control group was migraine (OR 16) or posttraumatic headache (OR 10.3; 95% CI, 2.3–46.7).[64] In the presence of hypothyroidism, headache can also be a manifestation of pituitary adenoma.[66]

HEADACHE ATTRIBUTED TO FASTING

Headache attributed to fasting is a diffuse nonmigrainous headache that begins during a fast of at least 8 hours and is relieved after eating (**Box 15**).[2] Even though the typical headache attributed to fasting is diffuse, nonpulsating, and mild to moderate in intensity, in those with a prior history of migraine the headache may resemble migraine without aura.[67]

One of the most commonly reported migraine triggers is hypoglycemia. Headache attributed to fasting is significantly more common in people who have a prior history of headache. In individuals without a well-defined history of headache, however, prolonged fasting may also be associated with the development of headaches. This is often seen in prolonged religious fasting and has been documented as Yom Kippur headache[68] and first-of-Ramadan headache.[69] Fasting headache can occur, however, in the absence of hypoglycemia, suggesting that other factors play an important role (eg, caffeine withdrawal, duration of sleep, and circadian factors). The likelihood of headache developing as a result of a fast increases with the duration of the fast. Nevertheless, this type of headache does not seem related to duration of sleep, caffeine withdrawal, or hypoglycemia. Although headache may occur under conditions of hypoglycemia-induced brain dysfunction, there is no conclusive evidence to support a causal association.

In terms of treatment, a recent study suggested that preemptive cyclooxygenase-2 (COX-2) inhibitor treatment (rofecoxib, 50 mg just before the onset of fasting) is effective in reducing these forms of headache, similar to its effect in menstrual migraine.[67] Because COX-2 inhibitors are not available in many countries, preemptive treatment with NSAIDs or long-acting triptans may be a reasonable option.

CARDIAC CEPHALALGIA

Cardiac cephalalgia is migraine-like headache, usually but not always aggravated by exercise, occurring during an episode of myocardial ischemia that is relieved by nitroglycerin (**Box 16**).[2] Lipton and colleagues[70] proposed that this type of headache is a rare and treatable form of exertional headache. During stress test in 2 subjects, typical headaches were correlated with electrocardiogram changes indicative of myocardial ischemia. In both patients, coronary angiography revealed 3-vessel disease, and

---

Box 15
Headache attributed to fasting

A. Diffuse headache not fulfilling the criteria for 1. Migraine or any of its subtypes but fulfilling criterion C.

B. The patient has fasted for ≥8 hours.

C. Evidence of causation demonstrated by both of the following:

   1. Headache has developed during fasting.

   2. Headache has significantly improved after eating.

D. Not better accounted for by another *ICHD-3* diagnosis.

Box 16
Cardiac cephalalgia

A. Any headache fulfilling criterion C.

B. Acute myocardial ischemia has been demonstrated.

C. Evidence of causation demonstrated by at least 2 of the following:

1. Headache has developed in temporal relation to onset of acute myocardial ischemia.

2. Either or both of the following:

   a. Headache has significantly worsened in parallel with worsening of the myocardial ischemia.

   b. Headache has significantly improved or resolved in parallel with improvement in or resolution of the myocardial ischemia.

3. Headache has at least 2 of the following 4 characteristics:

   a. Moderate to severe intensity

   b. Accompanied by nausea

   c. Not accompanied by phototophia or phonophobia

   d. Aggravated by exertion

4. Headache is relieved by nitroglycerine or derivatives of it.

D. Not better accounted for by another *ICHD-3* diagnosis.

---

myocardial revascularization procedures were followed by complete resolution of headaches.

ICHD-3 states that diagnosis must include careful documentation of headache and simultaneous cardiac ischemia during treadmill or nuclear cardiac stress testing. Cardiac cephalalgia occurring at rest, however, has been described.[71] Several case reports documented that this type of headache may be the sole manifestation of myocardial ischemia.[71–74] Failure to recognize and correctly diagnose cardiac cephalalgia can have serious consequences.[75,76] Therefore, distinguishing this disorder from migraine without aura is of crucial importance, particularly because vasoconstrictor medications (eg, triptans and ergots) are indicated in the treatment of migraine but contraindicated in patients with ischemic heart disease. Both disorders can produce severe head pain accompanied by nausea, and both can be triggered by exertion.

The mechanisms involved in cardiac cephalalgia remain unclear. Possible mechanisms reported, however, are related to neural convergence, including somatic and sympathetic impulses that converge in the posterior horn of the spinal cord, mixing neural supply to cervical area and cranial vessels; transient increases of intracardiac pressure that cause intracranial pressure elevation and severe headache; and the functioning ventricular pacemaker, which can also produce the headache.[72]

HEADACHE ATTRIBUTED TO OTHER DISORDER OF HOMEOSTASIS

Headache attributed to other disorder of homeostasis is a headache caused by any disorder of homeostasis not described previously (**Box 17**). Although relationships between headache and a variety of systemic and metabolic diseases have been proposed, systematic evaluation of these relationships has not been performed and there is insufficient evidence on which to build operational diagnostic criteria.[2]

> **Box 17**
> **Headache attributed to other disorder of homeostasis**
>
> A. Any headache fulfilling criterion C.
> B. A disorder of homeostasis other than those described previously and known to be able to cause headache has been diagnosed.
> C. Evidence of causation demonstrated by either or both of the following:
>   1. Headache has developed in temporal relation to the onset of the disorder of homeostasis.
>   2. Either or both of the following:
>   a. Headache has significantly worsened in parallel with worsening of the disorder of homeostasis.
>   b. Headache has significantly improved or resolved in parallel with improvement in or resolution of the disorder of homeostasis.
> D. Not better accounted for by another *ICHD-3* diagnosis.

SUMMARY

The metabolic headaches are secondary headaches that appear as a consequence of metabolic disturbances. Treatment of the underlying disease is associated with headache improvement.

REFERENCES

1. Headache Classification Subcommittee of the International Headache Society: classification and diagnostic criteria for headache disorders, cranial neuralgia, and facial pain. Cephalalgia 1988;8(Suppl 7):1–96.
2. Headache Classification Subcommittee of the International Headache Society. The International classification of headache disorders, 3rd edition beta version. Cephalalgia 2013;33(9):629–808.
3. Headache Classification Subcommittee of the International Headache Society. The International classification of headache disorders, 2nd edition. Cephalalgia 2004;24(Suppl 1):1–15.
4. Queiroz LP, Rapoport AM. High-altitude headache. Curr Pain Headache Rep 2007;11:293–6.
5. Bian SZ, Zhang JH, Gao XB, et al. Risk factors for high-altitude headache upon acute high-altitude exposure at 3700 m in young Chinese men: a cohort study. J Headache Pain 2013;14:35.
6. Alizadeh R, Ziaee V, Aghsaeifard Z, et al. Characteristics of Headache at Altitude among Trekkers; A comparison between acute mountain sickness and non- acute mountain sickness headache. Asian J Sports Med 2012;3(2):126–30.
7. Hackett PH, Roach RC. High-altitude illness. N Engl J Med 2001;345:107–14.
8. Kallenberg K, Bailey DM, Christ S, et al. Magnetic resonance imaging evidence of cytotoxic cerebral edema in acute mountain sickness. J Cereb Blood Flow Metab 2006;27:1064–71.
9. Silber E, Sonnenberg P, Collier DJ, et al. Clinical features of headache at altitude: a prospective study. Neurology 2003;60:1167–71.
10. Lawley J, Oliver S, Mullins P, et al. Investigation of whole-brain white matter identifies altered water mobility in the pathogenesis of high-altitude headache. J Cereb Blood Flow Metab 2013;33(8):1286–94.

11. Appenzeller O, Minko T, Qualls C, et al. Migraine in the Andes and headache at sea level. Cephalalgia 2005;25:1117–21.
12. Carlsten C, Swenson ER, Ruoss S. A dose-response study of acetazolamide for acute mountain sickness prophylaxis in vacationing tourists at 12,000 feet (3630 m). High Alt Med Biol 2004;5:33–9.
13. Bärtsch P, Swenson E. Acute high-altitude illnesses. N Engl J Med 2013; 368(24):2294–302.
14. Burtscher M, Likar R, Nachbauer W, et al. Aspirin for prophylaxis against headache at high altitudes: randomised, double blind, placebo controlled trial. BMJ 1998;316:1057–8.
15. Gertsch JH, Corbett B, Holck PS, et al. Altitude sickness in climbers and efficacy of NSAIDs trial (ASCENT): randomized, controlled trial of ibuprofen versus placebo for prevention of altitude illness. Wilderness Environ Med 2012;23:307–15.
16. Lipman GS, Kanaan NC, Holck PS, et al. Ibuprofen prevents altitude illness: a randomized controlled trial for prevention of altitude illness with nonsteroidal anti-inflammatories. Ann Emerg Med 2012;59:484–90.
17. Mainardi F, Maggioni F, Lisotto C, et al. Headache attributed to airplane travel ('airplane headache'): clinical profile based on a large case series. Cephalalgia 2012;32(8):592–9.
18. Mainardi F, Maggioni F, Lisotto C, et al. Diagnosis and management of headache attributed to airplane travel. Curr Neurol Neurosci Rep 2013;13:335.
19. Cherian A, Mathew M, Iype T, et al. Headache associated with airplane travel: a rare entity. Neurol India 2013;61(2):164.
20. Berilgen MS, Müngen B. A new type of headache, headache associated with airplane travel: preliminary diagnostic criteria and possible mechanisms of aetiopathogenesis. Cephalalgia 2011;31(12):1266–73.
21. Chesire WP. Headache and facial pain in scuba divers. Curr Pain Headache Rep 2004;8:315–20.
22. Di Fabiio R, Vanacore N, Davassi C, et al. Scuba diving is not associated with high prevalence of headache: a cross-sectional study in men. Headache 2012;52:385–92.
23. Cheshire WP Jr, Ott MC. Headache in divers. Headache 2001;41:235–47.
24. Englund M, Risberg J. Self-reported headache during saturation diving. Aviat Space Environ Med 2003;74(3):236–41.
25. Arieli R, Shochat T, Adir Y. CNS toxicity in closed-circuit oxygen diving: symptoms reported from 2527 dives. Aviat Space Environ Med 2006;77(5): 526–32.
26. Tobis MJ, Azarbal B. Does patent foramen ovale promote cryptogenic stroke and migraine headache? Tex Heart Inst J 2005;32:362–5.
27. Rains JC, Poceta JS. Headache and sleep disorders: review and clinical implications for headache management. Headache 2006;46:1344–63.
28. Loh NK, Dinner DS, Foldvary N, et al. Do patients with obstructive sleep apnea wake up with headaches? Arch Intern Med 1999;159:1765–8.
29. Poceta JS. Sleep-related headache. Curr Treat Options Neurol 2002;4:121–8.
30. Scher AI, Stewart WF, Lipton RB. Factors associated with the onset and remission of chronic daily headache in a population-based study. Pain 2003;106: 81–9.
31. Graff-Radford SB, Newman A. Obstructive sleep apnea and cluster headache. Headache 2004;44:607–10.
32. Chen PK, FUh JL, Lane HY, et al. Morning headache in habitual snorers: frequency, characteristics, predictors and impacts. Cephalalgia 2011;31(7):829–36.

33. Kristiansen HA, Kvaerner KJ, Akre H, et al. Sleep apnoea headache in the general population. Cephalalgia 2011;32(6):451–8.
34. Goksan B, Gunduz A, Karadeniz D, et al. Morning head- ache in sleep apnoea: clinical and polysomnographic evaluation and response to nasal continuous positive airway pressure. Cephalalgia 2009;29:635–41.
35. Alberti A, Mazzotta G, Gallinela E, et al. Headache characteristics in obstructive sleep apnea syndrome and insomnia. Acta Neurol Scand 2005;111:309–16.
36. Bana DS, Yap AU, Grahan JR. Headache during hemodialysis. Headache 1972; 12:1–14.
37. Antoniazzi AL, Bigal ME, Bordini CA, et al. Headache associated with dialysis: the International Headache Society criteria revisited. Cephalalgia 2003;23:146–9.
38. Goksel BK, Torun D, Karaca S, et al. Is low magnesium level associated with hemodialysis headache? Headache 2006;46:40–5.
39. Goksan B, Karaali-Savrun F, Ertan S, et al. Hemodialysis-related headache. Cephalalgia 2004;24:284–7.
40. Antoniazzi AL, Bigal ME, Bordinic CA, et al. Headache and hemodialysis: a prospective study. Headache 2003;43:99–102.
41. Antoniazzi AL, Corrado AP. Dialysis headache. Curr Pain Headache Rep 2007; 11:297–303.
42. Dahlke EL, Wilcke TS, Krämer BK, et al. Improvement of dialysis headache after treatment with ACE-inhibitors but not angiotensin II receptor blocker: a case report with pathophysiological considerations. Cephalalgia 2004;25:71–4.
43. Kruszewski P, Bieniaszewski L, Neubauer J, et al. Headache in patients with mild to moderate hypertension is generally not associated with simultaneous blood pressure elevation. J Hypertens 2000;18:437–44.
44. Gus M, Fuchs FD, Pimentel M, et al. Behavior of ambulatory blood pressure surrounding episodes of headache in mildly hypertensive patients. Arch Intern Med 2001;161:252–5.
45. Cooper WD, Glover DR, Hormbrey JM, et al. Headache and blood pressure: evidence of a close relationship. J Hum Hypertens 1989;3:41–4.
46. Dodick DW. Recurrent short-lasting headache associated with paroxysmal hypertension: a clonidine-responsive syndrome. Cephalalgia 2000;20:509–14.
47. Gipponi S, Venturelli E, Rao R, et al. Hypertension is a factor associated with chronic daily headache. Neurol Sci 2010;31(Suppl 1):171–3.
48. Thomas JE, Rooke ED, Kvale WF. The neurologists experience with pheochromocytoma. JAMA 1966;197:754–8.
49. Mannelli M, Ianni L, Cilotti A, et al. Pheochromocytoma in Italy: a multicentric retrospective study. Eur J Endocrinol 1999;141:619–24.
50. Lance JW, Hinterberger H. Symptom of pheochromocytoma with particular reference to headache, correlated with catecho- lamine production. Arch Neurol 1976;33:281–8.
51. Loh KC, Shlossberg AH, Abbott EC, et al. Phaeochromocytoma: a ten-year survey. QJM 1997;90:51–60.
52. Vaughan CJ, Delanty N. Hypertensive emergencies. Lancet 2000;356:411–7.
53. Zampaglione B, Pascale C, Marchisio M, et al. Hypertensive urgencies and emergencies. Prevalence and clinical presentation. Hypertension 1996;27:144–7.
54. Walker JJ. Pre-eclampsia. Lancet 2000;56:1260–5.
55. Land SH, Donovan T. Pre-eclampsia and eclampsia headache: classification recommendation. Cephalalgia 1999;19:67–9 [letter].
56. Furlan JC. Headache attributed to autonomic dysreflexia. Neurology 2011;77: 792–8.

57. Immink R, van den Born BJ, van Montfrans G, et al. Impaired cerebral autoregulation in patients with malignant hypertension. Circulation 2004;110:2241–5.
58. Schwartz R, Jones K, Kalina P, et al. Hypertensive encephalopathy: findings on CT, MR imaging and SPECT imaging in 14 cases. Am J Roentgenol 1992;159(2): 379–83.
59. Amraoui F, van Montfrans GA, van den Born BJ. Value of retinal examination in hypertensive encephalopathy. J Hum Hypertens 2010;24:274–9.
60. Facchinetti F, Allais G, D'Amico R, et al. The relationship between headache and preeclampsia: a case–control study. Eur J Obstet Gynecol Reprod Biol 2005; 121:143–8.
61. Kewalramani LS. Autonomic dysreflexia in traumatic myelopathy. Am J Phys Med 1980;59:1–21.
62. Lindan R, Joiner E, Freehafer AA, et al. Incidence and clinical features of autonomic dysreflexia in patients with spinal cord injury. Paraplegia 1980;18:285–92.
63. Moreau T, Manceau E, Giraud L. Headache in hypothyroidism. Prevalence and outcome under thyroid hormone therapy. Cephalalgia 1998;18:687–9.
64. Bigal ME, Sheftell FD, Tepper S. Chronic daily headache: identification of factors associated with induction and transformation. Headache 2002;42:575–81.
65. Tepper DE, Tepper SJ, Sheftell FD, et al. Headache attributed to hypothyroidism. Curr Pain Headache Rep 2007;11:304–9.
66. Arafah B, Prunty D, Ybarra J, et al. The dominant role of increased intrasellar pressure in the pathogenesis hypopituitarism, hyperprolactinemia, and headache in patients with pituitary adenomas. J Clin Endocrinol Metab 2000;85: 1789–93.
67. Drescher MJ, Elstein Y. Prophylactic COX-2 inhibitor: an end to the Yom Kippur headache. Headache 2006;46:1487–91.
68. Kundin JE. Yom Kippur headache. Neurology 1996;47:854.
69. Awada A, al Jumah M. The first-of-Ramadan headache. Headache 1999;39: 490–3.
70. Lipton RB, Lowenkopf T, Bajwa ZH, et al. Cardiac cephalgia: a treatable form of exertional headache. Neurology 1997;49:813–6.
71. Chen SP, Fuh JL, Yu WC, et al. Cardiac cephalalgia: case series and review of the literature with new ICDH-II criteria revisited. Eur Neurol 2004;24:231–4.
72. Wei JH, Wang HF. Cardiac cephalalgia: case reports and review. Cephalalgia 2008;28:892–6.
73. Martinez H, Rangel-Guerra R, Canut-Martinez L, et al. Cardiac headache: hemicranial cephalalgia as the sole manifestation of coronary ischemia. Headache 2002;42:1029–32.
74. Seow VK, Chong CF, Wang TF, et al. Severe explosive headache: a sole presentation of acute myocardial infarction in a young man. Am J Emerg Med 2007; 25(2):250–1.
75. Bini A, Evangelista A, Castellini P, et al. Cardiac cephalalgia. J Headache Pain 2009;10:3–9.
76. Bigal M, Gladstone J. The Metabolic headaches. Curr Pain Headache Rep 2008;12:292–5.

The Neck and Headaches

Nikolai Bogduk, MD, PhD, DSc

KEYWORDS

- Headache • Cervical • Cervicogenic • Diagnosis • Treatment

KEY POINTS

- The mechanism of cervicogenic headache is convergence between cervical afferents and trigeminal or cervical afferents in the dorsal horn of the C1-3 segments of the spinal cord.
- No clinical features have been validated for the diagnosis of cervicogenic headache.
- Definitive diagnosis requires evidence of a cervical source of pain, usually by the application of controlled, diagnostic blocks.
- The C2-3 zygapophysial joint is the most common source of cervicogenic headache to have been identified.
- Of conservative therapies, the best evidence supports exercise, with or without manual therapy.
- Headache stemming from the C2-3 or C3-4 zygapophysial joint can be successfully treated with thermal radiofrequency neurotomy.

CASE STUDY

Patient 001 was a 23-year-old female nurse, who attributed the onset of her headaches to prolonged periods of wearing heavy lead aprons in a radiology suite. Her headache was constant and centered on the right occipital region, spreading to the forehead and right orbit. The headaches had persisted for 3 years and were not relieved by physical therapy or analgesics. The patient could not work and was involved in a worker's compensation claim. Examination revealed tenderness maximal over the C2-3 region of the cervical spine; headache was aggravated by rotation of the head. The headache was completely relieved by anesthetizing the right third occipital nerve. Repeat blocks, on 3 occasions, consistently relieved the headache completely, in accordance with the duration of action of the agents used: lignocaine or bupivacaine. Intra-articular injection of steroids temporarily relieved her headache for a few weeks, whenever they were used as a palliative measure. Thermal radiofrequency third occipital neurotomy completely relieved her headaches, for 9 months in the first instance. On recurrence of the headache, repeat neurotomy relieved the headache for 12 months after the first repeat, and then 14 months after the second repeat.

Disclosure: The author has nothing to declare.
Newcastle Bone and Joint Institute, Royal Newcastle Centre, University of Newcastle, PO Box 664J, Newcastle, New South Wales 2300, Australia
E-mail address: vicki.caesar@hnehealth.nsw.gov.au

Neurol Clin 32 (2014) 471–487
http://dx.doi.org/10.1016/j.ncl.2013.11.005   **neurologic.theclinics.com**

Having been relieved of her headache, the patient completed a university entrance examination, and then a university degree, before returning to full-time employment. Yearly repeat neurotomy has kept her free of headache.

DEFINITION

Pain arising from the upper cervical spine may be referred into regions of the head. The patient may be unaware of a cervical problem, and headache becomes the presenting feature. Technically, such headaches should be classified as referred pain from the cervical spine, but the term of reference that has largely been adopted in the literature, and in clinical practice, is cervicogenic headache.[1–4]

MECHANISM

The anatomic basis of cervicogenic headache is convergence, onto second-order neurons in the C1-C3 segments of the spinal cord, between nociceptive afferents of the first division of the trigeminal nerve and nociceptive afferents of the C1, C2, and C3 spinal nerves.[5] Convergence between trigeminal and cervical afferents explains referral of pain from cervical sources to the forehead, orbit, and temporal regions of the head. Convergence between other cervical afferents and those of C2 explains referral of pain to the occiput and parietal regions.

Physiologic convergence has been shown in laboratory animals, between trigeminal afferents from the dura mater of the skull and cervical afferents in the greater occipital nerve.[6–9] The convergence largely involves Aδ and C fibers, onto neurons in laminae I, II, V, and VI of the dorsal horn at C2. Stimulation of trigeminal afferents sensitizes the response to cervical input, and stimulation of cervical afferents sensitizes trigeminal input.

In human volunteers, pain in the head has been evoked experimentally by electrical stimulation of the dorsal rootlets of C1[10] and by noxious stimulation of the greater occipital nerve[11] or the suboccipital muscles of the neck.[12–15] Noxious stimulation of the C2-3 intervertebral disk, but not lower disks, produces pain in the occipital region.[16,17] Distending the C2-3 zygapophysial joint with injections of contrast medium produces pain in the occipital region,[18] as does distending the lateral atlantoaxial joint or the atlanto-occipital joint.[19] All segments from the occiput to C4-5 are capable of producing referred pain to the occiput, but referral to the forehead and orbital regions more commonly occurs from segments C1 and C2.[13]

In patients with suspected cervicogenic headache, headache can be relieved by anesthetizing the C2-3 zygapophysial joint[20–22] or the lateral atlantoaxial joint.[23–28] The C2-3 zygapophysial joint is the most common source,[22,27–29] followed by the lateral atlantoaxial joint,[27,28] and occasionally, the C3-4 zygapophysial joint.[27,29,30]

From a given joint, pain can be perceived in various regions of the head, but certain trends are evident (**Fig. 1**).[27] Pain from C2-3 tends to be perceived across the lateral occipital region and into the forehead and orbital region. Pain from C1-2 also tends to gravitate to the orbital region but otherwise more often occurs in the vertex or around the ear. Pain from C3-4 tends to focus in the suboccipital region and upper cervical spine; when it does spread to the head, it is largely restricted to the posterior regions, sparing the forehead and orbit.

CLINICAL FEATURES

The essential clinical feature of cervicogenic headache is dull, aching pain perceived in some combination of the occipital, temporal, parietal, frontal, or orbital regions of

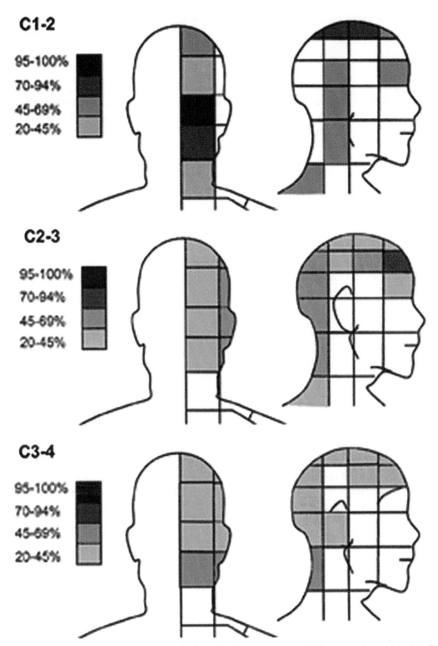

Fig. 1. Maps of the frequency with which pain from the synovial joints indicated is distributed to various regions of the head. (*From* Cooper G, Bailey B, Bogduk N. Cervical zygapophysial joint pain maps. Pain Med 2007;8:344–53; with permission.)

the head. Although a cervical source of pain is necessary for the diagnosis, its features may be cryptic or elusive. Certain, putatively distinctive, clinical features have been listed,[31–33] but none has been validated,[1–4] and none has been accepted by the International Headache Society in its taxonomy.[34] As a result, cervicogenic headache is essentially a headache for which a cervical source of pain needs to be shown.

DISTINCTIONS

Although technically a form of cervicogenic headache, because they involve a cervical nerve, 2 conditions are distinguished from common, or idiopathic, cervicogenic headache, by their unique, clinical features and pathology. Both involve the C2 spinal nerve.

Headache is a feature of neck-tongue syndrome, but its cardinal and distinctive feature is numbness of the tongue on rotating the head.[35] The numbness is caused by stretching of cervical afferents from the hypoglossal nerve by a subluxating lateral atlantoaxial joint; the temporary headache is probably caused by strain of the joint.[36]

C2 neuralgia is distinguished by intermittent, lancinating pain into the occiput, which may be accompanied by lacrimation and ciliary injection.[37] The condition can be caused by various disorders that affect the C2 spinal nerve where it runs behind the lateral atlantoaxial joint. Inflammatory disorders of the joint may result in the nerve becoming incorporated in the fibrotic changes of chronic inflammation.[38–40] Otherwise, the C2 spinal nerve can be affected by meningioma,[41] neurinoma,[42] anomalous vertebral arteries,[39] and venous abnormalities, ranging from single to densely interwoven, dilated veins surrounding the C2 spinal nerve and its roots[43] to U-shaped arterial loops or angiomas compressing the C2 dorsal root ganglion.[38,39,43]

So-called occipital neuralgia is a variously and poorly defined entity that was a popular, anecdotal diagnosis of occipital headache in the past. However, no explanation has been provided for why a disorder of a cutaneous nerve should cause deep, dull, aching pain; no pathology has been proved; and no controlled studies of diagnosis or treatment have been published.[2–4] Some cases in the past may have been instances of C2 neuralgia before that entity was defined; other cases may have been examples of referred pain from upper cervical skeletal structures.

SOURCES

The neuroanatomy of cervicogenic headache dictates that any of the structures innervated by the C1-C3 spinal nerves could be a source of headache.[2–4] These structures include the posterior neck muscles, the C2-3 and C3-4 zygapophysial joints, the atlantoaxial joints, the C2-3 and C3-4 intervertebral disks, the dura mater of the upper cervical spine, and the vertebral artery. Importantly, the dura mater and vessels of the posterior cranial fossa are innervated by cervical nerves, and disorders of these structures are critical in the differential diagnosis of cervicogenic headache. Similarly, for present purposes, the common carotid artery can also be considered a cervical structure.

From time to time, structures below C3 have been implicated as a source of cervicogenic headache, but the evidence is indirect. The structures for which there is the most abundant and most rigorous evidence lie within the catchment of the C1-C3 spinal nerves.

CAUSES

In conventional pathology terms, many causes of cervicogenic headache have been reported, but each in small numbers. Pathologically specific causes underlie only a few cases.

Accepted as possible causes of cervicogenic headache are tumors and infections of the upper cervical spine,[34] but these are rare. Also accepted is rheumatoid arthritis of the upper cervical joints, but this diagnosis arises in patients with manifest arthritis elsewhere in the limbs. Theoretically, rheumatoid arthritis or gout might present initially in the neck, but such cases have not been reported in the headache literature. A case report warns that metastasis to a cervical lymph node can cause cervicogenic headache.[44]

Although, in the past, congenital anomalies have been listed in the differential diagnosis of cervicogenic headache, there is no evidence to implicate them so.[2–4] Likewise, trigger points in the upper cervical muscles have been advanced as a cause of cervicogenic headache, but no controlled studies have vindicated this contention.

The C2-3 intervertebral disk has been implicated in several studies,[16,17,45] as a source of cervicogenic headache, but the pathology that renders a cervical disk painful has not been established. Several studies have implicated the lateral atlantoaxial joint as a source.[23–26] In posttraumatic cases, the responsible lesions might include capsular rupture, intra-articular hemorrhage, and bruising of intra-articular meniscoids, or small fractures through the superior articular process of the axis.[46]

The most extensively, and most rigorously, studied form of cervicogenic headache is pain from the C2-3 zygapophysial joint, mediated by the third occipital nerve, and therefore known as third occipital headache.[20] Studies in experimental animals have shown that zygapophysial joints can become a source of persistent, nociceptive pain when subject to submaximal strain injuries, such as whiplash.[47,48] The lesion affects the capsule of the joint, but is not manifest radiographically as arthopathy. Studies using controlled diagnostic blocks have shown that in 53% of patients with headache after whiplash, their pain can be traced to a C2-3 zygapophysial joint.[22] This figure renders the C2-3 zygapophysial joint the most common source of cervicogenic headache, with microscopic capsular injury being the pathology.

DIAGNOSIS

The essential requirement for the diagnosis of cervicogenic headache is a cervical source or cervical cause for the pain. The International Headache Society explains that this diagnosis is typically not possible using a conventional approach to the diagnosis of headache, relying on history, physical examination, or medical imaging (**Box 1**).[34] Controlled diagnostic blocks are required to establish a cervical source of pain.[34]

Certain clinical features can be used to suspect cervicogenic headache with different certainties of diagnosis (**Box 2**).[49] A diagnosis of possible cervicogenic headache can be entertained if patients have unilateral headache and pain starting in the neck. Satisfying any 3 additional criteria promotes the diagnosis to probable cervicogenic headache. The clinical features that most strongly indicate cervicogenic headache are pain radiating to the shoulder and arm; varying duration or fluctuating continuous pain; moderate, nonthrobbing pain; and history of neck trauma.[49]

A definitive diagnosis can be established using controlled, diagnostic blocks, protocols for which have been defined.[50–52] Such blocks include intra-articular blocks of the lateral atlantoaxial joint (**Fig. 2**), blocks of the third occipital nerve to anesthetize the C2-3 zygapophysial joint (**Fig. 3**), and blocks of the medial branches of the C3 and C4 dorsal rami, which innervate the C3-4 zygapophysial joint. Suitable controls include using local anesthetic agents with different durations of action, or injections of normal saline, or anesthetizing an adjacent structure that is not the source of pain.[50–52] To be convincing, diagnostic blocks should completely relieve the headache whenever the target structure is anesthetized with an active agent, with relief lasting for the duration of action of the agent used, and no relief if normal saline is used, or if an alternate structure is anesthetized.

> **Box 1**
> **Diagnostic criteria for cervicogenic headache, as proposed by the International Headache Society**
>
> *Diagnostic Criteria*
>
> A. Pain referred from a source in the neck and perceived in 1 or more regions of the head and/or face, fulfilling criteria C and D
>
> B. Clinical, laboratory, and/or imaging evidence of a disorder or lesion within the cervical spine or soft tissues of the neck known to be, or generally accepted as, a valid cause of headache[1]
>
> C. Evidence that the pain can be attributed to the neck disorder or lesion based on at least 1 of the following:
>
>   1. Demonstration of clinical signs that implicate a source of pain in the neck[2]
>
>   2. Abolition of headache following diagnostic blockade of a cervical structure or its nerve supply using placebo- or other adequate controls[3]
>
> D. Pain resolves within 3 months after successful treatment of the causative disorder or lesion
>
> *Notes*
>
> 1. Tumors, fractures, infections, and rheumatoid arthritis of the upper cervical spine have not been validated formally as causes of headache, but are nevertheless accepted as valid causes when demonstrated to be so in individual cases. Cervical spondylosis and osteochondritis are NOT accepted as valid causes fulfilling criterion B. When myofascial tender spots are, the headache should be coded under 2. *Tension-type headache*.
>
> 2. Clinical signs acceptable for criterion C1 must have demonstrated reliability and validity. The future task is the identification of such reliable and valid operational tests. Clinical features such as neck pain, focal neck tenderness, history of neck trauma, mechanical exacerbation of pain, unilaterality, coexisting shoulder pain, reduced range of motion in the neck, nuchal onset, nausea, vomiting, photophobia, and so forth are not unique to cervicogenic headache. These may be features of cervicogenic headache, but they do not define relationship between the disorder and the source of the headache.
>
> 3. Abolition of headache means complete relief of headache, indicated by a score of zero on a visual analogue scale (VAS). Nevertheless, acceptable as fulfilling criterion C2 is ≥90% reduction in pain to a level of <5 on a 100-point VAS.
>
> *From* Headache Classification Committee of the International Headache Society (IHS). The International Classification of Headache Disorders, 3rd edition (beta version). Cephalgia 2013;33(9):629–808; with permission.

Target structures can be selected from epidemiologic data. Contemporary data implicate the C2-3 zygapophysial joint as the most common, and therefore most likely, source of cervicogenic headache.[22,27–30] Next most likely are the lateral atlantoaxial joint and the C3-4 zygapophysial joint. These pretest probabilities may change in the future as diagnostic blocks of the lateral atlantoaxial joints become more widely used. If synovial joints prove not to be the source of pain, the C2-3 intervertebral disk can be tested using diskography.[16,17,45]

A significant feature of patients in whom third occipital nerve blocks have been positive is that all had a history of trauma. This finding reinforces history of trauma as a cardinal clinical feature for probable cervicogenic headache (see **Box 2**). No studies have shown that third occipital headache occurs without a history of trauma.

Differential Diagnosis

Certain serious conditions need to be considered in the differential diagnosis of cervicogenic headache. These conditions include space-occupying lesions of the posterior

---

Box 2
Criteria for identifying possible and probable cervicogenic headache, as proposed by Antonaci and colleagues

1. Unilateral headache without side-shift

2. Symptoms and signs of neck involvement:

   Pain triggered by neck movement or sustained awkward posture and/or external pressure of the posterior neck or occipital region

   Ipsilateral neck, shoulder, and arm pain

   Reduced range of motion

3. Pain episodes of varying duration or fluctuating continuous pain

4. Moderate, nonexcruciating pain, usually of a nonthrobbing nature

5. Pain starting in the neck, spreading to oculofrontotemporal areas

6. Anesthetic blockades abolish the pain transiently provided complete anesthesia is obtained or sustained neck trauma a relatively short time prior to the onset

7. Various attack-related phenomena: autonomic symptoms and signs, nausea, vomiting, ispilateral edema, and flushing in the periocular area, dizziness, photophobia, phonophobia, blurred vision in the ipsilateral eye

From Antonaci F, Ghirmai S, Bono S, et al. Cervicogenic headache: evaluation of the original diagnostic criteria. Cephalalgia 2001;21:573–83; with permission.

---

cranial fossa and aneurysms of the vertebral artery or internal carotid artery. Technically, these conditions constitute a form of cervicogenic headache, in that the pain is mediated by cervical nerves, and early in their evolution, these conditions can cause headache that is indistinguishable clinically from other forms of cervicogenic headache. However, they are distinguished from conventional cervicogenic headache by having detectable lesions that can have serious neurologic sequelae.

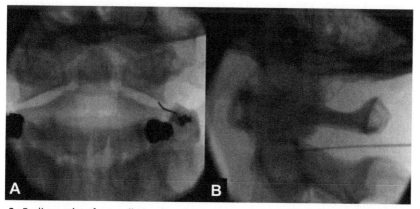

Fig. 2. Radiographs of a needle in place for performing an intra-articular block of the right lateral atlantoaxial joint. (*A*) Anteroposterior view. (*B*) Lateral view. (*From* International Spine Intervention Society. Lateral atlantoaxial joint blocks. In: Bogduk N, editor. Practice guidelines for spinal diagnostic and treatment procedures. 2nd edition. San Francisco (CA): International Spinal Intervention Society; 2013. p. 43; with permission.)

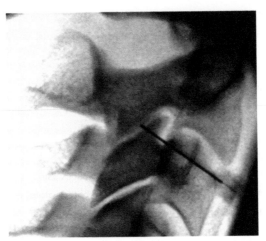

Fig. 3. A lateral radiograph of a needle in place for performing a third occipital nerve block. (*From* International Spine Intervention Society. Third occipital nerve blocks. In: Bogduk N, editor. Practice guidelines for spinal diagnostic and treatment procedures. 2nd edition. San Francisco (CA): International Spinal Intervention Society; 2013. p. 155; with permission.)

Space-occupying lesions of the posterior cranial fossa are distinguished from cervicogenic headache by the neurologic signs and increased intracranial pressure that they cause. However, early in the presentation, these signs might still be developing. Therefore, practitioners need to be alert to the subsequent onset of neurologic signs that declare these conditions.

Sixty percent of patients with aneurysms of the vertebral artery or the internal carotid artery present with headache as the sole feature.[53–56] Within a matter of a few days, aneurysms typically declare themselves by the onset of neurovascular features. However, during this period, the headache may be misdiagnosed as common cervicogenic headache, unless the practitioner is alert to the possibility of aneurysm. This dilemma is particularly relevant for practitioners who perform manipulative therapy for the neck. In the event of a subsequent stroke, it is impossible to determine if the aneurysm and stroke were caused by the manipulation or if it was a spontaneous aneurysm that would have caused stroke irrespective of the aneurysm.

Imaging

There is no evidence that medical imaging is diagnostic of any cause of cervicogenic headache. Imaging is indicated only in patients who show neurologic signs. However, in that context, the indication for imaging is the neurologic signs, not the pain.

In patients with cardiovascular risk factors or a history of neck distortion or cervical manipulation, aneurysm needs to be considered. For this entity, magnetic resonance angiography is the appropriate investigation.

Manual Examination

Manual therapists contend that they can diagnose symptomatic joints by examining the cervical spine. Previously, this belief was based on 1 small study, which ostensibly validated manual examination of the cervical spine.[57] However, that study has now been refuted by a larger study,[58] using more rigorous diagnostic criteria and more rigorous statistical analysis. Manual examination, therefore, lacks a proven foundation as a diagnostic test for cervicogenic headache.

TREATMENT

Two approaches have been used for the treatment of cervicogenic headache. Conservative therapies have been used in patients in whom a clinical diagnosis of cervicogenic headache was made, based on diagnostic criteria that have not been validated. Consequently, not all patients who were treated may have had a cervical source of headache. Furthermore, these therapies were applied without a specified source of pain being treated. Targeted treatments have been used in patients in whom the putative source of pain was identified with various degrees of rigor, ranging from clinical suspicion to single diagnostic blocks or controlled diagnostic blocks.

CONSERVATIVE THERAPY

No drugs have been proved to be effective for cervicogenic headache. Infliximab has been tested but not in a controlled study.[59] Eighty percent of patients treated with transcutaneous electrical nerve stimulation reported at least 60% reduction in their headache index, at 1 month,[60] but no longer-term data are available, and none from controlled studies. Injections of onabotulinum toxin are no more effective than placebo.[61]

Manual therapy has been advocated for headache believed to be of cervical origin, but most of the literature consists of case reports or case series.[62] The few randomized controlled studies have provided follow-up of only 1 or 3 weeks, and systematic reviews[62–64] have variously found the evidence for manual therapy to be limited, or of varying quality, with conflicting results, rendering the efficacy of manual therapy uncertain.

The largest and strongest study of conservative therapy for cervicogenic headache[65] showed that treatment with manual therapy, specific exercises, or manual therapy plus exercises were each significantly more effective at reducing headache frequency and intensity than was no specific care by a general practitioner. However, manual therapy alone was not more effective than exercises alone, and combining the 2 interventions did not achieve better outcomes. Seventy-six percent of patients achieved greater than 50% reduction in headache frequency at the 7-week follow-up, and 35% achieved complete relief. At 12 months, 72% had greater than 50% reduction in headache frequency, but the proportion who had complete relief was not reported. Corresponding figures for reduction in pain intensity were not reported.

Targeted Treatment

Various interventions have targeted the greater occipital nerve in the treatment of cervicogenic headache. These interventions include injections and various surgical procedures.

Greater occipital nerve

Ninety percent of patients treated with an injection of 160 mg of depot methylprednisolone onto the greater occipital nerve obtained relief, but only for 10 to 77 days.[66] Surgical liberation of the nerve initially relieved headache in 80% of cases but the relief had a median duration of only 3 to 6 months.[67] Excision of the greater occipital nerve provided relief in some 70% of patients, but for a median duration of only 244 days.[68]

In 1 study, patients were selected for surgery if they satisfied the clinical criteria for cervicogenic headache and obtained relief of headache from diagnostic blockade of the C2 spinal nerve.[69] They underwent decompression and microsurgical neurolysis of the C2 spinal nerve, with excision of scar and ligamentous and vascular elements that compressed the nerve. Fourteen of 31 patients were rendered pain-free. Details on the remaining patients are incomplete, but ostensibly, 51% gained what was called adequate relief and 11% suffered a recurrence.

Pulsed radiofrequency therapy applied to the greater occipital nerve is no more effective than an injection of methylprednisolone and bupivacaine onto the nerve, with 9 of 15 patients reporting 50% relief at 9 months after pulsed radiofrequency and 5 of 15 patients having the same outcome after injection.[70] Otherwise, the application of pulsed radiofrequency to the C2 ganglion has been described only in case reports.[71,72]

A novel intervention has recently been reported. It involves the injection of 3 to 10 mL of processed, autologous adipose tissue onto the greater occipital nerve.[73] Nineteen of 24 patients were said to have had a good clinical response (not otherwise defined) at 3 months, with 7 suffering a recurrence by 6 months.

Lateral atlantoaxial joint

In 1 study, 32 patients with headache suspected to arise from a lateral atlantoaxial joint were treated with intra-articular injection of 1 mL of a mixture of bupivacaine and triamcinolone.[74] At 3 months, 25% had at least 50% relief of pain, and 16.6% had sustained relief at 9 months. In the absence of controls, a placebo effect cannot be excluded.

Another study did not indicate how patients were selected but 86 were treated with intra-articular pulsed radiofrequency.[75] At least 50% relief was reported by 43 patients at 6 months and by 38 patients at 12 months.

For patients whose headache can be relieved by lateral atlantoaxial joint blocks, an option for treatment is arthrodesis of the joint. The surgical literature attests to complete relief of pain being achieved, albeit in small numbers of patients, for more than 2 years.[76–78]

C2-3 disk

In those patients in whom the source of headache can be traced to the C2-3 intervertebral disk, disk excision and anterior cervical fusion reportedly can be effective.[45] Because this intervention is surgical in nature and uncommonly used for headache, controlled trials are unlikely to be conducted. Anecdotal data, therefore, will remain the highest level of evidence available.

Zygapophysial joints

For headache stemming from the C2-3 zygapophysial joint, 1 study reported that at 19 months after an intra-articular injection of steroids into the joint, 11% of patients were free of pain.[79] Otherwise, most studies of third occipital headache and headache from C3-4 have addressed the effectiveness of thermal radiofrequency neurotomy.

Radiofrequency Neurotomy

Thermal radiofrequency neurotomy is a procedure in which conduction along a nerve is blocked by coagulating it with an electrode inserted percutaneously. The rationale for the procedures is that if pain can be relieved temporarily by anesthetizing a nerve, the relief can be prolonged by coagulating the nerve. The critical indication for thermal radiofrequency neurotomy is, therefore, complete relief of pain after controlled, diagnostic blocks of the target nerve or nerves. In the context of cervicogenic headache, the target nerve is the third occipital nerve (**Fig. 4**) or the medial branches of the C3-4 dorsal rami, in patients whose headache can be relieved by anesthetizing one or other of these nerves. A randomized, placebo-controlled trial[80] has shown that responses to thermal

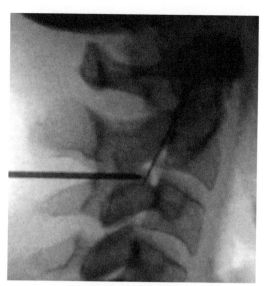

Fig. 4. A lateral radiograph of an electrode in place for performing thermal radiofrequency neurotomy of a right third occipital nerve.

radiofrequency neurotomy are not caused by placebo effects. Its success in the treatment of headache, therefore, cannot be dismissed as a placebo effect.

Three studies purport to show that radiofrequency neurotomy is not effective.[81–83] However, they do not provide evidence to this effect, for several reasons. In all of these studies, patients were selected on clinical criteria. So, it is not evident if all patients had cervicogenic headache, and if they did, what the source of pain was. Second, the neurotomy technique used has never been validated. So, it is not evident if treatment was technically adequate. Third, neurotomy was performed at segmental levels (C3-C6) that have never been incriminated as a common source of headache. So, even if technically adequate, the treatment may have been at a clinically irrelevant segmental level and, therefore, tantamount to a sham treatment. Jointly and several, these features preclude these studies from providing valid evidence on the treatment of cervicogenic headache.

Totally opposite results are obtained if a diagnosis is carefully established using controlled diagnostic blocks, and meticulous surgical technique is used. For patients in whom diagnostic blocks indicate that the C2-3 zygapophysial joint is the source of pain, it is possible to denervate that joint by radiofrequency neurotomy of the third occipital nerve. If the source of pain lies in the C3-4 joint, diagnostic blocks of the medial branches of C3 and C4 should relieve the headache, and those nerves can be coagulated. The procedure involves placing an electrode parallel to the target nerve (see **Fig. 4**) and using it to coagulate the nerve.

If patients are selected using controlled, third occipital nerve blocks, with the diagnostic criterion being complete relief of headache, and if meticulous technique is carefully used to coagulate the nerve, complete relief of headache can be achieved in 88% of patients after thermal radiofrequency neurotomy.[84] The median duration of relief was 297 days, with some patients still having continuing relief at the time of review. These results have been corroborated by a second[85] and third study.[86]

Similar outcomes have been reported in patients whose headache could be relieved by controlled blocks of the C3-4 medial branches.[87] After thermal radiofrequency

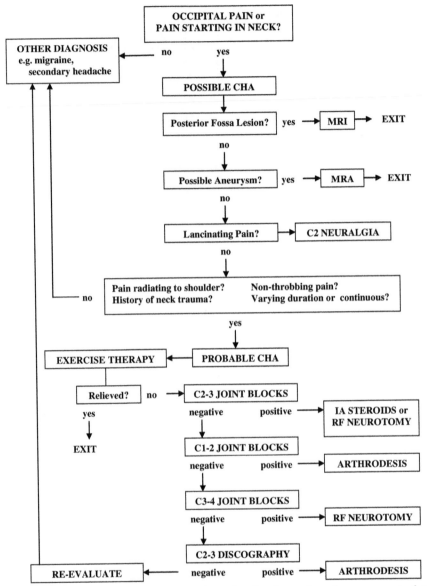

Fig. 5. A flow chart depicting a clinical pathway for the diagnosis and management of cervicogenic headache. CHA, cervicogenic headache; IA steroids, intra-articular steroids; MRA, magnetic resonance angiography; MRI, magnetic resonance imaging; RF neurotomy, radiofrequency neurotomy.

neurotomy of these nerves, more than 70% of patients maintained at lest 75% relief of their headache at 6 months and 12 months.

For patients in whom headaches recur, relief can be reinstated by repeating the neurotomy. By repeating neurotomy as required, some patients have been able to maintain relief of their headache for longer than 2 years.[84]

CLINICAL PATHWAY

A clinical pathway has been recommended for the management of cervicogenic headache.[3,4] The pathway embraces interventions for which there is at least reasonable evidence of efficacy coupled with safety but abjures interventions that are anecdotal or for which there is little or trivial evidence (**Fig. 5**).

The first half of the pathway pertains to formulating a diagnosis. Occipital pain or pain in the neck invites a diagnosis of possible cervicogenic headache. Thereafter, important differential diagnoses should be considered and excluded. Subsequently, additional clinical features can promote the diagnosis to one of probable cervicogenic headache, which is sufficient to pursue conservative therapy.

Of conservative therapies, there is strong evidence for only 1 intervention, which is exercise therapy, coupled or not with manual therapy. Most patients in primary care should benefit from this intervention.

Patients who do not benefit can be investigated more intensively. Because the pretest probability is highest for C2-3 zygapophysial joint pain, investigations should start with third occipital nerve blocks to test for this condition. If controlled blocks are positive, the patient can be treated with radiofrequency neurotomy. Intra-articular injection of steroids is a plausible, less destructive option, but lacks a definitive evidence-base.

If C2-3 blocks are negative, the next step is to test for lateral atlantoaxial joint pain with C1-2 blocks. If these blocks are positive, treatment by arthrodesis can be considered, because this is the only treatment of lateral atlantoaxial joint pain that has been found to provide complete relief of pain. Palliative treatment, in the form of intra-articular injections of steroids, or pulsed radiofrequency, might be an alternative, but with the understanding that these interventions may be no more than a placebo.

If C1-2 blocks are negative, the C3-4 zygapophysial joint should be tested. If blocks are positive, treatment is possible with C3-4 medial branch radiofrequency neurotomy. If C3-4 blocks are negative, the only remaining option is to test for C2-3 disk pain by diskography. If diskography is positive, treatment by arthrodesis can be considered.

If diskography and blocks of the joints of the upper 3 cervical segments all prove negative, there are no further, established investigations to pursue. The patient and their management should be revaluated. Either the diagnosis is not cervicogenic headache, or the patient has a cervical cause of pain that cannot be pinpointed using available technology. The options may be to treat the patient palliatively, by providing nonspecific pain relief, or to enroll them in whatever ethics-approved study is available of procedures that have experimental or investigational status. Ethics-approved studies guarantee patient safety and protect them from unwittingly being subjects to practitioners who are no more than experimenting with untested and unproven procedures, without disclosing to the patient that they are doing so.

REFERENCES

1. Bogduk N. Distinguishing primary headache disorders from cervicogenic headache: clinical and therapeutic implications. Headache Current 2005;2:27–36.
2. Bogduk N, Bartsch T. Headaches of cervical origin: focus on anatomy and physiology. In: Goadsby PJ, Silberstein SD, Dodick DW, editors. Chronic daily headache for clinicians. London: BC Decker; 2005. p. 369–81.
3. Bogduk N, Bartsch T. Cervicogenic headache. In: Silberstein SD, Lipton RB, Dodick DW, editors. Wolff's headache. 8th edition. New York: Oxford University Press; 2008. p. 551–70.

4. Bogduk N, Govind J. Cervicogenic headache: an assessment of the evidence on clinical diagnosis, invasive tests, and treatment. Lancet Neurol 2009;8:959–68.
5. Kerr FW. Structural relation of the trigeminal spinal tract to upper cervical roots and the solitary nucleus in the cat. Exp Neurol 1961;4:134–48.
6. Kerr FW. Trigeminal nerve volleys. Arch Neurol 1961;5:171–8.
7. Angus-Leppan H, Lambert GA, Michalicek J. Convergence of occipital nerve and superior sagittal sinus input in the cervical spinal cord of the cat. Cephalalgia 1997;17:625–30.
8. Bartsch T, Goadsby PJ. Stimulation of the greater occipital nerve induces increased central excitability of dural afferent input. Brain 2002;125:1496–509.
9. Bartsch T, Goadsby PJ. Increased responses in trigeminocervical nociceptive neurons to cervical input after stimulation of the dura mater. Brain 2003;126:1801–13.
10. Kerr FW. A mechanism to account for frontal headache in cases of posterior fossa tumors. J Neurosurg 1962;18:605–9.
11. Piovesan EJ, Kowacs PA, Tatsui CE, et al. Referred pain after painful stimulation of the greater occipital nerve in humans: evidence of convergence of cervical afferences on trigeminal nuclei. Cephalalgia 2001;21:107–9.
12. Cyriax J. Rheumatic headache. Br Med J 1938;193(2):1367–8.
13. Campbell DG, Parsons CM. Referred head pain and its concomitants. J Nerv Ment Dis 1944;99:544–51.
14. Feinstein B, Langton JB, Jameson RM, et al. Experiments on referred pain from deep somatic tissues. J Bone Joint Surg Am 1954;36A:981–97.
15. Wolff HG. Headache and other head pain. 2nd edition. New York: Oxford University Press; 1963. p. 582–616.
16. Schellhas KP, Smith MD, Gundry CR, et al. Cervical discogenic pain: prospective correlation of magnetic resonance imaging and discography in asymptomatic subjects and pain sufferers. Spine 1996;21:300–12.
17. Grubb SA, Kelly CK. Cervical discography: clinical implications from 12 years of experience. Spine 2000;25:1382–9.
18. Dwyer A, Aprill C, Bogduk N. Cervical zygapophysial joint pain patterns I: a study in normal volunteers. Spine 1990;15:453–7.
19. Dreyfuss P, Michaelsen M, Fletcher D. Atlanto-occipital and lateral atlanto-axial joint pain patterns. Spine 1994;19:1125–31.
20. Bogduk N, Marsland A. On the concept of third occipital headache. J Neurol Neurosurg Psychiatr 1986;49:775–80.
21. Bogduk N, Marsland A. The cervical zygapophysial joints as a source of neck pain. Spine 1988;13:610–7.
22. Lord S, Barnsley L, Wallis B, et al. Third occipital headache: a prevalence study. J Neurol Neurosurg Psychiatr 1994;57:1187–90.
23. Ehni G, Benner B. Occipital neuralgia and the C1-2 arthrosis syndrome. J Neurosurg 1984;61:961–5.
24. McCormick CC. Arthrography of the atlanto-axial (C1-C2) joints: technique and results. J Intervent Radiol 1987;2:9–13.
25. Busch E, Wilson PR. Atlanto-occipital and atlanto-axial injections in the treatment of headache and neck pain. Reg Anesth 1989;14(Suppl 2):45.
26. Aprill C, Axinn MJ, Bogduk N. Occipital headaches stemming from the lateral atlanto-axial (C1-2) joint. Cephalalgia 2003;22:15–22.
27. Cooper G, Bailey B, Bogduk N. Cervical zygapophysial joint pain maps. Pain Med 2007;8:344–53.

28. Yin W, Bogduk N. The nature of neck pain in a private pain clinic in the United States. Pain Med 2008;9:196–203.
29. Lord SM, Bogduk N. The cervical synovial joints as sources of post-traumatic headache. J Musculoskel Pain 1986;4:81–94.
30. Govind J, King W, Giles P, et al. Headaches and the cervical zygapophysial joints: a prevalence study. Syllabus of the 14th Annual Scientific Meeting of the International Spine Intervention Society. Salt Lake City, July 13–15, 2006. p. 169–71.
31. Sjaastad O, Saunte C, Hovdahl H, et al. "Cervicogenic" headache. An hypothesis. Cephalalgia 1983;3:249–56.
32. Sjaastad O, Fredriksen TA, Pfaffenrath V. Cervicogenic headache: diagnostic criteria. Headache 1990;30:725–6.
33. Sjaastad O, Fredriksen TA, Pfaffenrath V. Cervicogenic headache: diagnostic criteria. Headache 1998;38:442–5.
34. International Headache Society. The international classification of headache disorders, 2nd edition. Cephalalgia 2004;24(Suppl 1):115–6.
35. Lance JW, Anthony M. Neck tongue syndrome on sudden turning of the head. J Neurol Neurosurg Psychiatr 1980;19(43):97–101.
36. Bogduk N. An anatomical basis for neck tongue syndrome. J Neurol Neurosurg Psychiatr 1981;44:202–8.
37. Bogduk N. Pain of cranial nerve and cervical nerve origin other than primary neuralgias. In: Olesen J, Goadsby PJ, Ramadan NM, et al, editors. The headaches. 3rd edition. Philadelphia: Lippincott Williams & Wilkins; 2006. p. 1043–51.
38. Jansen J, Markakis E, Rama B, et al. Hemicranial attacks or permanent hemicrania–a sequel of upper cervical root compression. Cephalalgia 1989;9:123–30.
39. Jansen J, Bardosi A, Hildebrandt J, et al. Cervicogenic, hemicranial attacks associated with vascular irritation or compression of the cervical nerve root C2. Clinical manifestations and morphological findings. Pain 1989;39:203–12.
40. Poletti CE, Sweet WH. Entrapment of the C2 root and ganglion by the atlanto-epistrophic ligament: clinical syndrome and surgical anatomy. Neurosurgery 1990;27:288–91.
41. Kuritzky A. Cluster headache-like pain caused by an upper cervical meningioma. Cephalalgia 1984;4:185–6.
42. Sharma RR, Parekh HC, Prabhu S, et al. Compression of the C-2 root by a rare anomalous ectatic vertebral artery. J Neurosurg 1993;78:669–72.
43. Hildebrandt J, Jansen J. Vascular compression of the C2 and C3 roots–yet another cause of chronic intermittent hemicrania? Cephalalgia 1984;4:167–70.
44. Kim HH, Kim YC, Park YH, et al. Cervicogenic headache arising from hidden metastasis to cervical lymph node adjacent to the superficial cervical plexus–a case report. Korean J Anesthesiol 2011;60:134–7.
45. Schofferman J, Garges K, Goldthwaite N, et al. Upper cervical anterior diskectomy and fusion improves discogenic cervical headaches. Spine 2002;27:2240–4.
46. Schonstrom N, Twomey L, Taylor J. The lateral atlanto-axial joints and their synovial folds: an in vitro study of soft tissue injuries and fractures. J Trauma 1993;35:886–92.
47. Bogduk N. On cervical zygapophysial joint pain after whiplash. Spine 2011;36:S194–9.
48. Curatolo M, Bogduk N, Ivancic PC, et al. The role of tissue damage in whiplash-associated disorders. Spine 2011;36:S309–15.

49. Antonaci F, Ghirmai S, Bono S, et al. Cervicogenic headache: evaluation of the original diagnostic criteria. Cephalalgia 2001;21:573–83.

50. International Spine Intervention Society. Lateral atlanto-axial joint blocks. In: Bogduk N, editor. Practice guidelines for spinal diagnostic and treatment procedures. 2nd edition. San Francisco (CA): International Spinal Intervention Society; 2013. p. 35–62.

51. International Spine Intervention Society. Third occipital nerve blocks. In: Bogduk N, editor. Practice guidelines for spinal diagnostic and treatment procedures. 2nd edition. San Francisco (CA): International Spinal Intervention Society; 2013. p. 141–63.

52. International Spine Intervention Society. Cervical medial branch blocks. In: Bogduk N, editor. Practice guidelines for spinal diagnostic and treatment procedures. 2nd edition. San Francisco (CA): International Spinal Intervention Society; 2013. p. 101–39.

53. Biousse V, D'Anglejan-Chatillon J, Massiou H, et al. Head pain in non-traumatic carotid artery dissection: a series of 65 patients. Cephalalgia 1994;14:33–6.

54. Silbert PL, Makri B, Schievink WI. Headache and neck pain in spontaneous internal carotid and vertebral artery dissections. Neurology 1995;45:1517–22.

55. Sturzenegger M. Headache and neck pain: the warning symptoms of vertebral artery dissection. Headache 1994;34:187–93.

56. Mokri B, Houser W, Sandok BA, et al. Spontaneous dissections of the vertebral arteries. Neurology 1988;38:880–5.

57. Jull G, Bogduk N, Marsland A. The accuracy of manual diagnosis for cervical zygapophysial joint pain syndromes. Med J Aust 1988;148:233–6.

58. King W, Lau P, Lees R, et al. The validity of manual examination in assessing patients with neck pain. Spine J 2007;7:22–6.

59. Martelletti P, van Suijlekom H. Cervicogenic headache. Practical approaches to therapy. CNS Drugs 2004;18:793–805.

60. Farina S, Granella F, Malferrari G, et al. Headache and cervical spine disorders: classification and treatment with transcutaneous electrical nerve stimulation. Headache 1986;26:431–3.

61. Linde M, Hagen K, Salvesen Ø, et al. Onabotulinum toxin A treatment of cervicogenic headache: a randomised, double-blind, placebo-controlled crossover study. Cephalalgia 2011;31:797–807.

62. Haldeman S, Dagenais S. Cervicogenic headaches: a critical review. Spine J 2001;1:31–46.

63. Posadzki P, Ernst E. Systematic reviews of spinal manipulations for headaches: an attempt to clear up the confusion. Headache 2011;51:1419–25.

64. Chaibi A, Russell MB. Manual therapies for cervicogenic headache: a systematic review. J Headache Pain 2012;13:351–9.

65. Jull G, Trott P, Potter H, et al. A randomized controlled trial of exercise and manipulative therapy for cervicogenic headache. Spine 2002;27:1835–43.

66. Anthony M. Cervicogenic headache: prevalence and response to local steroid therapy. Clin Exp Rheumatol 2000;18(Suppl 19):S59–64.

67. Bovim G, Fredriksen TA, Stolt-Nielsen A, et al. Neurolysis of the greater occipital nerve in cervicogenic headache. A follow up study. Headache 1992;32:175–9.

68. Anthony M. Headache and the greater occipital nerve. Clin Neurol Neurosurg 1992;94:297–301.

69. Pikus HJ, Phillips JM. Characteristics of patients successfully treated for cervicogenic headache by surgical decompression of the second cervical root. Headache 1995;35:621–9.

70. Garbhelink T, Michálek P, Adamus M. Pulsed radiofrequency therapy versus greater occipital nerve block in the management of refractory cervicogenic headache–a pilot study. Prague Med Rep 2011;112:279–87.

71. Zhang J, Shi DS, Wang R. Pulsed radiofrequency of the second cervical ganglion (C2) for the treatment of cervicogenic headache. J Headache Pain 2011;12:569–71.

72. Bovaira M, Peñarrocha M, Peñarrocha M, et al. Radiofrequency treatment of cervicogenic headache. Med Oral Patol Oral Cir Bucal 2013;18:e293–7.

73. Gaetani P, Klinger M, Levi D, et al. Treatment of chronic headache of cervical origin with lipostructure: an observational study. Headache 2013;53:507–13.

74. Narouze SN, Casanova J, Maekhail N. The longitudinal effectiveness of lateral atlantoaxial intra-articular steroid injection in the treatment of cervicogenic headache. Pain Med 2007;8:184–8.

75. Halim W, Chua NH, Vissers KC. Long-term pain relief of patients with cervicogenic headaches after pulsed radiofrequency application into the lateral atlantoaxial (C1-2) joint using an anterolateral approach. Pain Pract 2010;10:267–71.

76. Ghanayem AJ, Leventhal M, Bohlman HH. Osteoarthrosis of the atlanto-axial joints–long-term follow-up after treatment with arthrodesis. J Bone Joint Surg Am 1996;78A:1300–7.

77. Joseph B, Kumar B. Gallie's fusion for atlantoaxial arthrosis with occipital neuralgia. Spine 1994;19:454–5.

78. Schaeren S, Jeanneret B. Atlantoaxial osteoarthritis: case series and review of the literature. Eur Spine J 2005;14:501–6.

79. Slipman CW, Lipetz JS, Plastara CT, et al. Therapeutic zygapophyseal joint injections for headache emanating from the C2-3 joint. Am J Phys Med Rehabil 2001;80:182–8.

80. Haspeslagh SR, van Suijlekom HA, Lame IE, et al. Randomised controlled trial of cervical radiofrequency lesions as a treatment for cervicogenic headache. BMC Anesthesiol 2006;6:1.

81. Stovner LJ, Kolstad F, Helde G. Radiofrequency denervation of facet joints C2-C6 in cervicogenic headache: a randomised, double-blind, sham-controlled study. Cephalalgia 2004;24:821–30.

82. van Suijlekom HA, van Kleef M, Barendse GA, et al. Radiofrequency cervical zygapophyseal joint neurotomy for cervicogenic headaches: a prospective study of 15 patients. Funct Neurol 1998;13:297–303.

83. Govind J, King W, Bailey B, et al. Radiofrequency neurotomy for the treatment of third occipital headache. J Neurol Neurosurg Psychiatr 2003;74:88–93.

84. Barnsley L. Percutaneous radiofrequency neurotomy for chronic neck pain: outcomes in a series of consecutive patients. Pain Med 2005;6:282–6.

85. MacVicar J, Borowczyk J, MacVicar AM, et al. Cervical medial branch radiofrequency neurotomy in New Zealand. Pain Med 2012;13:647–54.

86. Lord SM, Barnsley L, Wallis BJ, et al. Percutaneous radio-frequency neurotomy for chronic cervical zygapophysial-joint pain. N Engl J Med 1996;335:1721–6.

87. Lee JB, Park JY, Park J, et al. Clinical efficacy of radiofrequency cervical zygapophyseal neurotomy in patients with chronic cervicogenic headache. J Korean Med Sci 2007;22:326–9.

An Update on Eye Pain for the Neurologist

Andrew G. Lee, MD[a,b,c,d,e,f,g,*], Nagham Al-Zubidi, MD[a],
Hilary A. Beaver, MD[a,b], Paul W. Brazis, MD[h,i]

KEYWORDS

- Eye pain • Headache syndromes • Ophthalmic neurologic syndromes
- Ocular and orbital disorders

KEY POINTS

- The practicing neurologist should be aware of the common causes of primary or referred eye pain.
- These entities include (1) ocular and orbital disorders that produce eye pain with a normal examination, (2) neurologic syndromes with predominantly ophthalmologic presentations, and (3) ophthalmologic presentations of selected headache syndromes.
- The neurologist should screen for specific symptoms and signs that should prompt ophthalmologic consultation.

INTRODUCTION

Pain in and around the eye with or without an associated headache is a relatively common presenting complaint to the neurologist. Although the main causes for eye pain are easily diagnosed by simple examination techniques that are readily available to a neurologist, sometimes the etiology is not as obvious and may require a referral to an ophthalmologist. This article summarizes and updates our prior review in *Neurologic Clinics*[1] on this topic and includes (1) ocular and orbital disorders that produce

The authors declare no conflict of interest.
[a] Department of Ophthalmology, The Methodist Hospital, Houston, TX, USA; [b] Department of Ophthalmology, Weill Cornell Medical College, New York, NY, USA; [c] Department of Neurology, Weill Cornell Medical College, New York, NY, USA; [d] Department of Neurosurgery, Weill Cornell Medical College, New York, NY, USA; [e] Department of Ophthalmology, The University of Texas Medical Branch, Galveston, TX, USA; [f] Department of Ophthalmology, The University of Iowa Hospitals and Clinics, Iowa City, IA, USA; [g] Department of Ophthalmology, Baylor College of Medicine, Houston, TX, USA; [h] Department of Ophthalmology, Mayo Clinic, Jacksonville, FL, USA; [i] Department of Neurology, Mayo Clinic, Jacksonville, FL, USA
* Corresponding author. The Department of Ophthalmology, The Methodist Hospital, 6560 Fannin Street, Scurlock 450, Houston, TX 77030.
E-mail address: AGLee@HoustonMethodist.org

Neurol Clin 32 (2014) 489–505
http://dx.doi.org/10.1016/j.ncl.2013.11.007
0733-8619/14/$ – see front matter © 2014 Elsevier Inc. All rights reserved.

neurologic.theclinics.com

Box 1
Red flags prompting ophthalmic referral for a patient who has eye pain

- New visual acuity, color vision defect, or visual field loss
- Relative afferent pupillary defect
- Extraocular muscle abnormality, ocular misalignment, or diplopia
- Proptosis
- Lid retraction or ptosis
- Conjunctival chemosis, injection, or redness
- Corneal opacity
- Hyphema or hypopyon
- Iris irregularity or nonreactive pupil
- Fundus abnormality (eg, retinal hemorrhages, optic disc edema, or optic atrophy)
- Recent intraocular surgery (<3 months)
- Recent ocular trauma

---

eye pain with a normal examination; (2) neurologic syndromes with predominantly ophthalmologic presentations; and (3) ophthalmologic presentations of selected headache syndromes.

A basic eye history and simple eye examination are critical for appropriate triage and referral purposes for the neurologist confronted by eye pain **Box 1**.[1] **Box 2** lists the common red flags that should prompt ophthalmologic referral.[1] In addition, specific characteristics of the eye pain, including onset, duration, timing, frequency, severity, and quality. **Box 3** lists some potentially urgent or emergent ocular conditions in the medical history that should prompt consideration for ophthalmologic referral.[1]

Most of the basic outpatient eye examinations for eye pain can be performed by the neurologist with a minimum of additional specialized equipment and the goal is to determine if any specific findings are present that should prompt ophthalmologic

---

Box 2
Specific history taking in eye pain

- Onset (acute, subacute, or chronic)
- Location (intraocular, retrobulbar, periocular, or frontal)
- Severity (on a scale of 1–10)
- Exacerbating or precipitating (eg, eye movement, sounds, lights, or position) factors
- Palliating factors (eg, lying down in a dark room)
- Radiation
- Quality and description of pain (eg, throbbing, sharp, or dull)
- Duration (seconds, minutes, hours, or days)
- Associated symptoms (eg, tearing, loss of vision, double vision, photophobia, discharge)
- Frequency (eg, once per day or once per year)

Box 3
Eye pain in patients who have a superficially normal eye examination ("white eye")

- Glaucoma
- Corneal disease
- Uveitis
- Posterior scleritis
- Intraocular or intraorbital tumor
- Optic neuropathy
- Orbital myositis

---

referral. **Box 4** lists some specific ophthalmologic conditions where an eye examination might help to confirm the diagnosis of the eye pain. **Box 5** lists a short checklist for the neurologist evaluating eye pain in making the decision to triage and refer.[1]

OCULAR AND ORBITAL ETIOLOGIES OF EYE PAIN

If the basic eye history is nonspecific and the basic eye examinations are normal, then the likelihood for an intraocular cause for the pain is diminished but not excluded completely. The ocular etiologies for eye pain with a quiet eye ("white eye"), however, are listed in **Box 3**.[1] The associated findings with eye pain that might suggest an orbital lesion are listed in **Box 5** and some specific examples of orbital processes that might cause eye pain are listed in **Box 6**. Specific ocular symptoms may be elicited or distinctive eye findings may be detected that should prompt urgent ophthalmologic referral (eg, angle-closure glaucoma, anterior or posterior uveitis, intraocular tumors, optic neuropathy, and orbital disorders). These are listed in **Table 1**.[2–46]

In addition to corneal abrasions, dry eye syndrome, blepharitis, allergic and infectious conjunctivitis, inflamed pterygia or pingueculae, and episcleritis may produce mild ocular pain. In general, however, any visible corneal pathology prompts ophthalmologic referral. We recommend against giving patients topical anesthetics, as this can lead to abuse and can mask serious underlying pathology.[6]

Headache syndromes can present with eye findings or ocular symptoms. These are listed in **Table 2**.[47–69]

Box 4
Painful optic neuropathy

- Optic neuritis (pain with eye movement)
- Optic perineuritis
- Inflammatory optic neuropathy (eg, sarcoidosis)
- Infiltrative optic neuropathy
- Ischemic optic neuropathy (eg, giant cell arteritis)
- Acute compressive optic neuropathy (eg, pituitary apoplexy)

Box 5
Findings suggesting orbital disease

- Optic neuropathy (eg, visual loss, relative afferent pupillary defect, or optic disc edema)
- Optociliary (retinochoroidal venous collateral) vessels on the optic disc head (compressive lesion of the optic nerve and central retinal vein)
- Limitation of ocular movements (extraocular muscle involvement)
- Proptosis (eg, orbital mass, thyroid eye disease, or orbital pseudotumor)
- Enophthalmos (scirrhous breast carcinoma)
- Gaze-evoked amaurosis (orbital mass compresses optic nerve during gaze)
- Conjunctival chemosis or injection (orbital inflammation or infection)
- Arterialization of episcleral or conjunctival vessels (carotid cavernous fistula)
- Pulsation of the globe (sphenoid wing dysplasia)

Box 6
Causes of pain and proptosis

1. Trauma
   - Orbital fracture
   - Orbital hemorrhage
   - Subperiosteal hematoma
2. Infectious
   - Orbital cellulites
   - Septic cavernous sinus thrombosis
3. Inflammation
   - Tolosa-Hunt syndrome
   - Orbital inflammatory pseudotumor
   - Sarcoidosis, granulomatosis with polyangiitis (ie, Wegener granulomatosis), systemic lupus erythematosus
4. Vascular
   - Orbital arteriovenous malformation
   - Carotid-cavernous fistula
5. Neoplastic
   - Orbital tumors (eg, rhabdomyosarcoma, dermoid, hemangioma)
   - Metastatic
   - Lymphoma
   - Contiguous or perineural spread of sinus neoplasm
6. Thyroid ophthalmopathy

Table 1
Ocular and orbital etiologies of interest to neurology

Etiology	Distinctive Symptoms and Signs	Comment
Eye strain (asthenopia)	Common cause of mild eye pain and headache with reading. Patients complain, of sore, tired eyes, burning, tearing, blurred vision and light sensitivity. Normal eye examination.	This complaint may rarely be the presenting sign of more serious underlying eye condition (eg, intermittent angle closure, ocular or orbital inflammation) but in general mild symptoms are likely to be benign.
Dry eye (**Fig. 1A&B**)	Very common cause of eye pain. Affects 10%–15% of adults. May simulate headache conditions. Chronic use of medications with anticholinergic side effects may be contributory.	The cornea is richly innervated by the ophthalmic division of the trigeminal nerve and corneal surface dryness may therefore be painful. Other ocular symptoms include burning, blurred vision, photophobia, and monocular diplopia. A short treatment trial with lubrication, occlusion of punctual tear outflow or other topical agents might be diagnostic and therapeutic.
Meibomianitis (chalazion) (**Fig. 2A&B**)	An inflammation of the oil glands or Meibomian glands along the upper and lower eyelid margins. Meibomianitis does not cause serious visual problems, but it can cause discomfort and eye pain and the eye may become dry, burning, itchy, watery, and red.	When they become inflamed, they no longer produce nice smooth clean oil. The oil can come out bubbly or thick, thus improperly coating the front of the eye.
Cornea (**Fig. 3**)	Corneal foreign bodies, abrasions, or erosions can be painful. They may be visible with fluorescein dye and cobalt blue light on the cornea.	Ophthalmic referral is generally recommended.
Acute angle closure glaucoma	Severe pain, blurred vision, markedly elevated intraocular pressure, or cloudy cornea. May have acute nausea or vomiting mimicking an acute abdomen or migraine attack.	Differs from the more common painless, and slowly progressive primary open-angle glaucoma. Acute angle closure requires urgent ophthalmic referral.
Uveitis (**Fig. 4**A, B, &C)	Pain, halos around lights, blurred vision, and a "red eye" may be present. Layered white cells may be present in the anterior chamber in severe cases (ie, hypopyon).	Urgent ophthalmic referral recommended.
Hyphema (**Fig. 5A&B**)	Layered red blood cells seen in the anterior chamber. Typically follows trauma but may occur in patients on anticoagulation. Pain and blurred vision common.	Urgent ophthalmic referral recommended.

(continued on next page)

Table 1
(continued)

Etiology	Distinctive Symptoms and Signs	Comment
Conjunctivitis	Conjunctival injection and irritation. Typically not severely painful. May have purulent or nonpurulent discharge.	Ophthalmic referral recommended.
Episcleritis and scleritis (**Fig. 6A&B**)	Often more injected and more painful than simple allergic or viral infectious conjunctivitis. Deeper involvement of vessels may be apparent and may have violaceous hue to sclera (ie, scleromalacia).	Urgent ophthalmic referral recommended. The eye may not be that "red" in posterior scleritis and the pain is typically more severe and boring in sensation in scleritis.
Optic neuritis and perineuritis	Visual loss is the predominant complaint, with pain with eye movement as a secondary symptom.	Ophthalmologic consultation recommended. Neuroimaging (eg, MRI) might show contrast enhancement of optic nerve (optic neuritis) or the optic nerve sheath (optic perineuritis).
Trochlear pain (trochleitis)	Localized superomedial pain and tenderness in orbit is characteristic and the pain may be exacerbated with eye movement.	Some patients complain of diplopia and erythema near the superior oblique tendon. Palpation of the trochlear region might reproduce the pain. Localized inflammation is the presumed mechanism for trochleitis. Treatment with local injection of lidocaine or local or systemic corticosteroids is often helpful.
Myositis and orbital inflammatory pseudotumor	Conjunctival redness or chemosis, pain with eye movement, proptosis, or diplopia.	Orbital imaging might show extraocular muscle enlargement or enlargement or enhancement of orbital structures. Urgent ophthalmologic consultation recommended.
Giant cell arteritis (**Fig. 7**)	Isolated eye pain is an unusual presenting symptom. Visual loss typically predominates. Headache, scalp tenderness, and jaw claudication are additional classic symptoms.	Serum stat erythrocyte sedimentation rate, platelet count, and C-reactive protein are often elevated. Temporal artery biopsy may be diagnostic. Start empiric corticosteroids immediately. Urgent ophthalmologic consultation recommended.
Orbital masses and vascular malformation	Rapid painful expanding orbital mass, proptosis, lid or conjunctival edema, vision loss, ophthalmoplegia, and elevated intraocular pressure are red flags for diagnosis.	Ophthalmic consultations is recommended.

(continued on next page)

Table 1 (continued)		
Etiology	**Distinctive Symptoms and Signs**	**Comment**
Abscess and cellulitis Preseptal and orbital cellulitis) (Fig. 8A&B)	Orbital cellulitis typically produces eyelid edema, erythema, exophthalmos, partial or total ophthalmoplegia, pain with eye movement, chemosis, decreased visual function, and relative afferent pupillary defect.	Urgent ophthalmic referral is recommended.
Thyroid eye disease (TED) or Graves orbitopathy (Fig. 9)	The characteristic signs are eyelid retraction and lid lag, proptosis, chemosis, periorbital edema, corneal exposure, diplopia, and sometimes a compressive optic neuropathy. Pain and ocular discomfort are often present early in the disease process. The pain may be caused by dry eyes and corneal exposure.	Orbital imaging (eg, CT, MRI) looking for enlargement of the extraocular muscle enlargement with sparing of the tendons is the distinctive radiographic sign. Typically the inferior and medial recti are affected first. Ophthalmic referral is recommended.
Microvascular ocular motor cranial mononeuro pathies	Ocular motor nerve palsies produce diplopia. Third nerve palsy may have ptosis and pupil involvement. The pain is often localized around the eye and in the ipsilateral ophthalmic nerve in ischemic palsies.	Ophthalmic consultation is generally recommended.
Pituitary tumor or apoplexy	Acute, severe headache is typical, especially in the setting of ophthalmoplegia, visual loss, endocrine dysfunction, or alteration in consciousness. Pituitary apoplexy typically occurs with hemorrhage or infarction of a preexisting pituitary tumor.	CT scan of the sella might show the suprasellar mass with a hyperdense acute hemorrhage and MRI is the preferred imaging study for pituitary apoplexy. Ophthalmic consultation is recommended.
Carotid artery dissection	Ipsilateral head, neck, face, or jaw. Pain may be located in the forehead or periocular region. The pain may precede the neurologic symptoms (eg, ipsilateral Horner syndrome, transient monocular visual loss, contralateral limb numbness or weakness, or stroke).	The potential confounding diagnosis is idiopathic cluster headache, as both conditions may present with a unilateral headache and a Horner syndrome. Neuroimaging is generally recommended of the head and neck to exclude carotid dissection. Ophthalmic consultation is recommended.

Abbreviations: CT, computed tomography; MRI, magnetic resonance imaging.
Data from Refs.[2–46,55,62]

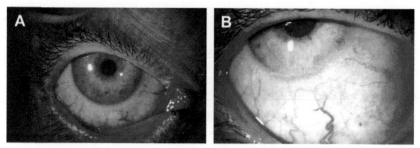

Fig. 1. (*A, B*) Severe dry eye with visible Rose Bengal staining of the corneal epithelium before (*A*) and after (*B*) staining.

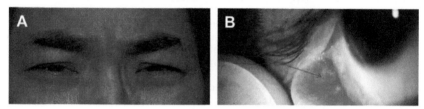

Fig. 2. (*A, B*) Meibomian gland disease with secondary eye pain and a small chalazion of the lid.

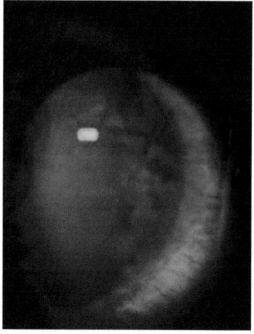

Fig. 3. Corneal epithelial defect with loss of luster of the corneal light reflex. Fluorescein dye (*green*) outlines the epithelial defect centrally.

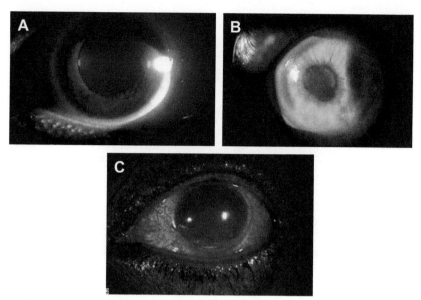

Fig. 4. (*A*) Uveitis showing keratic participitates on the corneal endothelium. (*B*) Uveitis with fibrin in the anterior chamber and posterior synechiae of the iris. (*C*) Uveitis patient with bloody hypopyon (red blood cells in the anterior chamber).

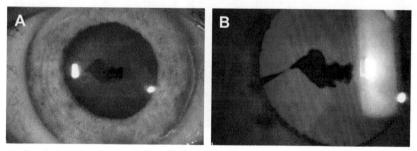

Fig. 5. (*A, B*) Spontaneous hyphema (red blood cells in the anterior chamber).

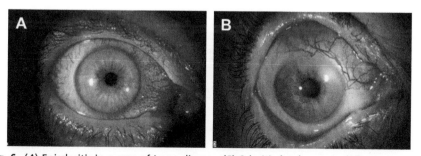

Fig. 6. (*A*) Episcleritis in a case of Lyme disease. (*B*) Scleritis (under upper lid).

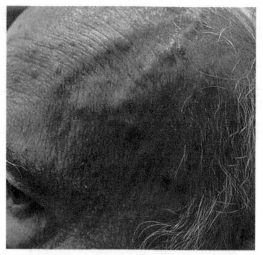

Fig. 7. Temporal artery nodularity in patient with giant cell arteritis.

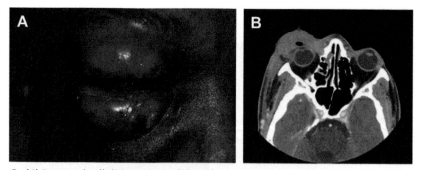

Fig. 8. (*A*) Preseptal cellulitis acute eyelid erythema and edema. (*B*) Computed tomography of the orbit with contrast showing soft tissue edema.

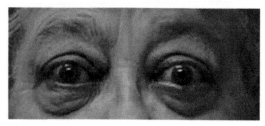

Fig. 9. Thyroid eye disease.

Table 2
Headache syndromes with eye findings or ocular symptoms

Etiology	Distinctive Finding	Comments
Raeder paratrigeminal syndrome	Unilateral oculosympathetic paresis (Horner syndrome). Ipsilateral trigeminal pain. Facial anhidrosis. Cranial nerve (eg. third, fourth, or sixth) palsy.	Idiopathic diagnosis of exclusion. Neuroimaging (typically a postcontrast MRI of brain) is recommended to exclude cavernous sinus pathology.
Gradenigo syndrome	Facial pain and sensory disturbance in the ophthalmic nerve distribution. Ipsilateral lateral rectus palsy (petrous apex of the temporal bone disease, including tumor, inflammation, or infection). Leptomeningitis and otitis media. Occasionally a Horner syndrome.	Neuroimaging is recommended to exclude inflammatory, infiltrative, or neoplastic etiology.
Post herpetic neuralgia following cutaneous herpes zoster virus (HZV)	Dermatomal vesicular eruption. In the ophthalmic nerve distribution (ie, herpes zoster ophthalmicus). Trigeminal pain may precede the rash in some cases of herpes zoster. Pain severe, constant, burning or gnawing pain with superimposed paroxysms of stabbing or shocklike pain. Hyperpathia (pain from nonpainful stimuli).	Eye pain can result from ipsilateral corneal involvement or uveitis. Ophthalmologic consultation is warranted in these patients. Some patients do not have the herpetic vesicular cutaneous rash (herpes zoster sine herpete).
Cluster and cluster-tic syndrome	Cluster headache presents with unilateral eye or orbital pain. Ipsilateral autonomic dysfunction (eg, Horner syndrome, lacrimation, nasal congestion, rhinorrhea, forehead and facial sweating, eyelid edema, ptosis, miosis, conjunctival injection).	Episodes are brief but severe and may be excruciating. A male predominance to the disorder. Attacks may be precipitated by alcohol use. Cluster-tic syndrome is a clusterlike headache associated with episodes of stabbing and ice pick–like pain. Cluster and other vascular headaches can be mimicked by intracranial lesions (eg, meningioma or aneurysm) and imaging may be necessary.

(continued on next page)

Table 2
(continued)

Etiology	Distinctive Finding	Comments
SUNCT syndrome	Short-lasting unilateral neuralgiform pain with conjunctival injection and tearing. Short (seconds to minutes) but frequent (up to 30 attacks per hour) attacks of eye pain. Autonomic features (eg, conjunctival injection and tearing, sweating of the forehead, or rhinorrhea) are variable.	Secondary SUNCT syndrome has been reported with ipsilateral cerebellopontine angle and brainstem AVM or cerebellopontine angle cavernous hemangioma.
Trigeminal neuralgia (tic douloureux)	Sudden, excruciating, lancinating, paroxysmal, brief (seconds), and unilateral facial pain. The maxillary or mandibular divisions of the trigeminal nerve most commonly are affected and involvement of the ophthalmic division is uncommon. Supraorbital nerve pain (supraorbital neuralgia) also may occur.	Trigeminal neuralgia can be caused by numerous intracranial lesions and neuroimaging is recommended.
Sphenopalatine neuralgia (Sluder neuralgia) and vidian neuralgia	Paroxysms of severe, unilateral pain localized to the middle third of the face, behind the eye, upper jaw, teeth, nose, and soft palate. The pain may be referred to the temple, occiput, and neck. No trigger points are evident. Autonomic features usually are absent.	Vidian neuralgia is a similar entity in which the pain is localized to the face, neck, and shoulder.
Ice-pick headache	Idiopathic stabbing headache (jabs and jolts syndrome, ice-pick headache, or needle-in-the-eye syndrome) refers to short-lived jabs of pain. Pain confined to the head, face, or eye that last for a fraction of a second and occur in single stabs or as a series of stabs.	These pains recur at irregular intervals from hours to days.
Ice cream headache	Eating ice cream or drinking iced drinks rapidly may precipitate severe pain (cold stimulus or ice cream headache). Pain typically is brief (25–60 s) and may be referred to the eye.	It may be bifrontal or unilateral. More common in migraineurs, and is benign.

Hypnic headache	Hypnic headache is a rare, nocturnal headache disorder affecting the elderly. Pain usually is throbbing in quality and bilateral and affects the frontal and facial areas. Episodes occur 2 to 4 h after sleep onset and are short lived (15–30 min but occasionally several hours).	Nausea may occur but other autonomic symptoms usually are absent.
Eye pain and lung cancer	Lung cancer can produce facial pain in the absence of intracranial or orbital metastasis. Facial pain is severe, aching, and aural-temporal, but occasionally orbital. The pain has been ipsilateral to the lung cancer in all of the reported patients.	The proposed mechanism is local invasion of the vagus nerve with referred pain (afferents traveling with visceral pain afferents that synapse with somatic sensory afferents within the descending tract and nucleus of the trigeminal nerve). This is a rare cause of eye pain.
Nonorganic pain	Pain with no objective examination findings may have nonorganic pain.	The etiologies of nonorganic pain include secondary gain (eg, malingering), exaggeration of pain (nonorganic overlay, hypochondriasis), and psychiatric disorders (eg, conversion disorder or somatization). Patients who have organic pain may have nonorganic overlay nonorganic pain syndrome, a diagnosis of exclusion.
Epicrania fugax	A paroxysmal head pain starting in a focal area located at a posterior cranial region and rapidly spreading forward to the ipsilateral eye or nose along a linear or zigzag trajectory. In some patients the pain is followed by ocular or nasal autonomic features. Pain described as stabbing or electric in quality. Pain intensity usually moderate or severe.	The pain almost always stems from a particular focal area located in the posterior scalp. Most attacks are spontaneous, but touch stimuli on the trigger point can elicit an attack. The paroxysms are brief, lasting just 1–10 s.

Abbreviations: AVM, arteriovenous malformation; MRI, magnetic resonance imaging; SUNCT, short-lasting unilateral neuralgiform headache attacks with conjunctival injection and tearing.
Data from Refs.[47–69]

SUMMARY

The practicing neurologist should be aware of the common causes of primary or referred eye pain. These entities include (1) ocular and orbital disorders that produce eye pain with a normal examination, (2) neurologic syndromes with predominantly ophthalmologic presentations, and (3) ophthalmologic presentations of selected headache syndromes. The neurologist should screen for specific symptoms and signs that should prompt ophthalmologic consultation.

REFERENCES

1. Lee AG, Beaver HA, Brazis PW. Painful ophthalmologic disorders and eye pain for the neurologist. Neurol Clin 2004;22(1):75–97.
2. White J. Diagnosis and management of acute angle-closure glaucoma. Emerg Nurse 2011;19(3):27.
3. Chien KH, Lu DW, Chen YH, et al. Relief of periorbital pain after acute angle closure glaucoma attack by botulinum toxin type A. J Glaucoma 2010;19(8): 546–50.
4. Dargin JM, Lowenstein RA. The painful eye. Emerg Med Clin North Am 2008; 26(1):199–216.
5. Turner A, Rabiu M. Patching for corneal abrasion. Cochrane Database Syst Rev 2006;(2):CD004764.
6. Wilson SA, Last A. Management of corneal abrasions. Am Fam Physician 2004; 70(1):123–8.
7. Yagci A, Bozkurt B, Egrilmez S, et al. Topical anesthetic abuse keratopathy: a commonly overlooked health care problem. Cornea 2011;30(5):571–5.
8. Ramamurthi S, Rahman MQ, Dutton GN, et al. Pathogenesis, clinical features and management of recurrent corneal erosions. Eye (Lond) 2006;20(6):635–44.
9. Powdrill S. Ciliary injection: a differential diagnosis for the patient with acute red eye. JAAPA 2010;23(12):50–4.
10. Pierce RG, Wong M, Skalet AB. More to mutton than meets the eye. J Gen Intern Med 2010;25(9):989.
11. Ertam I, Kitapcioglu G, Aksu K, et al. Quality of life and its relation with disease severity in Behçet's disease. Clin Exp Rheumatol 2009;27(2 Suppl 53):S18–22.
12. Rasić DM, Stanković Z, Terzić T, et al. Primary extranodal marginal zone lymphoma of the uvea associated with massive diffuse epibulbar extension and focal infiltration of the optic nerve and meninges, clinically presented as uveitis masquerade syndrome: a case report. Med Oncol 2010;27(3):1010–6.
13. Scherer JR. Inflammatory bowel disease: complications and extraintestinal manifestations. Drugs Today (Barc) 2009;45(3):227–41.
14. Bakri SJ, Larson TA, Edwards AO. Intraocular inflammation following intravitreal injection of bevacizumab. Graefes Arch Clin Exp Ophthalmol 2008;246(5): 779–81.
15. Sivaraj RR, Durrani OM, Denniston AK, et al. Ocular manifestations of systemic lupus erythematosus. Rheumatology (Oxford) 2007;46(12):1757–62.
16. Ephgrave K. Extra-intestinal manifestations of Crohn's disease. Surg Clin North Am 2007;87(3):673–80.
17. Bonfioli AA, Orefice F. Toxoplasmosis. Semin Ophthalmol 2005;20(3):129–41.
18. Zink JM, Singh-Parikshak R, Johnson CS, et al. Hypopyon uveitis associated with systemic lupus erythematosus and antiphospholipid antibody syndrome. Graefes Arch Clin Exp Ophthalmol 2005;243(4):386–8.

19. Heiner JD, Kalsi KS. Eye pain after blunt ocular trauma. Traumatic mydriasis with hyphema. Ann Emerg Med 2012;59(6):456–68.
20. Bagnis A, Lai S, Iester M, et al. Spontaneous hyphaema in a patient on warfarin treatment. Br J Clin Pharmacol 2008;66(3):414–5.
21. Arthur SN, Wright MM, Kramarevsky N, et al. Uveitis-glaucoma-hyphema syndrome and corneal decompensation in association with cosmetic iris implants. Am J Ophthalmol 2009;148(5):790–3.
22. Pokharel A, Subedi S, Bajracharya M. Peripheral ulcerative keratitis triggered by bacterial conjunctivitis. Nepal J Ophthalmol 2010;2(1):71–3.
23. Richards AL, Patel VS, Simon JW, et al. Eye pain in preschool children: diagnostic and prognostic significance. J AAPOS 2010;14(5):383–5.
24. García DP, Alperte JI, Cristóbal JA, et al. Topical tacrolimus ointment for treatment of intractable atopic keratoconjunctivitis: a case report and review of the literature. Cornea 2011;30(4):462–5.
25. Rudloe TF, Harper MB, Prabhu SP, et al. Acute periorbital infections: who needs emergent imaging? Pediatrics 2010;125(4):e719–26.
26. Kim SJ, Flach AJ, Jampol LM. Nonsteroidal anti-inflammatory drugs in ophthalmology. Surv Ophthalmol 2010;55(2):108–33.
27. Cronau H, Kankanala RR, Mauger T. Diagnosis and management of red eye in primary care. Am Fam Physician 2010;81(2):137–44.
28. Tarabishy AB, Jeng BH. Bacterial conjunctivitis: a review for internists. Cleve Clin J Med 2008;75(7):507–12.
29. Sainz de la Maza M, Molina N, Gonzalez-Gonzalez LA, et al. Clinical characteristics of a large cohort of patients with scleritis and episcleritis. Ophthalmology 2012;119(1):43–50.
30. Anshu A, Chee SP. Posterior scleritis and its association with HLA B27 haplotype. Ophthalmologica 2007;221(4):275–8.
31. Barnett MH, Chohan G, Davies L. Blurred vision and pain in the eye. Med J Aust 2011;195(6):329–32.
32. Abou Zeid N, Bhatti MT. Acute inflammatory demyelinating optic neuritis: evidence-based visual and neurological considerations. Neurologist 2008;14(4):207–23.
33. Germann CA, Baumann MR, Hamzavi S. Ophthalmic diagnoses in the ED: optic neuritis. Am J Emerg Med 2007;25(7):834–7.
34. Protti A, Spreafico C, Frigerio R, et al. Optic neuritis: diagnostic criteria application in clinical practice. Neurol Sci 2004;25(Suppl 3):S296–7.
35. Costa RM, Dumitrascu OM, Gordon LK. Orbital myositis: diagnosis and management. Curr Allergy Asthma Rep 2009;9(4):316–23.
36. Ramalho J, Castillo M. Imaging of orbital myositis in Crohn's disease. Clin Imaging 2008;32(3):227–9.
37. Isobe K, Uno T, Kawakami H, et al. Radiation therapy for idiopathic orbital myositis: two case reports and literature review. Radiat Med 2004;22(6):429–31.
38. Pemberton JD, Fay A. Idiopathic sclerosing orbital inflammation: a review of demographics, clinical presentation, imaging, pathology, treatment, and outcome. Ophthal Plast Reconstr Surg 2012;28(1):79–83.
39. Mendenhall WM, Lessner AM. Orbital pseudotumor. Am J Clin Oncol 2010;33(3):304–6.
40. Swamy BN, McCluskey P, Nemet A, et al. Idiopathic orbital inflammatory syndrome: clinical features and treatment outcomes. Br J Ophthalmol 2007;91(12):1667–70.

41. Fiore DC, Pasternak AV, Radwan RM. Pain in the quiet (not red) eye. Am Fam Physician 2010;82(1):69–73.
42. Borchers AT, Gershwin ME. Giant cell arteritis: a review of classification, pathophysiology, geoepidemiology and treatment. Autoimmun Rev 2012;11(6–7): A544–54.
43. Kermani TA, Warrington KJ. Recent advances in diagnostic strategies for giant cell arteritis. Curr Neurol Neurosci Rep 2012;12(2):138–44.
44. Keller DL. Giant cell arteritis. Cleve Clin J Med 2011;78(8):512.
45. Schmidt J, Warrington KJ. Polymyalgia rheumatica and giant cell arteritis in older patients: diagnosis and pharmacological management. Drugs Aging 2011;28(8):651–66.
46. Murphy MA, Szabados EM, Mitty JA. Lyme disease associated with postganglionic Horner syndrome and Raeder paratrigeminal neuralgia. J Neuroophthalmol 2007;27(2):123–4.
47. Shoja MM, Tubbs RS, Ghabili K, et al. Johan Georg Raeder (1889-1959) and paratrigeminal sympathetic paresis. Childs Nerv Syst 2010;26(3):373–6.
48. Loretan S, Duvoisin B, Scolozzi P. Unusual fatal petrositis presenting as myofascial pain and dysfunction of the temporal muscle. Quintessence Int 2011;42(5): 419–22.
49. Tornabene S, Vilke GM. Gradenigo's syndrome. J Emerg Med 2010;38(4): 449–51.
50. Kanai A, Okamoto T, Suzuki K, et al. Lidocaine eye drops attenuate pain associated with ophthalmic postherpetic neuralgia. Anesth Analg 2010;110(5):1457–60.
51. Gilden D, Cohrs RJ, Mahalingam R, et al. Neurological disease produced by varicella zoster virus reactivation without rash. Curr Top Microbiol Immunol 2010;342:243–53.
52. Opstelten W, Eekhof J, Neven AK, et al. Treatment of herpes zoster. Can Fam Physician 2008;54(3):373–7.
53. Pavan-Langston D. Herpes zoster antivirals and pain management. Ophthalmology 2008;115(Suppl 2):S13–20.
54. Volpi A. Severe complications of herpes zoster. Herpes 2007;14(Suppl 2):35–9.
55. Friedman DI, Gordon LK, Quiros PA. Headache attributable to disorders of the eye. Curr Pain Headache Rep 2010;14(1):62–72.
56. Wolfe S, Van Stavern G. Characteristics of patients presenting with ocular pain. Can J Ophthalmol 2008;43(4):432–4.
57. Leroux E, Ducros A. Cluster headache. Orphanet J Rare Dis 2008;3:20.
58. May A. Cluster headache: pathogenesis, diagnosis, and management. Lancet 2005;366(9488):843–55.
59. Jansen J, Sjaastad O. Hemicrania with massive autonomic manifestations and circumscribed eyelid erythema. Acta Neurol Scand 2006;114(5):334–9.
60. Bichuetti DB, Yamaoka WY, Bastos JR, et al. Bilateral SUNCT syndrome associated to chronic maxillary sinus disease. Arq Neuropsiquiatr 2006;64(2B):504–6.
61. Rozen TD, Haynes GV, Saper JR, et al. Abrupt onset and termination of cutaneous allodynia (central sensitization) during attacks of SUNCT. Headache 2005;45(2):153–5.
62. Friedman DI. Headache and the eye. Curr Pain Headache Rep 2008;12(4): 296–304.
63. Harooni H, Golnik KC, Geddie B, et al. Diagnostic yield for neuroimaging in patients with unilateral eye or facial pain. Can J Ophthalmol 2005;40(6):759–63.
64. Obermann M, Holle D. Hypnic headache. Expert Rev Neurother 2010;10(9): 1391–7.

65. Holle D, Wessendorf TE, Zaremba S, et al. Serial polysomnography in hypnic headache. Cephalalgia 2011;31(3):286–90.
66. Evans RW. Hemicrania Continua-like headache due to nonmetastatic lung cancer—a vagal cephalalgia. Headache 2007;47(9):1349–51.
67. Guerrero AL, Cuadrado ML, Porta-Etessam J, et al. Epicrania fugax: ten new cases and therapeutic results. Headache 2010;50(3):451–8.
68. Cuadrado ML, Gómez-Vicente L, Porta-Etessam J, et al. Paroxysmal head pain with backward radiation: will epicrania fugax go in the opposite direction? J Headache Pain 2010;11(1):75–8.
69. Colombo B, Dalla Libera D, Comi G. Ocular pain: a neurological perspective. Neurol Sci 2010;31(Suppl 1):S103–5.

Headaches Caused by Nasal and Paranasal Sinus Disease

Michael J. Marmura, MD, Stephen D. Silberstein, MD*

KEYWORDS

- Headache • Rhinosinusitis • Sphenoid sinusitis • Contact-point headache

KEY POINTS

- Headache and rhinosinusitis are 2 of the most common conditions seen in clinical practice.
- In general, chronic and disabling headaches, especially if migraine features are present, are not due to sinus abnormality.
- In suspected cases of bacterial sinusitis, computed tomography and magnetic resonance imaging are both effective in demonstrating the infection.
- Although most cases of sinusitis are fairly easy to diagnose, sphenoid sinusitis may be overlooked, and can present with progressive or thunderclap headache in adults.
- Contact-point headache should be considered in patients with focal headaches and a contact point on the lateral nasal wall.

SINUSITIS

Sinus infections are much less common today than they were in the preantibiotic era, but are still overdiagnosed. Acute sinusitis, a relatively uncommon cause of headache, is the result of infection of 1 or more of the cranial sinuses (**Fig. 1**). Acute sinusitis usually is characterized by purulent discharge in the nasal passages and a pain profile determined by the site of infection. Sinusitis is overdiagnosed as a cause of headache because of the belief that pain over the sinuses must be related to the sinuses. In fact, frontal head pain more often is caused by migraine or tension-type headache. Whether nasal obstruction can lead to chronic headache is controversial.[1] Paradoxically, serious sinus disease also tends to be underdiagnosed, as sphenoid sinus infection frequently is missed.[2]

Because sphenoid sinusitis differs from other forms of sinusitis in clinical features and treatment, it is considered separately in this article. Although it represents only 3% of sinusitis cases, because it is potentially life threatening its importance is out

Department of Neurology, Thomas Jefferson University Hospital, Jefferson Headache Center, 900 Walnut Street, Suite 2000, Philadelphia, PA 19107, USA
* Corresponding author.
E-mail address: stephen.silberstein@jefferson.edu

Neurol Clin 32 (2014) 507–523
http://dx.doi.org/10.1016/j.ncl.2013.11.001   **neurologic.theclinics.com**
0733-8619/14/$ – see front matter © 2014 Elsevier Inc. All rights reserved.

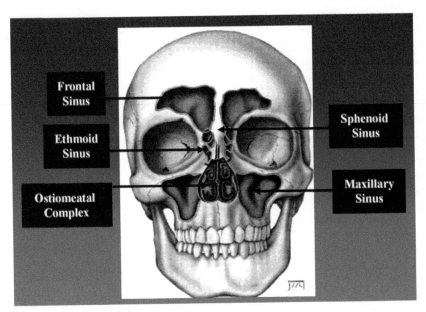

Fig. 1. Location of cranial sinuses.

of proportion to its prevalence. Sinusitis affects more than 32 million people in the United States annually, and resulted in 13 million physician visits in 2000.[3] A National Health Interview Survey conducted in the United States between 1990 and 1992 found that chronic sinusitis was the second most frequent disease after orthopedic deformities, with an annual average of 33.1 million cases.[3] Approximately 0.5% of upper respiratory infections in adults are complicated by sinusitis.[4] As many as 38% of patients who have symptoms of sinusitis in adult general medicine clinics may have acute bacterial rhinosinusitis. In otolaryngology practices, the prevalence was higher (50%–80%). Although sinusitis generally is more common in children than in adults, frontal and sphenoid sinusitises are rare in children. In the primary care setting, between 6% and 18% of children presenting with upper respiratory infections may have acute bacterial sinusitis.[5] In the preantibiotic era, the sphenoid sinus was involved in as many as 33% of cases of sinusitis. Its incidence today is approximately 3%.[2]

The maxillary and ethmoid sinuses, both present at birth, are the most common sites of clinical infection in children. The sphenoid sinus develops after the age of 2 years and starts to pneumatize at the age of 8 years. The frontal sinuses develop from the anterior ethmoid sinus at approximately 6 years of age. The frontal and sphenoid sinuses become clinically important in the teenage years, and frequently become infected in pansinusitis. Isolated sphenoid sinusitis is rare.[6] The clinical diagnosis of sinusitis usually is based on symptoms that suggest maxillary or frontal sinus involvement. Ethmoid sinusitis frequently is a cause of frontal and maxillary sinusitis.[7,8] Obstruction of the ostiomeatal complex, the common drainage pathway for the ethmoid, frontal, and maxillary sinuses, is the usual precursor to sinus disease.[9]

Anatomy and Physiology

The ethmoid bone, a T-shaped structure that supports the bilateral ethmoid labyrinth, forms the lateral nasal wall. The horizontal limb of the T is formed by the cribriform plate, from which the ethmoid labyrinth is suspended. This complex structure has multiple bony septa and the medial projections of the superior and middle turbinates. Lateral to the uncinate process, which is a secondary projection of the ethmoid bone, is the infundibulum, a recess into which the maxillary sinus drains. The infundibulum drains into the hiatus semilunaris, which in turn drains into the middle meatus, located between the uncinate process and the middle turbinate. The frontal sinus drains into the frontal recess, which may drain into either the middle meatus or the ethmoidal infundibulum. This region is known as the ostiomeatal complex[9] (maxillary sinus ostium, infundibulum, hiatus semilunaris, middle turbinate, ethmoidal bulla, and frontal ostium). The sphenoidal sinus and posterior ethmoidal cells drain into the sphenoethmoidal recess.

The primary functions of the nasal passages are to warm, humidify, and filter inspired air. The paranasal sinuses are air-filled cavities that connect with the nasal airway. These cavities are lined with pseudostratified ciliated epithelial tissue, which is covered by a thin layer of mucus. Large inhaled particulate matter passes over this constantly moving ciliated epithelial layer and is deposited there. The cilia and the mucous layer are in constant motion in a predetermined direction. Mucus and debris are transported toward the ostia by the beating of the cilia and are expelled into the nasal airway.[6,9,10] Any bacterial contamination of the sinuses is effectively cleared by this mechanism. If the sinus ostia are obstructed, mucociliary flow is interrupted. Obstruction causes the oxygen tension within the sinus to decrease and the carbon dioxide tension to increase. This anaerobic, stagnant environment, high in carbon dioxide, can facilitate bacterial growth.[9]

For many years surgical drainage of the sinuses, avoiding the region of the natural ostia, was the treatment of choice for sinus infections. This procedure alleviated the acute sinus infection but did not prevent reaccumulation of mucus within the sinus. The normal beat of the cilia transports mucus toward the natural ostium. Surgically creating a new ostium at a site distant from the natural ostium fails to direct the flow of mucus to the new opening.[9]

All sinuses normally contain anaerobic bacteria, and more than one-third harbor a mixed environment of aerobic and anaerobic organisms. Ciliary dysfunction and retention of secretions that are the result of ostial obstruction can result in bacterial proliferation and sinus infection. Aerobes that are present in normal and disease states include the gram-positive streptococci (α, β, and *Streptococcus pneumoniae*) and *Staphylococcus aureus*, and gram-negative *Moraxella catarrhalis*, *Haemophilus influenzae*, and *Escherichia coli*. Anaerobic organisms include the gram-positive peptococci and *Propionibacterium* species. The *Bacteroides* and *Fusobacterium* species also play a role in chronic sinusitis.[6,11]

Systemic diseases that predispose to sinusitis include cystic fibrosis, immune deficiency, bronchiectasis, and the immobile cilia syndrome. Local factors include upper respiratory infections (usually viral), allergic rhinitis, overuse of topical decongestants, hypertrophied adenoids, deviated nasal septum, nasal polyps, tumors, and cigarette smoke.[6] The most common predisposing factor is mucosal inflammation from a viral upper respiratory infection or allergic rhinitis.[5] The sinuses are involved in nearly 90% of viral upper respiratory infections. Eighty-seven percent of patients who have a common cold and no previous history of rhinosinusitis have maxillary sinus abnormalities, 65% have ethmoid sinus abnormalities, and 30% to 40% have frontal or sphenoid sinus abnormalities on computed tomography (CT). The abnormalities are most likely the result of highly viscid secretions in the sinuses. Seventy-seven percent of patients have an occluded infundibulum. These abnormalities usually resolve spontaneously, but some patients develop secondary bacterial infections.[12] Foreign bodies are a common cause of obstruction in children, and 10% of sinus infections have a dental origin.[5] Loss of immunocompetence related to human immunodeficiency virus (HIV) infection, chemotherapy, posttransplant immunosuppression, insulin-dependent diabetes mellitus, or some connective tissue disorders predisposes patients to rhinosinusitis and increases the likelihood of its persistence. Rhinosinusitis is common in the intensive care unit (ICU), because prolonged supine positioning compromises mucociliary clearance and adds to the problems created by mucosal drying from transnasal supplemental oxygenation and sinus ostial obstruction from nasotracheal or nasogastric tubes. Rhinosinusitis occurs in 95.5% of bedridden ICU patients who have a nasogastric or nasotracheal tube in place for at least a week.[13] Unobstructed flow through the sinus ostia and its narrow communicating passage within the ostiomeatal complex is integral to mucociliary clearance and ventilation. Persistent low-grade inflammation in the ethmoid sinus may cause few localizing symptoms, but can predispose to recurrent maxillary and frontal sinus infections (**Table 1**).[6,9]

Diagnostic Testing

The physical examination may not be helpful, particularly in sphenoid sinusitis. Not all patients are febrile, and sinus tenderness is not always present. Pus is not always seen in sphenoid sinusitis. Kibblewhite and colleagues[14] found purulent exudate in only 3 of 14 patients. Transillumination of the sinuses has low sensitivity and specificity,[15] and routine anterior rhinoscopy performed with a headlight and nasal speculum allows only limited inspection of the anterior nasal cavity.

Standard radiography

Standard radiography is inadequate for the clinical evaluation of sinusitis because it does not evaluate the anterior ethmoid air cells, the upper two-thirds of the nasal cavity, or the infundibular, middle meatus, or frontal recess air passages.[10]

Neuroimaging

CT is the optimal radiographic study to assess the paranasal sinuses for evidence of disease. The mucosa of the normal, noninfected sinus approximates the bone so closely that it cannot be visualized on CT. Therefore, any soft tissue seen within a sinus is abnormal.[16] CT may demonstrate mucosal thickening, sclerosis, clouding, or air-fluid levels. Imaging must be performed in the coronal plane to adequately demonstrate the ethmoid complex. It can reveal the extent of mucosal disease in the ostiomeatal complex. The test-retest reliability of CT in the assessment of chronic rhinosinusitis

Table 1
Selected factors that affect the risk of sinusitis

Condition	Comments
Upper respiratory infection	Usually viral
Allergic rhinitis	Overuse of topical decongestants can make worse
Foreign bodies	Most common in children
Nasal polyps or tumors	
Cigarette smoking	
Deviated nasal septum	
Prolonged	
Cystic fibrosis	Suspect *Pseudomonas aeruginosa*
Diabetes mellitus	Suspect fungal or *Staphylococcus aureus*
Immunosuppression including human immunodeficiency virus infection	At higher risk for fungal, cytomegalovirus, mycobacterial, or parasitic infection

was high and stable in a prospective series of patients scheduled for endoscopic sinus surgery.[17] The prevalence of reversible sinus abnormalities on CT in patients who have the common cold is high.[12] This finding suggests that CT may not be specific for bacterial infections. Middle meatus involvement was present in 72 of 100 CT examinations of patients who had chronic sinusitis. Anterior ethmoid sinus infection was found in every patient who had frontal or maxillary sinusitis. Middle meatal disease was found in the rest of these patients; it extended to, and occluded, the frontal recess in the patients who had frontal sinusitis and extended to, and occluded, the infundibulum in all cases of maxillary mucoperiosteal disease.[3]

Incidental anatomic abnormalities within the paranasal sinuses are common. Incidental anatomic abnormalities on CT scans occur in 27% to 45% of asymptomatic individuals.[18] Patients undergoing endoscopic sinus surgery for chronic rhinosinusitis were evaluated with CT and staged according to the Lund system, whereby each paranasal sinus (anterior ethmoid, posterior ethmoid, maxillary, frontal, and sphenoid sinus for each side) was given a score of 0 for no opacification, 1 for partial opacification, or 2 for total opacification. The ostiomeatal complex was assigned a score of 0 for patent or 2 for obstructed. The Lund score ranged from 0 to 24. Controls were patients undergoing sinus CT for other reasons. In the disease-positive group of patients who had chronic rhinosinusitis, the mean Lund score was 9.8 (9.0–10.6). The mean Lund score of the control group (without disease) was 4.3 (3.5–5.0). The area under the curve for the receiver-operating characteristic was 0.802 ($P<.001$). Using a Lund score cutoff value of greater than 2 as abnormal, the sinus CT showed sensitivity and specificity of 94% and 41%, respectively. Increasing the cutoff value to 4 changed the sensitivity and specificity to 85% and 59%, respectively.[18]

Lund scores of 0 or 1 are unlikely to represent true chronic rhinosinusitis, whereas Lund scores of 4 or greater are highly likely to represent true chronic rhinosinusitis. Lund scores of 2 to 3 are ambiguous, and further clinical evaluation or follow-up is warranted.[18]

During the edematous phase of the nasal cycle, normal nasal mucosa on a T2-weighted image can resemble pathologic change. Despite these specificity problems, magnetic resonance imaging (MRI) is more sensitive than CT in detecting fungal infection.[10] Maxillary mucosal thickening of more than 6 mm, complete sinus opacification, and air-fluid levels on neuroimaging correlate with positive sinus cultures.[19] Thirty percent to 40% of the normal population, however, has mucosal thickening on CT evaluation.[20] The 1999 Agency for Healthcare Policy and Research meta-analysis of 6 studies showed that sinus radiography has moderate sensitivity (76%) and specificity (79%) compared with sinus puncture in diagnosing acute bacterial rhinosinusitis. CT or MRI is necessary to definitively diagnose sphenoid sinusitis, because plain radiographs are nondiagnostic in approximately 26% of cases.[18] CT scanning is the gold standard for the diagnosis of sphenoid sinus disease; MRI is an adjunct (**Table 2**).

Transillumination, ultrasonography, and anterior rhinoscopy

Transillumination of the sinuses has low sensitivity and specificity.[15] Ultrasonography has lower sensitivity and specificity than sinus radiography.[15] Routine anterior rhinoscopy performed with a headlight and nasal speculum allows only limited inspection of the anterior nasal cavity.

Diagnostic fiberoptic endoscopy

The flexible fiberoptic rhinoscope allows direct visualization of the nasal passages and sinus drainage areas (ostiomeatal complex), and is complementary to CT or MRI. A

Table 2	
Advantages of CT and MRI in the evaluation of sinusitis	
Advantages of CT	**Advantages of MRI**
Defines the bony anatomy better than MRI	Better visualization of the nasal mucosa
Gold standard for the diagnosis of sphenoid sinusitis	Better than CT in distinguishing between bacterial, viral, or fungal infection
Coronal imaging effectively diagnoses ethmoid sinusitis	Distinguishes between mucoceles and benign tumors
Adequately demonstrates mucosal thickening or air-fluid levels	Diagnosis of bone erosion, ie, due to neoplasm

trained operator can perform this procedure easily, and the patient tolerates it well. Infection is easily diagnosed if purulent material is seen emanating from the sinus drainage region. Mucosal sinus thickening frequently is present in normal, nonsymptomatic patients. In these cases, endoscopy should be positive before a diagnosis of sinusitis is made.[9,11] Sphenoid sinusitis is an exception to this generalization.

Endoscopy should be considered when a patient who is suspected of having a sinus-related problem fails conservative medical treatment and has an inconclusive CT or MRI. Some physicians use endoscopy before neuroimaging. Negative neuroimaging and endoscopy usually, but not always, rules out sinus disease.[10]

Castellanos and Axelrod[21] evaluated 246 patients who had undiagnosed headache and a negative neurologic evaluation. Ninety-eight had only rhinoscopic evidence of sinusitis, 84 had both rhinoscopic and standard radiographic evidence of sinusitis, and 64 had neither. Patients were treated with antibiotics for 4 weeks, at which time only those patients who had rhinoscopic or radiologic evidence of sinusitis reported headache improvement. This study was open and uncontrolled, but repeat rhinoscopic evaluation showed clearing of infection coincident with headache improvement.

Clinical Findings

In 1996, the American Academy of Otolaryngology—Head and Neck Surgery standardized the terminology for paranasal infections.[22] The term rhinosinusitis was believed more appropriate than sinusitis because rhinitis typically precedes sinusitis, purulent sinusitis without rhinitis is rare, the mucosa of the nose and sinuses are contiguous, and symptoms of nasal obstruction and discharge are prominent in sinusitis.[23] The diagnosis of rhinosinusitis usually is based on symptoms indicating maxillary or frontal sinus involvement, which may occur secondarily to, and is frequently a result of, ethmoid disease. Obstruction of the sinus ostia is the usual precursor of sinusitis.[10,24]

Rhinosinusitis is divided into 4 categories based on the temporal course and the signs and symptoms of the disease (see **Table 1**): (1) acute rhinosinusitis is sudden in onset; it lasts from 1 day to 4 weeks and there is complete resolution of the symptoms; (2) recurrent acute rhinosinusitis requires 4 or more episodes of acute rhinosinusitis, lasting at least 7 days each, in any 1-year period; (3) subacute rhinosinusitis is continuous with acute rhinosinusitis and lasts from 4 to 12 weeks[25]; and (4) chronic rhinosinusitis requires that signs or symptoms persist for 12 weeks or longer and may be punctuated by acute infectious episodes (**Table 3**).

Most cases of infectious rhinosinusitis that last less than 7 days are viral. In adults, acute bacterial sinusitis most often presents with 7 days or more of purulent anterior

Table 3
Classification of adult rhinosinusitis

Classification	Duration	Strong History	Include in Differential	Special Notes
Acute	≤4 wk	≥2 major factors, 1 major factor and 2 minor factors, or nasal purulence on examination	1 major factor or ≥2 minor factors	Fever or facial pain does not constitute a suggestive history in the absence of other nasal signs or symptoms; consider acute bacterial rhinosinusitis if symptoms worsen after 5 d, persist for >10 d, or are out of proportion to those typically associated with viral infection
Subacute	4–12 wk	Same as chronic	Same as chronic	Complete resolution after effective medical therapy
Recurrent acute	≥4 episodes per year, with each episode lasting ≥7–10 d and no intervening signs and symptoms of chronic rhinosinusitis	Same as acute		
Chronic	≥12 wk	≥2 major factors, 1 major factor and 2 minor factors, or nasal purulence on examination	1 major factor or ≥2 minor factors	Facial pain does not constitute a suggestive history in the absence of other nasal signs or symptoms
Acute exacerbations of chronic	Sudden worsening of chronic rhinosinusitis, with return to baseline after treatment			

Adapted from Lanza DC, Kennedy DW. Adult rhinosinusitis defined. Otolaryngol Head Neck Surg 1997;117:S1–7; with permission.

rhinorrhea, nasal congestion, postnasal drip, facial or dental pain/pressure, and cough, frequently with a nighttime component (**Box 1**).

Facial tenderness and pain, nasal congestion, and purulent nasal discharge are common manifestations of acute sinus infection. Other classic signs and symptoms include anosmia, pain on mastication, and halitosis. An upper respiratory infection or a history of one may be present.[15] Although fever is present in approximately 50% of adults and 60% of children, and headache is common, the symptoms of headache, facial pain, and fever often are of minimal value in the diagnosis of sinusitis. Williams and colleagues[26] looked at the sensitivity and specificity of individual symptoms in making the diagnosis of sinusitis. No single item was both sensitive and specific. Maxillary toothache was highly specific (93%), but only 11% of the patients had this symptom. Logistic regression analysis showed 5 independent predictions of sinusitis: maxillary toothache (odds ratio [OR] 2.9), abnormal transillumination (OR 2.7, sensitivity 73%, specificity 54%), poor response to decongestants (OR 2.4), purulent discharge (OR 2.9), and colored nasal discharge (OR 2.2). The data did not support the other textbook findings for sinusitis (an antecedent upper respiratory infection or history of facial pain). Headache had an odds ratio of 1.0, with 68% sensitivity and 30% specificity. The low specificity is because of the lack of descriptive features of the headache. Facial pain and itchy eyes had an OR of 1.0. Fever, sweats, or chills were found in 48% of patients, with an OR of 0.9 (sensitivity 45%, specificity 51%). It has been suggested that highly specific symptoms, such as facial erythema or maxillary toothache, or symptoms that persist for more than 10 days, warrant a

---

Box 1
Factors associated with the diagnosis of chronic rhinosinusitis

Major factors

  Facial pain/pressure[a]

  Facial congestion/fullness

  Nasal obstruction/blockage

  Nasal discharge/purulence/discolored postnasal discharge drainage

  Hyposmia/anosmia

  Purulence in nasal cavity on examination

  Fever (acute rhinosinusitis only)[b]

Minor factors

  Headache

  Fever (all nonacute)

  Halitosis

  Fatigue

  Dental pain

  Cough

  Ear pain/pressure/fullness

  [a] Facial pain/pressure alone does not constitute a suggestive history for rhinosinusitis in the absence of another major nasal symptom or sign.
  [b] Fever in acute sinusitis alone does not constitute a strongly suggestive history for acute sinusitis in the absence of another major nasal symptom or sign.

diagnosis and treatment.[27] Diagnostic accuracy may be similar to that of sinus radiography when 3 or 4 of the following symptoms are present: purulent rhinorrhea with unilateral predominance, local pain with unilateral predominance, bilateral purulent rhinorrhea, and pus in the nasal cavity.[28]

Naranch and colleagues[29] compared sinus and systemic tenderness in rhinosinusitis with other disorders. Cutaneous pressures (kg/cm^2) causing pain at 5 sinus and 18 systemic sites were measured. Lower sinus thresholds were found in the rhinosinusitis groups. Subjects with chronic fatigue syndrome had sinus and systemic thresholds that were 44% lower than those of subjects not with chronic fatigue syndrome, suggesting that systemic hyperalgesia contributes to chronic fatigue syndrome, sinus tenderness, and rhinosinusitis complaints.

Children with acute and chronic sinusitis almost always present with purulent nasal discharge and cough, which are not characteristic in adults with acute and chronic sinusitis. Fever is infrequent, even with acute sinusitis, and usually is associated with complicated acute sinusitis.[30]

Sinus infection can result in acute suppurative meningitis, subdural or epidural abscess, and brain abscess. In addition, osteomyelitis and subperiosteal abscess can occur. Infection of the ethmoid and, to a lesser extent, the sphenoid sinuses, is responsible for orbital complications, including edema, orbital cellulitis, and subperiosteal and orbital abscess.[6] A mucocele is a mucus-containing cyst located in the sinuses, most commonly (and mostly benign) in the maxillary sinus (mucus retention cyst). Those located in the frontal, sphenoid, or ethmoid sinus can enlarge and erode into the surrounding structures. A pyocele is an infected mucocele.[31]

Wolff[32] showed that the sinuses themselves are relatively insensitive to pain. The pain associated with sinusitis comes from engorged and inflamed nasal structures: nasofrontal ducts, turbinates, ostia, and superior nasal spaces. Headache associated with paranasal sinus disease usually has a deeper, dull, aching quality combined with a heaviness and fullness. It seldom is associated with nausea and vomiting.

The International Headache Society (IHS) has established criteria for acute headache caused by rhinosinusitis.[33] To qualify as rhinosinusitis headache, there must be clinical, nasal endoscopic, and/or imaging evidence of sinusitis and at least 2 of the following: (1) headache has significantly worsened in parallel with worsening of the rhinosinusitis; (2) headache has significantly improved or resolved in parallel with improvement in or resolution of the rhinosinusitis; (3) headache is exacerbated by pressure applied over the paranasal sinuses; (4) in the case of unilateral rhinosinusitis, the headache is ipsilateral to the rhinosinusitis. However, these criteria may not be valid for sphenoid sinusitis, as purulent discharge often is lacking, and headache may precede sinus drainage. Once drainage begins, obstruction is relieved and the headache may begin to abate.

All sinusitis pain is not the same. Maxillary sinusitis pain most typically is located in the cheek, the gums, and the teeth of the upper jaw. Ethmoid sinusitis pain is felt between the eyes. The eyeball may be tender, and pain may be aggravated by eye movement. Frontal sinusitis pain is felt mainly in the forehead. Sphenoid sinusitis pain is felt in the vertex, but has a more general localization. Ethmoid and maxillary sinusitis usually is associated with rhinitis.

Hypertrophic turbinates, atrophic sinus membranes, and nasal passage abnormalities resulting from septal deflection are other conditions that may cause headache; however, they are not sufficiently validated as a cause of headache. Migraine and tension-type headache often are confused with true sinus headache because of their similar location. To diagnose IHS sinus headache, the previously defined criteria must be fulfilled strictly.

Differential Diagnosis

Although hypertrophic turbinates, atrophic sinus membranes, and nasal passage abnormalities caused by septal deflection may cause headache, these conditions have not been validated as causes of chronic headache. Whether nasal obstruction can lead to chronic headache is controversial.[1] Septal deformations with a contact point on the lateral nasal wall may produce episodic or transient headache. These abnormalities may be ignored by radiologists and should be considered when headaches are refractory to standard therapy. Ear/nose/throat evaluation may be useful, and intranasal blockade with an anesthetic such as lidocaine may confirm the diagnosis. If diagnosed correctly, removing the contact point may improve the headaches.[34] Given that these radiologic abnormalities are common in patients without headache, it is unclear as to whether so-called contact-point headaches can occur without a central disorder, such as a genetic predisposition to migraine or headache.

Migraine and tension-type headache often are confused with true sinus headache because of their similar locations. Some patients, in addition to having all the features of migraine without aura, have head pain in the facial areas, associated congestion of the nose, and headaches triggered by weather changes. None of these patients has purulent nasal discharge or the other abnormalities seen in acute rhinosinusitis. It is necessary, therefore, to differentiate headaches caused by rhinosinusitis from so-called sinus headaches, which are headache attacks fulfilling the criteria of migraine without aura with prominent autonomic symptoms in the nose, or migraine without aura triggered by nasal changes.

Eross and colleagues[35] evaluated 100 consecutive patients with self-diagnosed sinus headache. The actual diagnoses were migraine (52%), probable migraine (23%), chronic migraine (11%), other unclassifiable headaches (9%), cluster headache (1%), and hemicrania continua (1%). Only 3% of patients were accurately diagnosed with headache attributable to rhinosinusitis. Nasal congestion was present in 73% of patients and postnasal drip in 56%. Most patients reported pain triggered by changes in weather or season, and many noted changes with allergies or altitude, which are common migraine triggers.

In a population-based headache study[36] of 23,564 subjects, 4967 individuals called their headache migraine and 3074 individuals had headache that met IHS migraine criteria. Among those with IHS migraine, only 53.4% recognized their headaches as migraine; stress headaches (n = 345) and sinus headaches (n = 365) were the most common erroneous labels reported.[36] People are confused by their headache location. Because the sinuses are close to the eyes, individuals may attribute headaches located in the frontal, supraorbital, or infraorbital region to the sinuses.

In another clinic-based study, headache symptoms, headache-associated disability, and response to therapy among patients who had self-described sinus headache were assessed.[37] Eligible patients had to have self-described sinus headaches and at least 1 migraine symptom: moderate to severe pain, nausea or vomiting, photophobia or phonophobia, unilateral pain, pain worsening with activity, or pulsating pain. Patients were excluded if they had a previous migraine diagnosis or exposure to triptans, headaches associated with fever or purulent nasal discharge, or radiographic evidence of a sinus infection. Patients who had self-described sinus headache had migraine (70%) or migrainous (28%) headache based on headache classification criteria.[33] Most had nasal symptoms, including stuffiness (74%) and runny nose, and 45% said their headaches were precipitated by changes in the weather. Thus, patients who believe they have sinus headache, have no signs or symptoms of rhinosinusitis, and have 1 symptom of migraine, have migraine.

The relationship between headache and subacute and chronic sinus disease is highly controversial. Radiographic evidence of sinus disease is common and does not establish the cause of the headache.[20] Headache associated with sinus disease usually is continuous, not intermittent. Chronic sinusitis frequently is associated with engorged and swollen nasal mucosa and a purulent or sanguinopurulent nasal discharge. A diagnosis of headache caused by chronic or recurring rhinosinusitis can only be made if there is clinical evidence of the disorder and if the headache waxes and wanes in parallel with the degree of sinus congestion.[33]

Faleck and colleagues[38] reported that 10% of 150 children and adolescents who presented with chronic, nonprogressive headache, clinically indistinguishable from muscle-contraction headache, had radiographic evidence of sinus abnormality. None had prominent respiratory symptoms. All improved with treatment directed toward the sinus disorder. Although some had complete sinus opacification, none had endoscopy performed to show active disease in the ostia.

Unusual headaches that do not meet criteria for migraine may also raise suspicion for sinus disease. Airplane headache, a sudden severe headache associated with airplane landings,[33] is often associated with sinus disorders.[39] There are also reports of maxillary and sphenoid sinus disease causing cluster headache syndrome with severe headache, ocular pain, and autonomic symptoms.[40]

Treatment

The following are the management goals for the treatment of sinusitis:

- Treat bacterial infection when present
- Reduce ostial swelling
- Drain the sinuses
- Maintain sinus ostia patency

Rhinitis and sinusitis may be difficult to distinguish from each other based on history alone. Most acute upper respiratory infections are viral and do not require antibiotic treatment. Symptoms that persist for 7 days or more make acute bacterial sinusitis more likely and the use of antibiotics appropriate. Chronic sinusitis may have an infectious or noninfectious basis. Underlying disorders that predispose to chronic sinusitis should be identified and treated as part of the treatment of chronic sinusitis.[41]

Uncomplicated bacterial sinusitis, other than sphenoid sinusitis, should be treated with a broad-spectrum oral antibiotic for 10 to 14 days. Because nasal culture does not correlate to sinus pathogens, initial treatment is empiric.[17] Steam and saline prevent crusting of secretions in the nasal cavity and facilitate mucociliary clearance. Locally active vasoconstrictor agents provide symptomatic relief by shrinking inflamed and swollen nasal mucosa. Their use should be limited to 3 to 4 days to prevent rebound vasodilation. Oral decongestants should be used if prolonged treatment (>3 days) is necessary. These agents are α-adrenergic agonists that reduce nasal blood flow without the risk of rebound vasodilation.[15]

Antihistamines are not effective in the management of acute rhinitis. Anti-inflammatory topical corticosteroids may help maintain ostial patency. Adding fluticasone to xylometazoline and antimicrobial therapy with cefuroxime improves clinical success rates and accelerates recovery when patients who have a history of chronic rhinitis or recurrent sinusitis present for treatment of acute rhinosinusitis.[42] Treatment failure and recurrent infections are indications for neuroimaging and endoscopy to search for a source of obstruction. Sinus sampling for culture should be considered. Endoscopic nasal surgery may be necessary to reopen and maintain the patency of the sinus ostia and ostiomeatal complex.[15]

Complications should be treated with high doses of intravenous antibiotics and surgical drainage, if appropriate, of any enclosed space.

SPHENOID SINUSITIS

Sphenoid sinusitis, because of its rarity, unique location, and complications, is discussed separately. Sphenoid sinusitis is an uncommon infection that accounts for approximately 3% of all cases of acute sinusitis. Usually accompanied by pansinusitis, it occurs alone less commonly. It frequently is misdiagnosed,[43] because the sphenoid sinus is not visualized adequately with routine sinus radiographs and is not accessible to direct clinical examination, even with the flexible endoscope. Although sphenoid sinusitis is an uncommon cause of headache, it is potentially associated with significant morbidity and mortality, and requires early identification and aggressive management.[2,14,43]

The sphenoid sinus is contained within the body of the sphenoid bone deep in the nasal cavity, and is divided in half by the intersphenoid septum. Each sinus communicates with the sphenoethmoidal recess, located at the posterior-superior aspect of the superior concha. The sphenoidal sinuses are present as minute cavities at birth, and their main development does not occur until puberty.[44]

The roof of the sphenoid sinus is related to the middle cranial fossa and the pituitary gland in the sella turcica: lateral is the cavernous sinus; posterior is the clivus and pons; anterior are the posterior nasal cavity, posterior ethmoid cells, and cribriform plate; and inferior is the nasopharynx. The cavernous sinus contains the internal carotid arteries and the third, fourth, fifth, and seventh cranial nerves. The maxillary division of the fifth nerve may indent the wall of the sphenoid sinus. The sphenoid walls can be extremely thin, and sometimes the sinus cavity is separated from the adjacent structure by just a thin mucosal barrier. Because of the close proximity to the cortical venous system, cranial nerves, and meninges, infection may spread to these structures and present as a central nervous system infection or neurologic catastrophe.[2,45]

Symptoms

Headache is the most common symptom of acute sphenoid sinusitis: it is present in all patients who are able to complain about it. The headache is aggravated by standing, walking, bending, or coughing, often interferes with sleep, and is poorly relieved by opioids. Its location is variable: vertex headache is rare; frontal, occipital, or temporal headache, or a combination of these locations, is most common.

Periorbital pain is common, in contrast to the common teaching that retro-orbital or vertex headache is the most common presenting symptom of sphenoid sinusitis.[46–48] Nausea and vomiting occur frequently, but nasal discharge, stuffiness, and postnasal drip are unusual. Fever occurs in more than half of patients who have acute sphenoid sinusitis.

Diagnosis

The diagnosis of sphenoid sinusitis frequently is delayed. Sphenoid sinusitis should be included in the differential diagnosis of acute or subacute headache. It may be mistaken for frontal or ethmoid sinusitis, aseptic meningitis, brain abscess, or septic thrombophlebitis. Sphenoid sinusitis can mimic trigeminal neuralgia, migraine, carotid artery aneurysm, or brain tumor.[2,14,43]

A severe, intractable, new-onset headache that interferes with sleep and is not relieved by simple analgesics should alert one to the diagnosis of sphenoid sinusitis.

The headache increases in severity and has no specific location. Pain or paresthesias in the facial distribution of the fifth nerve, and photophobia or eye tearing are also suggestive of sphenoid sinusitis.[2,14,41,46,47,49]

The physical examination may not be helpful. Not all patients are febrile, sinus tenderness rarely is present, and pus is not always seen, although Lew and colleagues[2] state that a careful examination of the nose and throat often demonstrates pus. Whether this reflects advanced disease or the presence of pansinusitis is uncertain. In a more recent series of 14 patients who had acute sphenoid sinusitis, Kibblewhite and colleagues[14] found purulent exudate in only 3 patients.

Neuroimaging is necessary to diagnose sphenoid sinusitis definitively. All of the cases in the series of Kibblewhite and colleagues[14] were diagnosed by radiography. Some cases can be diagnosed by plain sinus radiographs but, because of the superimposition of soft tissues, plain radiographs are nondiagnostic in approximately 25% of cases.[45] If sphenoid sinusitis is suspected and plain radiographs are nondiagnostic, CT or MRI is indicated.

In a high-risk group of 300 patients referred with a clinical diagnosis of sinusitis, 68% had abnormal plain radiographs but none had sphenoid sinus abnormalities, suggesting that the specificity of plain radiographs is very high.[50] The mucosa of the sinus approximates the bone so closely that it cannot be visualized on CT. Therefore, any soft-tissue bulge seen in the sinus is abnormal.[18] Digre and colleagues[51] reviewed 300 CT or MRI radiographic studies. The sphenoid sinus was visualized in all cases. Abnormalities were detected in 7% of routine CT scans, 8% of posterior fossa scans, and 6% of MRI scans. Of the 21 patients who had sphenoid abnormalities, 24% in their highly selected sample had important clinically related disease.

Complications

Major complications of sphenoid sinusitis include bacterial meningitis,[2] cavernous sinus thrombosis,[2,14,43,45] subdural abscess, cortical vein thrombosis, ophthalmoplegia, and pituitary insufficiency. Sphenoid sinusitis can present as aseptic meningitis because of the presence of a parameningeal focus.[52] Patients can present with the complications of sphenoid sinusitis, including visual loss mimicking optic neuritis, multiple cranial nerve palsies, or papilledema. Sudden onset, as a result of cavernous sinus thrombosis, can mimic a subarachnoid hemorrhage.[53]

Øktedalen and Lilleås[54] reported 4 patients admitted to an infectious disease department with meningitis, sepsis, and orbital cellulitis. Diagnosis was difficult in all cases. All 4 patients had fever and headache. Three of the 4 had normal plain sinus radiographs. CT diagnosed all cases. Six of Lew and colleagues'[2] 15 acute cases had meningitis, 5 had cavernous sinus thrombosis, 1 had cortical vein thrombosis, 1 had unilateral ophthalmoplegia, and 1 had orbital cellulitis. Eight of Kibblewhite and colleagues'[14] 14 patients had complications on admission. None of the patients studied by Goldman and colleagues[43] had complications. The difference in the complication rate is a result of selection bias: Goldman and colleagues'[43] patients were retrieved from emergency room records, whereas those in the series of Lew and colleagues,[2] Øktedalen and Lilleås,[54] and Kibblewhite and colleagues[14] came from inpatient records.

Treatment

Sphenoid sinusitis without complications may be managed with high-dose intravenous antibiotics and topical and systemic decongestants for 10 to 14 days.[14,43] If the fever (if present) and the headache do not start to improve within 24 to 48 hours, or if any complications are present or develop, drainage of the sphenoid sinus is indicated.[43] Rarely fungal infection can occur, even in immunocompetent persons.[55]

NASAL HEADACHE

Many rhinologists hold the controversial belief that septal deformation, especially of traumatic origin, may exert pressure on the sensitive structure of the lateral nasal wall, causing referred pain and chronic headache. McAuliffe and colleagues[56] studied the sensitivity of the nasal cavities and paranasal sinuses using touch, pressure, and faradic stimulation. The nasal turbinates and sinus ostia were much more sensitive than the mucosal lining of the septum and the paranasal sinuses. Most of the pain elicited was referred pain. It was of increased intensity, longer duration, and referred to larger areas in subjects who had swelling and engorgement of the nasal turbinates and the sinus ostia.

Schønsted-Madsen and colleagues[1] followed up 444 patients who had nasal obstruction, 157 of whom had headache. Treatment consisted of septoplastic surgery, reconstruction of the nasal pyramids, or submucosal conchotomy. The headache usually was localized to the forehead, glabella, or above and around the eyes. Thirty-six patients had constant headache, 48 daily headache, 56 weekly headache, and 17 monthly headache. Fifty-seven patients had mild headache, 66 had moderate headache, and 34 had severe headache. Many of these patients misused analgesics. Eighty percent of the patients who underwent surgery were relieved of nasal obstruction (the primary reason for surgery), and 60% of the patients who underwent surgery were relieved of chronic headache. If the surgery relieved the nasal obstruction, 80% had headache relief; however, if the surgery failed, only 30% had headache relief.

Clerico[57] reported 10 patients who had intractable migraine, tension-type headache, or cluster headache without significant nasal or sinus symptoms. Various intranasal and sinus abnormalities, such as anatomic variation or subclinical inflammation, were found on CT or nasal endoscopy. The patients were treated medically or surgically, and all improved. Low and Willatt[58] reported 106 patients who had a submucous resection for a deviated nasal septum. Almost half (47.4%) had recurring headaches preoperatively. Postoperatively, 63.6% had complete or partial relief at follow-up for as long as 18 months. Although 79.3% of patients had headache relief when evaluated before 1 year, only 46.2% had relief after 1 year.

These studies do not account for the historical relationship between headache onset and the development of nasal obstruction, or for the analgesic or decongestant overuse that may produce daily headache. In addition, any surgical procedure has a powerful placebo effect. The studies do suggest that some patients who have nasal obstruction have headache that is relieved by successful medical or surgical treatment. Because the prevalence of migraine in the population is approximately 12%, episodic tension-type headache prevalence approximately 90%, and chronic tension-type headache prevalence approximately 3%, these data are difficult to interpret. In addition, these studies had no control group and only responders were reported in Clerico's study.[57]

In a retrospective review of operative notes of 170 patients who underwent functional endoscopic sinus surgery, 50 patients (29%) who had a history of chronic headaches were identified. Thirty-seven met the predetermined inclusion criteria for this study, which were (1) a history of chronic headaches, (2) rhinologic cause for these headaches suggested by the presence of contact points (documented by nasal endoscopy or CT scans), (3) no other origin or cause of headaches after a thorough evaluation, and (4) surgical intervention that included relief of contact points by inferior, middle, or superior turbinoplasty. After surgery, 29 of the 34 patients (85%) in the study group reported a decrease in headache frequency. There were many patients who had severe contact points on CT, however, and did not complain of headaches. In fact, most patients who had headaches and contact points also had concurrent chronic sinusitis, which served as the primary indication for surgery in this patient population.[58]

Other open studies[59,60] and reviews[61] suggest that headache can be the only clinical presentation of sinus or nasal abnormality. These studies do not use established criteria for headache or the new diagnostic criteria for sinusitis.

REFERENCES

1. Schønsted-Madsen U, Stoksted P, Christensen PH, et al. Chronic headache related to nasal obstruction. J Laryngol Otol 1986;100:165–70.
2. Lew D, Southwick FS, Montgomery WW, et al. Sphenoid sinusitis: a review of 30 cases. N Engl J Med 1983;19:1149–54.
3. Sande MA, Gwaltney JM. Acute community-acquired bacterial sinusitis: continuing challenges and current management. Clin Infect Dis 2004; 39(Suppl 13):S151–8.
4. Collins JG. Prevalence of selected chronic conditions: United States 1990-1992. Vital Health Stat 10 1997;(984):1–89.
5. Diaz I, Bamberger DM. Acute sinusitis. Semin Respir Infect 1995;10:14–20.
6. Reilly JS. The sinusitis cycle. Otolaryngol Head Neck Surg 1990;103:856–62.
7. Hilding AC. Physiologic basis of nasal operations. Calif Med 1950;72:103–7.
8. Messerklinger W. Endoscopy of the nose. Baltimore (MD): Urban and Schwartzenberg; 1978.
9. McCaffrey TV. Functional endoscopic sinus surgery: an overview. Mayo Clin Proc 1993;68:675–7.
10. Zinreich SJ. Paranasal sinus imaging. Otolaryngol Head Neck Surg 1990;103: 863–9.
11. Kennedy DW. Surgical update. Otolaryngol Head Neck Surg 1990;103:884–6.
12. Gwaltney JM, Phillips CD, Miller RD, et al. Computed tomographic study of the common cold. N Engl J Med 1994;330:25–30.
13. Rouby J, Laurent P, Gosnach M, et al. Risk factors and clinical relevance of nosocomial maxillary sinusitis in the critically ill. Am J Respir Crit Care Med 1994;150:776–83.
14. Kibblewhite DJ, Cleland J, Mintz DR. Acute sphenoid sinusitis: management strategies. J Otolaryngol 1988;17:159–63.
15. Stafford CT. The clinician's view of sinusitis. Otolaryngol Head Neck Surg 1990; 103:870–5.
16. Schatz CJ, Becker TS. Normal CT anatomy of the paranasal sinuses. Radiol Clin North Am 1984;22:107–18.
17. Bhattacharyya N. Test-retest reliability of computed tomography in the assessment of chronic rhinosinusitis. Laryngoscope 1999;109:1055–8.
18. Bhattacharyya N, Fried MP. The accuracy of computed tomography in the diagnosis of chronic rhinosinusitis. Laryngoscope 2003;113:125–9.
19. Druce HM, Siavin RG. Sinusitis: a critical need for further study. J Allergy Clin Immunol 1991;88:675–7.
20. Havas TE, Motbey JA, Gullane PJ. Prevalence of incidental abnormalities on computed tomographic scans of the paranasal sinuses. Arch Otolaryngol 1988;114:856–9.

21. Castellanos J, Axelrod D. Flexible fiberoptic rhinoscopy in the diagnosis of sinusitis. J Allergy Clin Immunol 1989;83:91–4.
22. Benninger MS, Anon J, Mabry RL. The medical management of rhinosinusitis. Otolaryngol Head Neck Surg 1997;117:S41–9.
23. Slavin RG. Nasal polyps and sinusitis. JAMA 1997;278:1849–54.
24. Zinreich SJ, Kennedy DW, Rosenbaum AE, et al. Paranasal sinuses: CT imaging requirements for endoscopic surgery. Radiology 1987;163:769–75.
25. Lanza DC, Kennedy DW. Adult rhinosinusitis defined. Otolaryngol Head Neck Surg 1997;117:S1–7.
26. Williams JW, Simel DL, Roberts L, et al. Clinical evaluation of sinusitis. Ann Intern Med 1992;117:705–10.
27. International rhinosinusitis advisory board infectious rhinosinusitis in adults: classification, etiology, and management. Ear Nose Throat J 1997;76:S5–22.
28. Lau J, Zucker D, Engels EA, et al. Diagnosis and treatment of acute bacterial rhinosinusitis. Evid Rep Technol Assess (Summ). Rockville (MD): Agency for Health Care Policy and Research; 1999.
29. Naranch K, Park YJ, Ramirez MR, et al. A tender sinus does not always mean rhinosinusitis. Otolaryngol Head Neck Surg 2002;127:387–97.
30. Muntz HR, Lusk RP. Signs and symptoms of chronic sinusitis. In: Lusk RP, editor. Pediatric sinusitis. New York: Raven Press; 1992. p. 1–6.
31. Hilger PA. Diseases of the nose. In: Hilger PA, editor. Boie's fundamentals of otolaryngology; a textbook of ear, nose, and throat disease. Philadelphia: WB Saunders; 1989. p. 206–48.
32. Wolff HG. Wolff's headache and other head pain. 1st edition. New York: Oxford University Press; 1948.
33. Headache Classification Committee of the International Headache Society (IHS). The international classification of headache disorders, 3rd edition (beta version). Cephalalgia 2013;33(9):629–808.
34. Rozen TD. Intranasal contact point headache: missing the "point" on brain MRI. Neurology 2009;72(12):1107.
35. Eross E, Dodick D, Eross M. The Sinus, Allergy and Migraine Study (SAMS). Headache 2007;47(2):213–24.
36. Lipton RB, Stewart WF, Liberman JN. Self-awareness of migraine: interpreting the labels that headache sufferers apply to their headaches. Neurology 2002; 58:S21–6.
37. Cady RK, Schreiber CP. Sinus headache or migraine? Considerations in making a differential diagnosis. Neurology 2002;58:S10–4.
38. Faleck H, Rothner AD, Erenberg G, et al. Headache and subacute sinusitis in children and adolescents. Headache 1988;28:96–8.
39. Mainardi F, Maggioni F, Lisotto C, et al. Diagnosis and management of headache attributed to airplane travel. Curr Neurol Neurosci Rep 2013; 13(3):335.
40. Zanchin G, Rossi P, Licandro AM, et al. Clusterlike headache. A case of sphenoidal aspergilloma. Headache 1995;35(8):494–7.
41. Dykewicz MS. Allergic disorders: rhinitis and sinusitis. J Allergy Clin Immunol 2003;111:S520–9.
42. Dolor RJ, Witsell DL, Hellkamp AS, et al. Comparison of cefuroxime with or without intranasal fluticasone for the treatment of rhinosinusitis. The CAFFS trial: a randomized controlled trial. JAMA 2001;286:3097–105.
43. Goldman GE, Fontanarosa PB, Anderson JM. Isolated sphenoid sinusitis. Am J Emerg Med 1993;11:235–8.

44. Goss CM. Gray's anatomy of the human body. 27th edition. Philadelphia: Lea & Febiger; 1959.
45. Sofferman RA. Cavernous sinus thrombophlebitis secondary to sphenoid sinusitis. Laryngoscope 1983;93:797–800.
46. Deans JA, Welch AR. Acute isolated sphenoid sinusitis: a disease with complications. J Laryngol Otol 1991;105:1072–4.
47. Nordeman L, Lucid E. Sphenoid sinusitis, a cause of debilitating headache. J Emerg Med 1990;8:557–9.
48. Urquhart AC, Fung G, McIntosh WA. Isolated sphenoiditis: a diagnostic problem. J Laryngol Otol 1989;103:526–7.
49. Turkewitz D, Keller R. Acute headache in childhood: a case of sphenoid sinusitis. Pediatr Emerg Care 1987;3:155–7.
50. Axelsson A, Jensen A. The roentgenologic demonstration of sinusitis. Am J Roentgenol Radium Ther Nucl Med 1974;122:621–7.
51. Digre KB, Maxner CE, Crawford S, et al. Significance of CT and MR findings in sphenoid sinus disease. AJNR Am J Neuroradiol 1989;10:603–6.
52. Brook I, Overturf GD, Steinberg EA, et al. Acute sphenoid sinusitis presenting as aseptic meningitis: a pachymeningitis syndrome. Int J Pediatr Otorhinolaryngol 1982;4:77–81.
53. Dale BA, Mackenzie IJ. The complications of sphenoid sinusitis. J Laryngol Otol 1983;97:661–70.
54. Øktedalen O, Lilleås F. Septic complications to sphenoidal sinus infection. Scand J Infect Dis 1992;24:353–6.
55. Molnár-Gábor E, Dóczi I, Hatvani L, et al. Isolated sinusitis sphenoidalis caused by *Trichoderma longibrachiatum* in an immunocompetent patient with headache. J Med Microbiol 2013;62(Pt 8):1249–52.
56. McAuliffe GW, Goodell H, Wolff HG. Experimental studies on headache: pain from the nasal and paranasal structures. Res Publ Assoc Res Nerv Ment Dis 1943;23:185–206.
57. Clerico DM. Sinus headaches reconsidered: referred cephalgia of rhinologic origin masquerading as refractory primary headaches. Headache 1995;35:185–92.
58. Low WK, Willatt DJ. Headaches associated with nasal obstruction due to deviated nasal septum. Headache 1995;35:404–6.
59. Parsons DS, Batra PS. Functional endoscopic sinus surgical outcomes for contact point headaches. Laryngoscope 1998;108:696–702.
60. Chow JM. Rhinologic headaches. Otolaryngol Head Neck Surg 1994;111:211–8.
61. Salman SD, Rebeiz EE. Sinusitis and headache. J Med Liban 1994;42:200–2.

Temporomandibular Disorders and Headaches

Steven B. Graff-Radford, DDS[a,b], Jennifer P. Bassiur, DDS[c],*

KEYWORDS

- Temporomandibular disorder • Migraine • Tension-type headache • Bruxism

KEY POINTS

- Temporomandibular disorders (TMDs) and headache are common and may be reported as single or separate entities.
- There is no single cause for TMDs.
- Patients with asymptomatic clicking, often do not require treatment.
- Therapy is indicated if pain, significant limitation in mandibular range of motion, or both are present.
- The pain associated with TMD is frequently of muscular origin.
- Imaging alone should not dictate treatment.
- The symptoms of TMD are often self-limiting.

INTRODUCTION

Temporomandibular disorders (TMDs) are a major cause of nondental pain in the orofacial region, and may cause headache.[1] The International Classification of Headache Disorders, 3rd edition (ICHD-3) recognizes headache attributed to TMDs[2] but, because headache and TMD are prevalent, have multifactorial origins, and have similar or overlapping symptoms, diagnosis is often confused. It is often difficult to differentiate these disorders when they coexist.[3] Overlap may also result from shared environmental and genetic factors involving abnormal pain processing and trigeminal sensitization. The trigeminal nerve is the final conduit of face, neck, and head pain,[4] which may be generated by musculoskeletal, vascular, or neural structures. Once pain is established, referral anywhere in the trigeminal and cervical complex can occur through central sensitization. Management of TMD may reduce nociception, ameliorate sensitization, and reduce primary headache. However, this does not mean there

[a] The Pain Center, 444 South San Vicente #1101, Los Angeles, CA 90048, USA; [b] Section of Oral Medicine and Orofacial Pain, UCLA School of Dentistry, 10833 Leconte Avenue, Los Angeles, CA 90024, USA; [c] Columbia University College of Dental Medicine, Division of Oral & Maxillofacial Surgery, 630 West 168th Street, Vanderbilt Building, 7th Floor, New York, NY 10032, USA
* Corresponding author. Columbia University College of Dental Medicine, Division of Oral & Maxillofacial Surgery, 630 West 168th Street, Vanderbilt Building, 7th Floor, New York, NY 10032.
E-mail address: jpb2133@cumc.columbia.edu

Neurol Clin 32 (2014) 525–537
http://dx.doi.org/10.1016/j.ncl.2013.11.009
0733-8619/14/$ – see front matter © 2014 Elsevier Inc. All rights reserved.

is a direct cause-and-effect relationship between TMD and primary headache; they can coexist and relate to each other through common neural circuits. Understanding the relationship between TMD and primary headache, as well as headache secondary to TMD, is important. Management is best achieved by addressing each individually and realizing that one can perpetuate the other.

TEMPOROMANDIBULAR DISORDERS

TMDs include musculoskeletal and neuromuscular conditions that involve the temporomandibular joints (TMJs), the masticatory muscles, and all associated tissues.[5] Common painful TMDs are generated from myogenous and/or arthrogenous components. A painful TMD may occur in 10% of the population and other signs and symptoms of TMD (eg, clicking, limited range of motion, pain on function) have been reported in 46.1% of the United States population.[6,7] Studies of nonpatient populations have found that up to 75% of people studied have at least one sign of joint dysfunction and nearly one-third of the population has at least one TMD symptom.[8] These data may be affected by differences in diagnostic criteria and data collection methods in the cross-sectional epidemiologic studies on the prevalence of TMDs. In 1992, the Research Criteria for TMD (RDC/TMD) introduced the use of standardized diagnostic criteria to improve consistency among studies. The RDC/TMD has provided researchers with a standardized process for examining, diagnosing, and classifying patients with TMD for the most common TMD subtypes.[9] A systematic review including only those studies using RDC/TMD reported prevalences up to 12.9% for masticatory muscle pain, 15.8% for disc derangements, and 8.9% for inflammatory-degenerative or painful TMJ disorders.[10] Less than 7% of individuals with TMDs need therapeutic intervention,[11] and an even smaller percentage complain of headache.

Headache and TMD are common and may therefore be reported as a single or as separate entities. The TMJ, masticatory muscles, and associated orofacial structures may act as triggering or perpetuating factors for primary headache. A primary headache disorder may similarly trigger or perpetuate pain in the masticatory muscles or TMJ. Ciancaglini and Radaelli[3] reported that headache occurs significantly more frequently in patients with TMD symptoms (27.4% vs 15.2%). Individuals with myogenous TMDs are more likely than those with arthrogenous TMDs to have headache, and the prevalence of TMD in patients with migraine and tension-type headache is higher than in a nonheadache population.[12] According to Glaros and colleagues,[13] individuals with chronic headache were more likely than nonheadache controls to meet criteria for an RDC/TMD diagnosis of myofascial pain. The potential for headache secondary to TMDs is recognized in the ICHD-3 with diagnostic criteria for 11.7 Headache attributed to temporomandibular disorder (TMD) (**Box 1**). Jaw movement or pressure applied to the TMJ or surrounding musculature frequently exacerbates the secondary headache. The described pain typically manifests ipsilaterally when the TMJ is the pain generator, but may be bilateral with muscular involvement.[2] Peripheral and central mechanisms are likely involved in myogenous TMDs.[14] Painful TMDs may increase central sensitization, inducing, exacerbating, or contributing to the chronification of headache. Regardless of whether or not evidence of causation can be shown, ignoring TMDs as peripheral triggers of headache often results in a poor clinical outcome.

CAUSES OF TMD

There are many factors associated with TMDs but no universal cause has been identified. There is no single cause for all TMDs. Inflammation of the TMJs' synovial lining or capsule may account for joint pain, and may be associated with an incoordination of

---

Box 1
ICHD-3 (beta) criteria for headache attributed to TMD (11.7)

Description:

Headache caused by a disorder involving structures in the temporomandibular region

Diagnostic criteria:

A. Any headache fulfilling criterion C

B. Clinical and/or imaging evidence of a pathologic process affecting the TMJ, muscles of mastication, and/or associated structures

C. Evidence of causation shown by at least 2 of the following:

  1. Headache has developed in temporal relation to the onset of the TMD

  2. Either or both of the following:

     a. Headache has significantly worsened in parallel with progression of the TMD

     b. Headache has significantly improved or resolved in parallel with improvement in or resolution of the TMD

  3. The headache is produced or exacerbated by active jaw movements, passive movements through the range of motion of the jaw, and/or provocative maneuvers applied to temporomandibular structures such as pressure on the TMJ and surrounding muscles of mastication

  4. Headache, when unilateral, is ipsilateral to the side of the TMD

D. Not better accounted for by another ICHD-3 diagnosis

From the Headache Classification Committee of the International Headache Society (IHS). The International Classification of Headache Disorders, 3rd edition (beta version). Cephalgia 2013;33(9):629–808; with permission.

---

the disc-condyle complex. Bone degeneration or disc displacement may occur, resulting in the incoordination during movement. Predisposing, initiating, or perpetuating factors for TMD may include parafunctional behaviors (clenching, bruxism) causing microtraumas, direct or indirect trauma, changes in occlusion, and systemic, genetic, and psychosocial factors.

Although parafunctional habits have been implicated in TMD, their relationships with headache remain unknown. Of all the parafunctional activities of the stomatognathic system, bruxism is regularly, if incorrectly, assumed to be the most damaging and a major risk factor for TMDs.[15] Bruxism involves diurnal or nocturnal parafunctional activity, including clenching, bracing, gnashing, and grinding of the teeth. It is common, occurring in 5% to 8% of the population, and independent of frequency in 31% of the population.[16–20] The reported prevalence data are variable, subject to identification (sleep or awake bruxism or both). Sleep bruxism (SB) is an oromandibular sleep-related movement disorder of repetitive gnashing of the teeth that is usually nocturnal, occurs during sleep, and is associated with arousals.[18,19,21] SB is affected by smoking, the use of drugs such as antidepressants, caffeine, alcohol,[16,22] type A personality and/or anxiety, as well as sleep-related breathing disorders.[22] Up to 65% of patients with SB report frequent headache.[23,24] A systematic literature review from 1998 to 2008 by Mandfredini and Lobbezoo[15] supported an association between self-report/questionnaire-diagnosed bruxism and TMD symptoms. In most of the self-report studies reviewed, the association was with myofascial pain or symptoms of muscle disorders. The investigators also described a positive association between myofascial pain and clinically diagnosed bruxism, With the caution that the bruxism diagnosis was pain dependent,[15] but only some bruxers have facial pain. Neither tooth wear nor polysomnogram-confirmed bruxism was predictably associated with TMD.[15] In the absence of control for other causes, tooth wear cannot reliably predict bruxism.[20] Evidence of SB on polysomnographic or electomyographic recordings may not represent activity that fluctuates over time. Experimental, sustained clenching can cause muscle pain, but it is usually short-lived.[15] Clenching that is not experimentally induced has not been shown to cause muscle pain. Fernandes and colleagues[25] found a significant increase in the risk for chronic migraine, episodic migraine, and episodic tension-type headache when SB was associated with TMD; however, SB alone did not increase the risk for headache. Although a causal relationship is not evident, SB is associated with TMDs and headache and may exacerbate TMD and/ or headache symptoms.

Sensory innervation of the TMJ is mediated through the mandibular division of the trigeminal nerve. The TMJ capsule, posterior attachment, and discal ligaments are sensitive to pain. The articular disc, vital to maintaining condylar stability during mandibular movement, is not sensitive to pain because it is devoid of direct innervation or vascularization. The richly vascularized and innervated posterior attachment is often implicated in joint pain.

Trauma to the TMJ may result in capsulitis. This acute inflammatory process tends to resolve quickly and without complication. By comparison, painful derangements of the TMJ are more likely to be associated with chronic joint disorders. The cause may be multifactorial or unclear, but often involves articular disc displacement.

The TMJ is formed by the articular surfaces of the temporal bone and the mandibular condyle, bilaterally. Each TMJ is separated into an upper and lower compartment by a fibrocartilaginous disc. The TMJ is subject to the pathologic disorders that affect other synovial joints, but it is unique in several anatomic features. The TMJs move as a functional unit and, unlike most synovial joints, are lined by fibrocartilage, which is more resistant to degenerative change and has a greater capacity for repair than hyaline cartilage. The ability of the TMJ to adapt to various biomechanical stresses is well documented.[26] Failure of this adaptive capacity mechanism may lead to tissue destruction and disc displacement and may be affected by age, stress, sex, systemic illness, or previous trauma. Incoordination of the disc-condyle relationship is a major component of TMDs. Articular disc displacement is the most common temporomandibular arthropathy and is characterized by an abnormal relationship or misalignment of the articular disc relative to the condyle.[26] This condition, often referred to as an internal derangement, interferes with smooth movement of the TMJ, resulting in joint noises, brief sticking or catching, or locking. Disc displacements can be divided into disc displacement with reduction and disc displacement without reduction (**Boxes 2 and 3**).[11] In disc displacement with reduction, the disc reduces, or is recaptured, on opening of the mouth. The disc reduction is accompanied by a sound that is often described as clicking or popping. With mandibular closure, a second sound called a reciprocal click or closing click may be audible as the disc moves off the condyle just before the teeth come together. Clicking sounds are not necessarily a sign of degeneration or an indication for treatment. Moderate to severe derangements have been observed on imaging in greater than one-third of an asymptomatic population,[27] and as many as 25% of clicking joints show normal or slightly displaced discs.[28] Irrespective of whether it is acute or chronic, disc displacement is not necessarily painful. Patients with pain-free clicking often do not require treatment. Therapy is indicated if pain, significant limitation in mandibular range of motion, or both are present.

Box 2
Diagnostic criteria for disc displacement with reduction

All of the following must be present:

Reproducible joint noise that usually occurs at variable positions during opening and closing mandibular movements.

Soft tissue imaging reveals displaced disc that improves its position during mandibular opening, and hard tissue imaging shows the absence of extensive degenerative bone changes (although the diagnosis of disc displacement can only be confirmed with soft tissue imaging, the temperate nature of the disorder does not warrant routine soft tissue imaging).

Any of the following may accompany the preceding items:

Pain, when present, is precipitated by joint movement

Deviation during opening movement coincides with a click

No restriction in mandibular movement

Episodic and momentary catching during opening (<35 mm) that self-reduces with voluntary mandibular repositioning

A disc displacement without reduction, also referred to as a closed lock, occurs when the out-of-place disc remains out of place during movement of the mandible. This condition is usually, but not necessarily, associated with limited range of motion and deflection to the affected side, because translation of the condyle is limited by position of the disc. Patients may provide a history of joint noises or momentary catching before the onset of an acute closed lock. TMDs are usually self-limiting, occurring in girls and women between the ages of 15 and 30 years. The disorders last 7 to 10 years, often with clicking followed by locking and then healing.

Box 3
Diagnostic criteria for disc displacement without reduction

All of the following must be present:

Persistent, markedly limited mouth opening (<35 mm) with a history of sudden onset.

Deflection to the affected side on mouth opening.

Markedly limited laterotrusion to the contralateral side (if unilateral disorder). Reproducible joint noise that usually occurs at variable positions during opening and closing mandibular movements.

Soft tissue imaging reveals displaced disc without reduction (although the diagnosis of disc displacement can only be confirmed with soft tissue imaging, the temperate nature of the disorder does not warrant routine soft tissue imaging).

Any of the following may accompany the preceding items:

Pain, precipitated by forced mouth opening

History of clicking that ceases with locking

Pain with palpation of the affected joint

Ipsilateral hyperocclusion

No or mild osteoarthritic changes with hard tissue imaging

The pain associated with TMD is frequently of muscular origin. The most common diagnosis is myofascial pain (MFP). Characterized by a regional muscle pain, MFP is described as dull or achy and is associated with the presence of trigger points in muscles, tendons, or fascia.[29–33] Persistent regional pain of the neck, shoulder, head, and orofacial region is commonly caused by MFP. Developmental (eg, stress or oral habits) and perpetuating (eg, poor sleep, postural abnormalities, depression) factors have been identified in association with MFP; however, the precise cause remains unclear.[34,35] MFP is characterized by the presence of trigger points with local and referred pain. The trigger points may be active or latent. When palpated, active trigger points refer pain to distant sites. Digital palpation of latent trigger points may result in local tenderness, but no distant referral occurs. MFP is not confined to a single dermatomal, myotomal, or visceral division. The tender points develop in tense muscles in which active or passive stretching produces increased pain associated with decreased motion. Contracting the muscle against fixed resistance produces maximal pain. Clinical examination reveals nodular or ropelike bands under the skin that are associated with the tender points. Palpation may result in pain and a visible movement by the patient, called a jump sign.[36] Palpating over the band, opposite to the muscle fiber orientation, may elicit a twitch response. A characteristic referral pattern can be elicited for each muscle. The referred pain and tenderness may initiate further muscle pain and satellite trigger points.

IMAGING IN TMD

Patient history and clinical findings should be used to determine the need for diagnostic imaging and the type of imaging indicated. Additional factors to consider are the cost, amount of radiation exposure, and potential impact on treatment of the selected imaging. Hard tissues such as bony structures can be evaluated, to varying degrees, using panoramic, transcranial, and tomographic studies. Computed tomography (CT) can show soft tissue, but is most useful for visualization of osseous abnormalities. A disadvantage of CT imaging is exposure to high levels of radiation. Cone beam CT (CBCT) provides similar visualization of osseous abnormalities.[37] CBCT uses a lower radiation dose than traditional CT imaging, provides high-resolution multiplanar images, and allows computer reconstruction into two-dimensional and three-dimensional images. Magnetic resonance imaging (MRI) remains the gold standard of diagnostic imaging for soft tissue visualization and is the best method to accurately assess disc position and to show its movement.[38] Useful information may be gathered from evaluating the movement of the disc-condyle complex from open-mouth to closed-mouth positions. Fig. 1 shows the normal anatomy of the TMJ. The TMJ is located anterior to the external auditory meatus and provides the articulation between the mandibular condyles and the squamous temporal bone. The dense, avascular, fibrocartilaginous articulating surfaces of the condyle and fossa function against the fibrous interarticular disc. Medial and lateral collateral ligaments connect the disc to the condyle. The disc attaches anteriorly to the lateral pterygoid muscle. The disc attaches posteriorly to highly vascularized and richly innervated retrodiscal tissue. This tissue is a source for inflammatory pain. Normal disc position in the open-mouth and closed-mouth positions can be seen in Fig. 1. Fig. 2 shows disc displacement with recapture on opening. Fig. 3 shows disc displacement without recapture of the disc on opening, sometimes described as a closed lock. The presence or absence of joint effusion[39] and osseous changes[40] may also be assessed on MRI. Although MRI provides useful additional information, systematic review did not show clear evidence of a relationship between MRI and clinical diagnoses.[41] Imaging alone should not dictate treatment.

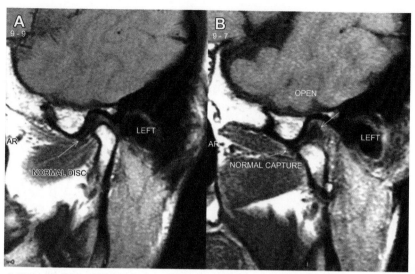

Fig. 1. Normal disc in the (*A*) closed-mouth and (*B*) open-mouth positions. The arrows point to the disc appearing as a dark bow tie shape. *Abbreviations:* AR, Anterior Right; PR, Posterior Right.

MANAGING TMD

TMD may cause headache[2] or may exacerbate headache symptoms. In contrast, a primary headache disorder may initiate pain in the masticatory muscles or TMJ.[8,42] A deficiency of many TMD-headache studies is the lack of a clear diagnosis. When headache is reduced following treatment of the TMD, uncertainty exists as whether or not it can be connected to, or correlated with, the TMD. Although providing

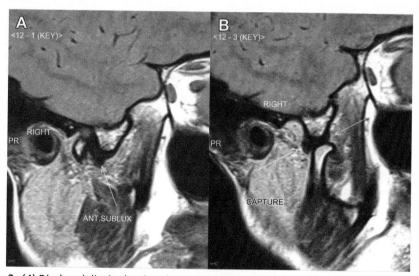

Fig. 2. (*A*) Displaced disc in the closed-mouth position. The arrow shows the disc anterior to the condyle. (*B*) Disc reduction to normal position on mouth opening. The arrows point to the disc seen as a dark bow tie shape. *Abbreviations:* AR, Anterior Right; PR, Posterior Right.

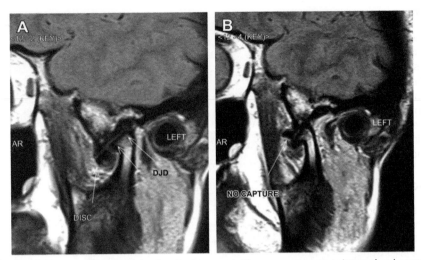

Fig. 3. (A) Degenerative condyle disc displacement. The upper arrows point to the degenerative condyle and the lower arrow points to the anteriorly positioned disc. (B) Open view shows no recapture. The arrow shows the nonreduced disc still anterior to the condyle on mouth opening.

treatment of a coexisting TMD may reduce headache pain intensity and frequency, it does not necessarily indicate a causal relationship. Nonetheless, in patients presenting with both TMD and headache, treatment outcomes may be improved by managing both disorders.

For most patients with TMD, initial conservative treatment is recommended and may include patient education and self-care, cognitive behavioral interventions, pharmacotherapy, physical therapy, and orthopedic appliances.[43] Surgical management may be effective for specific articular disorders and may include arthrocentesis (joint lavage), arthroscopy, open surgical procedures, and joint replacement. TMJ surgery is not indicated for asymptomatic or minimally symptomatic patients, and should only be considered when nonsurgical conservative therapy has proved ineffective.[44] Management strategies for TMD are summarized in **Box 4.**

Box 4
Basic principles of management of TMDs

Patient education and self-care

Cognitive behavioral interventions

Pharmacologic management

• Analgesics, antiinflammatories, muscle relaxants, sedatives, antidepressants

Physical therapies

• Posture training, stretching exercises, mobilization, physical modalities, appliance therapy, occlusal therapy

Surgery

PATIENT EDUCATION AND SELF-CARE

The symptoms of TMD are often self-limiting. The disorder resolves in most patients, usually within 7 years.[45,46] Conservative and noninvasive interventions typically yield positive results in most patients. Although this explanation alone is helpful in reducing fear in the patient, it is essential to educate the patient to rest the masticatory system, avoiding perpetuating factors such as eating hard, chewy foods or chewing gum. Patients should be taught to be aware of and avoid parafunctional habits like clenching when possible. In addition, a home physiotherapeutic program of heat or ice to the painful areas, massage, and range-of-motion exercises can reduce pain and improve function.[43]

COGNITIVE BEHAVIORAL INTERVENTIONS

A key component in the management of patients with TMD is behavioral modification of maladaptive habits. For some patients this may be achieved with simple instruction and exercise, whereas others may require a more structured program facilitated by a specialist in behavioral modification. More structured programs may include lifestyle counseling, progressive relaxation, biofeedback, hypnosis, and cognitive behavior therapy. Treatment should be tailored to individual patient needs and preferences.[47]

PHARMACOLOGIC THERAPY

For TMD, the most common pharmacologic agents include nonsteroidal antiinflammatory drugs and muscle relaxants. Tricyclic antidepressants, selective serotonin-norepinephrine reuptake inhibitors, and antiepileptic drugs are also important in pain management.[48] When included in comprehensive therapy, pharmacologic agents can enhance patient comfort and healing.

PHYSICAL THERAPIES

The goals of physical therapy include the reduction of pain and improvement of joint movement through the alteration of nociceptive input, reduction of inflammation, coordination and strengthening of muscle activity, and allowing the regeneration of tissues. Physical therapies that are frequently used include posture training, exercise, joint mobilization, and the use of various physical agents or modalities. Physical agents and modalities that are commonly used include electrotherapy, ultrasound, iontophoresis, laser therapy, acupuncture, and splint therapy. Each is controversial regarding efficacy, particularly splint therapy.

Splints, also known as interocclusal guards, orthotics, orthoses, bite guards, night-guards, bruxism appliances, or orthopedic appliances, are removable appliances that cover all (full coverage) or some (partial coverage) of the teeth of 1 arch, and may or may not reposition the mandible. They may be useful as combination of mechanical and behavioral therapies in the management of TMD. In a systematic review, Fricton and colleagues[49] reviewed 44 studies involving intraoral appliances. Compared with placebo or no treatment, a hard stabilization appliance (a splint that covers all maxillary or mandibular teeth, that repositions the jaw, and is general worn at night only) was most effective in improving TMD-associated pain. Other types of splints (partial coverage, mandibular repositioning) were associated with greater potential for adverse effects and were no more effective than the stabilization splint in reducing TMD pain and headache. Anterior positioning splints may be more effective than stabilization splints for the management of painful TMJ clicking or locking. However, because they are also more likely to be associated with potentially irreversible occlusal changes,[50] they must be used with caution.

Studies in headache are limited and regularly lacking specific diagnoses, but they show splint therapy to be as effective as physical medicine techniques, cognitive behavior therapies, or acupuncture, and more effective than pharmacotherapy in 1 study.[51] Current evidence does not support the use of partial-coverage anterior bite planes, such as the nociceptive trigeminal inhibition reflex device (a hard splint that covers only the upper central incisors and lower central and lateral incisors, and holds the mandible forward) in the management of tension-type headache or migraine, but does support its use in the management of bruxism and myogenous TMD.[42] Despite the evidence that splint therapy is beneficial, splints are not intended to be used in isolation, but should be included as part of an integrated therapy program.[52] The use of any type of splint has the potential for adverse effects, which can be minimized by judicious use in select patients, appropriate splint design and adjustment, and regular patient monitoring. Occlusal therapy devices should be used only in those patients who possess the clear understanding that they must be compliant for follow-up. The use of splint therapy in headache management remains appropriate when painful TMDs, including masticatory myalgia or TMJ arthralgia, initiate or exacerbate headache symptoms.[53]

SURGICAL TREATMENT

TMJ surgery is considered to be useful in certain TMDs. There are few studies that examine surgery and response to headache. Vallerand and Hall[54] reported on 50 patients diagnosed with internal TMJ derangements, myalgia, and headaches who had not responded to nonsurgical management. The surgical procedures they underwent included disc repositioning, repair of disc perforation, disc recontouring, lysis of adhesions, and discectomy. In the retrospective evaluation, most patients reported decreases in headache in addition to decreases in joint pain and noise. The surgeons offered the explanation that the change in head pain was a secondary result of decreased joint pain, which facilitates the patient's ability to cope with other pains. In another study, Montgomery and colleagues[55] reported significant changes in TMJ, ear, neck, and shoulder pains, whereas headaches were less consistently changed, following arthroscopy of the TMJ.

SUMMARY

When managing headache and TMD symptoms, it is suggested the headache and TMD be treated together but separately. The clinician should address the TMD if the patient presents with at least 3 of the following 4 signs and symptoms: (1) pain in the preauricular and temporal region brought on by functions such as chewing; (2) pain on palpation over the TMJ; (3) joint noise such as clicking, popping, or crepitus; and (4) limited range of motion. If there is marked limitation of opening (less than 25 mm, measured interincisally) imaging of the joint may be necessary. This imaging can help define whether the limitation is caused by displaced disc without reduction or by muscle spasm or splinting. The treatment should then include education regarding limiting jaw function, appliance therapy, instruction in jaw posture (keeping the teeth apart during the day), and stretching exercises, as well as medications to reduce inflammation and relax the muscles. Antiinflammatories should be taken time contingently not pain contingently, usually for a few weeks. The use of physical therapies, such as spray and stretch and trigger point injections, is helpful if there is a MFP problem.

In selecting the prophylaxis for the migraine headache, it may also be useful to keep in mind what the musculoskeletal problem entails. The tricyclic antidepressants and the new-generation antiepileptic drugs are effective in muscle pain conditions. Selection of one of these in place of the muscle relaxant may therefore reduce the migraine frequency as well as the TMD. If the TMD involves disc displacement with reduced range of motion, the use of arthrocentesis and/or arthroscopy is often helpful in restoring range of motion. There is little use for open joint surgery, orthognathic intervention, or occlusal modification. Behavioral strategies including relaxation training and cognitive therapy are also useful if stress is a perpetuating factor.

REFERENCES

1. Okeson JP. Bell's orofacial pain. 5th edition. Chicago: Quintessence; 2005.
2. Headache Classification Committee of the International Headache Society (IHS). The international classification of headache disorders, 3rd edition (beta version). Cephalalgia 2013;33:629–808.
3. Ciancaglini R, Radaelli G. The relationship between headache and symptoms of temporomandibular disorders in the general population. J Dent 2001;29:93–8.
4. Piovesan EJ, Kowacs PA, Tatsui CE, et al. Referred pain after painful stimulation of the greater occipital nerve in humans: evidence of convergence of cervical afferents on trigeminal nuclei. Cephalalgia 2001;21(2):107–9.
5. Greene CS. Managing the care of patients with temporomandibular disorders: a new guideline for care. J Am Dent Assoc 2010;141:1086–8.
6. Le Resche L. Epidemiology of temporomandibular disorders: implications for the investigation of etiologic factors. Crit Rev Oral Biol Med 1997;8:291–305.
7. Glass EG, McGlynn FD, Glaros AG, et al. Prevalence of temporomandibular disorder symptoms in a major metropolitan area. Cranio 1993;11:217–20.
8. Graff-Radford SB. Temporomandibular disorders and headache. Dent Clin North Am 2007;51:129–44.
9. Dworkin SF, Le Resche L. Research diagnostic criteria for temporomandibular disorders: review, criteria, examinations and specifications, critique. J Craniomandib Disord 1992;6:301–55.
10. Manfredini D, Guarda-Nardini L, Winocur E, et al. Research diagnostic criteria for temporomandibular disorders: a systematic review of axis I epidemiologic findings. Oral Surg Oral Med Oral Pathol Oral Radiol Endod 2011;112:453–62.
11. De Leeuw R, Klasser GD, editors. Orofacial pain: guidelines for assessment, diagnosis and management. 5th edition. Hanover Park (IL): American Academy of Orofacial Pain. Quintessence Publishing; 2013. p. 130. Chapter 8.
12. Bellegaard V, Thede-Schmidt-Hansen P, Svensson P, et al. Are headache and temporomandibular disorders related? A blinded study. Cephalalgia 2008;28:832–41.
13. Glaros AG, Urban D, Locke J. Headache and temporomandibular disorders: evidence for diagnostic and behavioral overlap. Cephalalgia 2007;27:542–9.
14. Fernándes de las Peñas C, Galán del Río F, Fernández-Carnero J, et al. Bilateral widespread mechanical pain sensitivity in women with myofascial temporomandibular disorder: evidence of impairment in central nociceptive processing. J Pain 2009;10:1170–8.
15. Mandfredini D, Lobbezoo F. Relationship between bruxism and temporomandibular disorders: a systematic review of literature from 1998 to 2008. Oral Surg Oral Med Oral Pathol Oral Radiol Endod 2010;109:e26–50.

16. Lobbezoo F, van der Zaag J, van Selms MK, et al. Principles for the management of bruxism. J Oral Rehabil 2008;35:509–23.
17. Bader G, Lavigne G. Sleep bruxism: an overview of an oromandibular disorder. Sleep Med Rev 2000;4:27–43.
18. Diagnostic Classification Steering Committee, Thorpy MJ. ICSD – International classification of sleep disorders diagnostic and coding manual. Rochester (MN): American Sleep Disorders Association; 1990.
19. Lavigne GJ, Khoury S, Abe S, et al. Bruxism physiology and pathology; an overview for clinicians. J Oral Rehabil 2008;35:476–94.
20. Manfredini D, Winocur E, Guarda-Nardini L, et al. Epidemiology of bruxism in adults: a systematic review of the literature. J Orofac Pain 2013;27:99–110.
21. American Academy of Sleep Medicine. International classification of sleep disorders. 2nd edition. Westchester (NY): American Academy of Sleep Medicine; 2005.
22. Ohayon MM, Li KK, Guilleminault C. Risk factors for sleep bruxism in the general population. Chest 2001;119(1):53–61.
23. Bader GG, Kampe T, Tagdea T, et al. Descriptive physiological data on a sleep bruxism population. Sleep 1997;20(11):982–90.
24. Camparis CM, Siqueira JT. Sleep bruxism: clinical aspects and characteristics in patients with and without chronic orofacial pain. Oral Surg Oral Med Oral Pathol Oral Radiol Endod 2006;101(2):188–93.
25. Fernandes G, Franco AL, Gonçalves DA, et al. Temporomandibular disorders, sleep bruxism and primary headaches are mutually associated. J Orofac Pain 2013;27:14–20.
26. Scapino RP. The posterior attachment: its structure, junction, and appearance in TMJ imaging studies, part 1. J Craniomandib Disord 1991;5:83–95.
27. Kirkos LT, Ortejndayhl DA, Mark AS, et al. Magnetic resonance imaging of the TMJ disc in asymptomatic volunteers. J Oral Maxillofac Surg 1987;45:852–4.
28. Devant YT, Greene CS, Perry HT, et al. A quantitative computer-assisted analysis of the disc displacement in patients with internal derangement using sagittal view and magnetic resonance imaging. J Oral Maxillofac Surg 1991; 49:1079–88.
29. Rivner MH. The neurophysiology of myofascial pain syndrome. Curr Pain Headache Rep 2001;5:432–40.
30. Gerwin RD. Classification, epidemiology, and natural history of myofascial pain syndrome. Curr Pain Headache Rep 2001;5:412–20.
31. Simons DG, Travell JG, Simons LS. 2nd edition. The trigger point manual, vol. 1. Baltimore (MD): Lippincott Williams & Wilkins; 1998.
32. Fricton JR. Masticatory myofascial pain: an explanatory model integrating clinical, epidemiological, and basic science research. Bull Group Int Rech Sci Stomatol Odontol 1999;41:14–25.
33. Graff-Radford SB. Myofascial pain diagnosis and management. Curr Pain Headache Rep 2004;8(6):463–7.
34. Fricton JR, Olsen T. Predictors of outcome for treatment of temporomandibular disorders. J Orofac Pain 1996;10:54–65.
35. Graff Radford SB, Reeves JL, Jaeger B. Management of chronic head and neck pain: effectiveness of altering factors perpetuating myofascial pain. Headache 1987;27:186–90.
36. Kraft GH, Johnson EW, Laban MM. The fibrositis syndrome. Arch Phys Med Rehabil 1968;49:155–62.
37. Honda K, Larheim TA, Maruhashi K, et al. Osseous abnormalities of the mandibular condyle: diagnostic reliability of cone beam computed tomography

compared with helical computed tomography based on an autopsy material. Dentomaxillofac Radiol 2006;35:152–7.

38. Emshoff R, Innerhofer K, Rudisch A, et al. Clinical versus magnetic resonance imaging with internal derangement of the temporomandibular joint. An evaluation of anterior disc displacement without reduction. J Oral Maxillofac Surg 2002;60:36–41.

39. Leidberg J, Panmekiate S, Petersson A, et al. Evidence-based evaluation of three imaging methods for the temporomandibular disc. Dentomaxillofac Radiol 1996;25:234–41.

40. Tasaki MM, Westesson PL. Temporomandibular joint: diagnostic accuracy with sagittal and coronal MR imaging. Radiology 1993;186:723–9.

41. Koh KJ, List T, Petersson A, et al. Relationship between clinical and magnetic resonance imaging diagnoses and findings in degenerative and inflammatory temporomandibular joint diseases: a systematic literature review. J Orofac Pain 2009;23:123–39.

42. Stapelmann H, Türp JC. The NTI-TSS device for the therapy of bruxism, temporomandibular disorder and headache – where do we stand? A qualitative systematic review of the literature. BMC Oral Health 2008;29:8–22.

43. McNeill C. Management of temporomandibular disorders: concepts and controversies. J Prosthet Dent 1997;77:510–22.

44. American Association of Oral and Maxillofacial Surgeons. Parameters of care for oral and maxillofacial surgery. A guide for practice, monitoring and evaluation (AAOMS parameters of care–2012). J Oral Maxillofac Surg 2012;70(11 Suppl 3): e204–31.

45. Apfelberg DB, Lavey E, Janetos G, et al. Temporomandibular joint disease: results of a ten year study. Postgrad Med 1979;65(5):167–9, 171–2.

46. Okeson JP, Hayes DK. Long-term results of treatment for temporomandibular disorders: an evaluation of patients. J Am Dent Assoc 1986;112(4):473–8.

47. Turner JA, Keefe FJ. Cognitive-behavioral therapy for chronic pain. In: Max M, editor. Pain 1999 – an updated review. Seattle (WA): IASP Press; 1999. p. 523–33.

48. Sharav Y, Singer E, Schmidt E, et al. The analgesic effect of amitriptyline on chronic facial pain. Pain 1987;31(2):199–209.

49. Fricton J, Look JO, Wright E, et al. Systematic review and meta-analysis of randomized controlled trials evaluating intraoral orthopedic appliances for temporomandibular disorders. J Orofac Pain 2010;24(3):237–54.

50. Widmalm SE. Use and abuse of bite splints. Compend Contin Educ Dent 1999; 20:249–54.

51. Schokker RP, Hansson TL, Ansink BJ. The result of treatment of the masticatory system of chronic headache patients. J Craniomandib Disord 1990;4(2):126–30.

52. Dao TT, Lavigne GJ. Oral splints: the crutches for temporomandibular disorders and bruxism? Crit Rev Oral Biol Med 1998;9(3):345–61.

53. Clark GT, Minakuchi H. Oral appliances. In: Laskin DM, Greene CS, Hylander WL, editors. TMDs. An evidence-based approach to diagnosis and treatments. Chicago: Quintessence Publishing; 2006. p. 377–90.

54. Vallerand WP, Hall MB. Improvement in myofascial pain and headaches following TMJ surgery. J Craniomandib Disord 1991;5:197–204.

55. Montgomery MT, Van Sickels JE, Harms SE, et al. Arthroscopic TMJ surgery: effects on signs, symptoms, and disc position. J Oral Maxillofac Surg 1989; 47:1263–71.

Trigeminal and Glossopharyngeal Neuralgia

Gaddum Duemani Reddy, MD, PhD, Ashwin Viswanathan, MD*

KEYWORDS

- Trigeminal neuralgia • Glossopharyngeal neuralgia • Medical treatment
- Surgical treatment

KEY POINTS

- Trigeminal neuralgia and glossopharyngeal neuralgia are debilitating forms of paroxysmal facial pain and are diagnosed based on history.
- First-line therapy for both pathologic conditions is medication. Carbamazepine is the drug of choice; however, there are other medical options for patients unable to tolerate the side effects of carbamazepine.
- Surgical therapy with either microvascular decompression and/or an ablative procedure is often successful for medically refractory cases and can be considered early in such cases.
- Radiosurgery is emerging as a potential treatment modality for medically refractory cases and it should be considered in patients who cannot undergo more invasive treatment modalities.

INTRODUCTION

Trigeminal neuralgia (TN) is a clinical condition characterized by agonizing paroxysmal pain occurring in one or more divisions of the trigeminal nerve. The characterization of the disease process we are familiar with today, with afflicted individuals complaining of lancinating pain when chewing, speaking, or swallowing, began in the seventeenth century with the work of John Locke.[1] Since that time, our understanding of the disease process has advanced significantly. Today, TN is a condition for which there are several treatment options. However, it cannot always be cured and a subset of patients remains refractory to multiple forms of treatment.

Glossopharyngeal neuralgia (GPN) is another paroxysmal pain condition that is characterized by pain in the throat, pharynx, and ears. Affected individuals can lose consciousness because of bradycardia or asystole. The treatment strategy parallels

Disclosures: None.
Department of Neurosurgery, Baylor College of Medicine, 1709 Dryden Street, Houston, TX 77030, USA
* Corresponding author.
E-mail address: ashwinv@bcm.edu

Neurol Clin 32 (2014) 539–552
http://dx.doi.org/10.1016/j.ncl.2013.11.008
0733-8619/14/$ – see front matter Published by Elsevier Inc.

that for TN; however, given its rarity, less is known about its pathogenesis and the efficacy of various treatment modalities.

TRIGEMINAL NEURALGIA

Epidemiology

The only estimate on the prevalence of TN is from Penman[2] in his 1968 contribution to the *Handbook of Clinical Neurology*, in which he approximated 107.5 per million men and 200.2 per million women are afflicted by this condition. The incidence, however, was more extensively studied with early studies reporting approximately 4.3 new cases per 100,000 people annually.[3] The female to male ratio was estimated in these studies to be roughly 1.5 to 1[4–6] and there is known age dependence, with an annual incidence of 17.5 per 100,000 in individuals aged 60 to 69 years and 25.6 per 100,000 for those older than 70 years.[7]

More recently, European studies have found significantly higher incidence rates for TN, ranging from 12.6 to 27 per 100,000.[8–10] Similar to the older studies, these rates vary significantly with age, with incidences of less than 0.5 per 100,000 in subjects younger than 18 years compared with upwards of 80 per 100,000 subjects in older age groups. The female to male ratios in these newer studies are also significantly higher, at approximately 2.3 to 1.

Recent definitions of TN have separated it into two categories: classic, which is idiopathic in nature, and symptomatic, which is associated with an identifiable structural lesion excluding vascular compression. In cases of symptomatic TN, the condition can be associated with a more generalized demyelinating disease process such as multiple sclerosis.[3] In studies evaluating subjects with multiple sclerosis, TN occurs in approximately 2% of subjects,[11,12] with an increased risk of bilateral symptoms. TN has also been associated with other cranial nerve neuralgias, most notably GPN,[13] in which approximately 11% of subjects have associated TN.[14]

Familial cases of TN are rare but have been reported with estimates of approximately 4% to 5%[3,15] in patients with unilateral TN. Bilateral TN, however, has a higher familial association of approximately 17%,[15] suggesting a stronger hereditary component in this subpopulation. Although the data are sparse, case reports on families with a strong history of TN suggest an autosomal dominant inheritance pattern.[16–19]

Pathogenesis

The cause of TN is unknown. It is suspected, however, that both central and peripheral nerve dysfunction play a role. In the case of the peripheral nerve, it is hypothesized that vascular compression of the trigeminal nerve root at the root entry zone leads to chronic focal demyelination and afferent hyperexcitability. This can lead to hyperexcitability in the trigeminal brainstem complex, which subsequently responds to both nonnoxious and noxious stimuli in the same manner leading to the symptoms seen in TN.[20] However, in what is termed the ignition hypothesis, the injured sensory root itself can become a site of ectopic firing.[21] This in turn leads to some neurons continuously firing, which could be the source of baseline burning pain found in some TN; however, other neurons are silent but respond to momentary stimulation for a prolonged period after discharges.

Notably, several aspects of TN suggest a central role for the central action of effective medications. In addition, gray matter in the anterior cingulated cortex, parahippocampus, and temporal lobe was diminished in correspondence with the duration of the disease in patients afflicted with TN[22] suggesting a mechanism by which the disease process can alter the central nervous system, which, in turn, could prolong the disease.

Diagnosis

In 2004, International Headache Society (IHS) established a set of guidelines for both classic and symptomatic TN.[23,24] Diagnosis for both conditions is primarily clinical and a diagnosis of either must be based on three fundamental components:

1. Durations lasting from fractions of a second to up to 2 minutes and involving one or more regions of the trigeminal nerve.
2. Characterizations as intense, sharp, superficial, stabbing, and/or precipitated by trigger areas or trigger factors.
3. Stereotyped in the individual patient.

In addition, for classic TN, there can be no clinically evident neurologic disorder and symptoms cannot be attributed to another disorder. Conversely, for symptomatic TN a causative lesion, other than vascular compression, has to be demonstrated.

According to the IHS guidelines, whereas classic TN can involve any distribution of the trigeminal nerve, most cases involve the second or third distribution. The ophthalmic division is involved in less than 5% of cases. In addition, pain never crosses midline. However, it can occur bilaterally. Although it is not part of the definition, a refractory period during which pain cannot be triggered usually follows a painful paroxysm.

The triggers areas are typically in the affected area and the nasolabial fold or chin may be particularly susceptible. The pain is commonly evoked by trivial stimuli such as brushing, shaving, smoking, or talking. However, as further stipulated by the IHS guidelines, it can occur with somatosensory stimulation outside the trigeminal area or with other strong sensory stimuli, such as bright lights or loud sounds.

Symptomatic TN typically demonstrates no refractory period, unlike the classic version. It also, by definition, requires the presence of a causative lesion, necessitating further evaluation, usually with imaging. In a recent set of management guidelines, it was estimated that routine neuroimaging with CT or MRI identifies a lesion, thus separating symptomatic from classic TN, in approximately 15% of cases.[25]

In several studies, special three-dimensional MRI reconstruction sequences have been shown useful in identifying vascular compression, including constructive interference in steady state (CISS), fast imaging employing steady-state acquisition (FIESTA), fast inflow with steady state procession (FISP), and spoiled gradient-recalled (SPGR).[26–29] However, vascular compression is also frequently seen in normal individuals[30] and the American Academy of Neurology and the European Federation of Neurological Societies (AAN-EFNS) recommendations are inconclusive on the usefulness of using these modalities to diagnose vascular compression.[25]

Although not discussed in the IHS diagnosis, the terms typical and atypical have been used to describe two forms of TN characterized by sporadic, burning, shocklike pain versus constant, aching, lower intensity pain, respectively. It is an often confusing classification because patients can have elements of both types. A new classification system that attempts to allay confusion was proposed in 2003. It describes two types of classic TN: (1) type I characterized by greater than 50% episodic pain, and (2) type II characterized by greater than 50% constant pain.[31] In addition, symptomatic TN is divided into five categories depending on mechanism.

Medical Treatment

Medical therapy remains the first-line treatment of TN. Since the first successful symptom reduction with Dilantin in 1958,[32] various degrees of success have been achieved with neuroleptic, muscle relaxant, and anticonvulsant medications, either alone or in conjunction with one another (**Table 1**).[33]

Table 1
Medical treatment of TN: commonly used medications

	Dosage (mg/d)	Duration to Relief	Side Effects
Carbamazepine	400–800	1–2 d	Leukopenia, aplastic anemia, drowsiness, ataxia
Oxcarbazepine	400–1200	1–2 d	Changes in vision, difficulty walking
Lamotrigine	150–400	1–2 d	Changes in vision, Stevens-Johnson syndrome
Baclofen	40–80	4–5 d	Confusion, withdrawal symptoms
Phenytoin	300–500	1–2 d	Confusion, decreased coordination
Gabapentin	900–2400	1–3 wk	Unsteadiness, rolling eye movements
Pregabalin	150–600	1–2 wk	Swelling, blurred vision

Carbamazepine

Since its first implementation for TN in 1962 by Blom,[34] carbamazepine has been the most extensively studied and validated medication for the treatment of TN. Within 10 years of Blom's first use, four randomized placebo-controlled clinical trials were published demonstrating its effectiveness[35–38] using dosages ranging from 100 mg to 2.4 g. Recently, after pooling these studies together, a Cochrane Database review further validated these results and with a number needed to treat of 1.8.[39] However, there is evidence that this effectiveness can be reduced over time.[40]

The overall use of carbamazepine, however, is limited by its adverse effects. These include its general side effects, such as ataxia, drowsiness, dizziness, rash, nausea, and vomiting, and its hematologic side effects, such as leukopenia and aplastic anemia. In the same Cochrane Database review, the frequency of these adverse effects was enough to give an overall number to harm of 3. In addition, it has extensive interactions with other drugs. It also has autoinduction of its own metabolism, making equilibrium levels difficult to assess before a grace period of 3 weeks.

Carbamazepine is generally started at 100 mg per day and increased slowly to avoid neurotoxicity. Typical increments are about 100 mg every 3 days until pain is relieved. Serum levels between 25 and 45 μmol/L are often used at optimal concentration ranges. Typical maintenance dosages are between 400 and 800 mg with maximum dosages of 1500 mg. No more than 400 mg should be given in one dose to avoid toxic effects. Given the propensity to drowsiness, it is optimally dosed at night and, given its potential hematologic side effects, a complete blood count is usually obtained before starting treatment and then every 2 weeks for the first few months. Liver and renal function tests should also be assessed before initiation of treatment and then at 2-month intervals. After approximately 1 month without symptoms, patients should be tapered off their medications by approximately 100 mg every week to avoid unnecessary potential side effects.

Oxcarbazepine

Oxcarbazepine is a derivative of carbamazepine, with similar mechanisms of actions, but with less complex pharmacokinetics and a better side-effect profile. Oxcarbazepine has shown to have a similar efficacy to carbamazepine. It was also shown to be efficacious in patients in whom carbamazepine was ineffective,[41] usually within the first month of treatment, but has decreased efficacy over time.[42] Practically, oxcarbazepine is started at 150 mg per day and increased by 150 mg per day every 3 days until pain relief is achieved. Maintenance doses range from 400 to 1200 mg per day.

Lamotrigine

Lamotrigine, a sodium channel modulator, was shown to be efficacious as treatment modality in case studies for both classic[43,44] and symptomatic[45] TN secondary to multiple sclerosis. Practically, lamotrigine is started at approximately 25 mg per day and increased by 25 mg per day every 3 days until pain relief is achieved. Typical maintenance doses range from 150 to 400 mg per day. Although lamotrigine has a favorable adverse-outcome profile in general, it has been known to lead to Stevens-Johnson syndrome, characterized by a severe rash that appears early in treatment, in which case it should be immediately discontinued.

Baclofen

Baclofen, a γ-aminobutyric acid (GABA) derivative, has also been shown effective as both monotherapy and in combination with other medications.[46] Baclofen is generally started at 15 mg per day; typically divided into 5 mg three times a day. The dosage is increased by 5 mg every other day until pain relief is achieved, which is typically at maintenance dosages of around 50 mg per day. If used as an adjuvant medication, the primary medication can be reduced and pain still controlled. Once pain relief is achieved, the dosage of baclofen should be tapered to reduce side effects. This is typically done in increments of 5 mg per week. Tapering can too quickly lead to withdrawal symptoms, including seizures and anxiety. The most common side effects of baclofen itself are gastrointestinal distress and drowsiness.

Phenytoin

Phenytoin, which works by stabilizing sodium channels, was the first widespread medication used in the treatment of TN. Now, because of newer medications, it is rarely used alone for chronic management. When used, it is typically started at dosages of 100 mg per day and increased to approximately 100 to 200 mg three times a day. Complications include gingival hyperplasia, hirsutism, and depression. It is also known to interact with several medications, including carbamazepine, which decreases the half-life and thereby increases the concentration. However, in some reports, intravenous phenytoin was shown to be effective at doses of 650 mg and rates of 25 mg per minute in managing acute exacerbations of otherwise medically refractory TN attacks.[47,48] This effect has also been appreciated in fosphenytoin,[49] which has a better parenteral tolerance than phenytoin. Treatment with intravenous fosphenytoin resulted in symptomatic improvement in 2 days, making it an ideal medication for acute treatments.

Gabapentin

Gabapentin, a GABA analogue, was shown effective in patients with both classic[50,51] and symptomatic[52,53] TN. Its primary advantage over other medications is its safer adverse-effects profile; the most common side effects are dizziness, fatigue, and weight gain. It is typically started at dosages of 100 mg three times a day and increased up to 2400 mg per day. Mean effective doses are typically around 900 mg.[54]

Pregabalin

Pregabalin, another GABA analogue, was also shown to be successful in the treatment of TN.[55,56] Like gabapentin, it has a relatively benign side-effect profile; most commonly dizziness, drowsiness, dry mouth, and weight gain. It is typically started at dosages of 75 mg twice a day and increased to 150 mg twice a day if no improvement is seen in 1 week and to 300 mg twice a day if no improvement is seen in 2 weeks. A mean dosage required for improvement is approximately 270 mg per day.[55]

Topiramate

Topiramate, an antiseizure medication, was shown effective in treating classic TN in dosages ranging from 50 mg to 100 mg per day.[57] It has also been effective in symptomatic TN secondary to multiple sclerosis[58] or postinjury.[59] In a meta-analysis of six randomized controlled trials out of China, topiramate was actually found to be more effective than carbamazepine after 2 months of treatment.[60] There was, however, no significant difference in adverse effects at 2 months.

Sumatriptan

Sumatriptan has also recently been shown to be effective in treating refractory TN when taken orally at dosages of 50 mg twice a day,[61] intranasally as an adjuvant,[62] or subcutaneously.[63] Subcutaneous delivery of 3 mg was shown to significantly improve symptoms within 15 minutes of delivery with effects lasting for approximately 8 hours, making it an ideal potential treatment of acute attacks. This can be combined with oral sumatriptan for both prompt and prolonged control.[64]

Surgical Treatment

Although medical therapy remains the first-line treatment of TN, patients who are refractory to medical therapy or cannot tolerate the side effects can be candidates for interventional therapies.[65] These procedures can be divided into two categories: (1) destructive, which includes percutaneous ablative techniques and radiosurgery, and (2) nondestructive or microvascular decompression (MVD) (**Table 2**).

Microvascular decompression

In 1967, Jannetta[66] described arterial compression of the trigeminal nerve at the pons as the source of TN, a theory that was postulated by Dandy around 30 years earlier.[1] Most neurosurgeons and neurologists now believe that microvascular compression is the source for most idiopathic TN. Largely, this stems from numerous studies demonstrating the effectiveness of MVD in which the contact between the compressing vascular structure and underlying trigeminal nerve is removed. In one of the largest series, Barker and colleagues[67] reviewed more than 1100 subjects who had undergone MVD over a 20-year period. At the 10-year evaluation, 70% were pain free

Table 2
Surgical treatments for trigeminal neuralgia

		Success Rates	
	Time to Relief	Immediate (%)	Long-term (%)
Nonablative			
MVD	Immediate	>90	70–80
Ablative			
Radiofrequency	Immediate	>95	57–75
Glycerol	Immediate	65–90	50–60
Balloon Compression	Immediate	85–95	35–70
Radiosurgery	1–2 wk	70–90	20–60

and another 4% were controlled with medications. Approximately 30% had recurrence and 11% underwent a second operation. The overall adverse-effect rate was low, with 1% having hearing loss, 1% having facial numbness, 0.2% dying within the postoperative period, and 0.1% having brain stem infarcts. Other studies have demonstrated similar findings of approximately a 70% long-term pain-free rate. This rate of long-term pain relief was seen in other studies, though initial success rates are higher.[68,69]

Most recurrence after MVD happens within the first 2 years. Although some factors, such as female gender and long pain duration, generally show a positive correlation with recurrence, other factors, such as age at surgery and character of TN, have been unequivocal.[68-70] Options for recurrence include repeat exploration; however, the potential for adverse effects is higher in these cases.[71]

Ablative techniques

Three percutaneous ablative techniques are commonly used to treat medically refractory TN: radiofrequency rhizotomy (RFL), percutaneous retrogasserian glycerol rhizotomy (PRGR), and balloon microcompression (BMC). Typically, only BMC requires general anesthesia. All three techniques rely on accurate cannulation of the trigeminal cistern through the medial portion of the foramen ovale. This uses three anatomic landmarks, originally described in 1912 by Hartel[72], in addition to C-arm fluoroscopic guidance. Using anterior or posterior radiographic views, the foramen oval can also be visualized just posterior to lateral pterygoid wing. A 20-gauge to 22-gauge spinal needle is passed from the entry point toward the foramen. Once the foramen is penetrated, the patient may experience a brief episode of pain and there is often jaw jerk elicited due to penetration of V3 and the semilunar ganglion. Once the cannula is inside the arachnoid of the trigeminal cistern, there is a spontaneous return of cerebrospinal fluid. In general, using lateral radiographs, the cannula should not extend past the clival control to avoid damage to critical neurovascular structures.

Radiofrequnecy rhizotomy

RFL involves inserting an electrode through the foramen ovale into the retrogasserian rootlets and thermally ablating conducting fibers. Stimulation before thermally ablation helps ensure that the desired distributions of the trigeminal nerve are targeted and that no side effects, such as extraocular movement involvement, are elicited. Results with RFL are effective, with almost 100% pain-free rates reported in multiple large series.[73,74] Recurrence rates in these trials range between 25% and 45% after a single session, but drop to almost zero after multiple sessions. Complications include depressed corneal reflex, which is reported in up to 20% of cases, and, less frequently, masseter weakness or dysesthesias. Patients with symptomatic TN from multiple sclerosis have good results with overall pain-free rates of approximately 70% after 5 years.[75] Some practitioners argue that the success of RFL shows that it should be used as a first-line surgical treatment except in individuals who specifically want to preserve sensation or have V1 and/or all three distribution involvements.[76] However, this has been controversial with some studies showing a significantly higher rate of recurrence after RFL versus MVD.[77]

Percutaneous retrogasserian glycerol rhizotomy (PRGR)

The technique of PRGR was first described by Hakanson[78] in 1982. It uses glycerol injection to destroy the retrogasserian fibers. Like RFL, it was shown effective for both symptomatic TN and classic TN, with initial pain resolution rates of approximately 90% in the first 2 months, which drops to 60% at 1 year, 50% at 3 years, and 40% at

5 to 6 years.[79,80] Complications are similar to those for RFL and occur in approximately 11% of cases.[81]

Balloon microcompression

BMC involves compression of the retrogasserian rootlets using an inflatable balloon. This procedure requires a larger cannula. Compression of the trigeminal ganglion can trigger bradycardia. It is commonly done under general anesthesia. Similar to other percutaneous methods, it has also proven effective. Immediate pain relief is seen in 85% to 99% of patients with recurrence rates ranging from 20% to 40% across multiple series.[82–84] Complication rates in these studies are also low and range from 4% to 8%.

Stereotactic radio surgery

Over the past 10 years, stereotactic radio surgery (SRS) has emerged as another treatment of refractory TN. Two SRS modalities have been investigated: Gamma Knife (Elekta, Atlanta GA), in which multiple beams of simultaneous radiation are used to create an isolated treatment area, and CyberKnife (Accuray, Sunnyvale CA), in which a single radiation beam is maneuvered in three-dimensional space to create a targeted treatment area.

Multiple retrospective series have been published analyzing the effectiveness of treatment with Gamma Knife. For all studies, typical isocenter areas are 4 mm and doses range from 70 to 90 Gy with doses higher than 90 Gy correlating with dysthesias.[85] Similar to other methods of treatment, immediate improvements are relatively high with values of 80% to 90% of patients being pain-free within the first year.[85–87] However, this value progressively declines to approximately 55% being pain-free at 3 years.[85] The percent of patients with significant pain reductions, characterized by pain adequately controlled with medication, also drop from approximately 60% to 80 % at 1 year[86,88] to 22% to 30% at 7 to 10 years.[86,88] Similar findings have been found in patients with symptomatic TN.[89] Comparison studies between Gamma Knife and MVD have found MVD to be significantly better in maintaining pain-free status,[90,91] but MVD is also associated with higher rates of cerebrospinal fluid leak, hearing loss, and persistent diplopia[90]; both modalities have equal rates of facial dysthesias.[91]

CyberKnife has also been shown efficacious in treating TN. Optimal treatment parameters were found to be a maximal median dose of 78 Gy and a median length of treated nerve of 6 mm.[92] Excellent pain relief was found in approximately 70% to 88% of patients with a median time to relief of 7 to 14 days[92,93] but, similar to other treatment modalities, this value drops progressively to roughly 50% at 2 years. Approximately 50% of patients have posttreatment numbness and approximately 18% have some form of complications.[92,93]

GLOSSOPHARYNGEAL NEURALGIA (GPN)

GPN is an uncommon facial pain syndrome typified by paroxysmal episodes of pain along the auricular and pharyngeal branches of the glossopharyngeal and vagus nerves. Patients typically complain of stabbing pain along one side of the throat, near the tonsillar area, with occasional radiation to the ear. When the parasympathetic functions of the vagus nerve are involved, patients also can have bradycardia, asystole, syncopal episodes, and convulsions.[94] It is often misdiagnosed as TN and can easily be confused with nervus intermedius neuralgia and/or superior laryngeal neuralgia.[95]

Incidence

Much less frequent than TN, the incidence of GPN is estimated to be approximately 0.2 to 0.7 per 100,000 patients.[6–8,96] Approximately a quarter of these will have bilateral presentations, which is appreciably higher than in TN, with most patients presenting older than 50 years of age. Also unlike TN, the female to male ratio is approximately equal.[7,8]

Diagnosis

Using the IHS diagnosis guidelines, GPN is also divided into classic and symptomatic GPN, in which the latter requires a causative lesion to be demonstrated by surgery and/or special investigation.[23,24] Both types require paroxysmal attacks of facial pain lasting from fractions of a second to up to 2 minutes that are stereotyped in the individual patient. The attacks must be (1) characterized as sharp, stabbing, and severe; (2) precipitated by swallowing, chewing, talking, coughing, or yawning; and (3) within the posterior part of the tongue, tonsillar fossa, pharynx, or beneath the angle of the lower jaw and/or in the ear. Symptomatic GPN may also have an aching pain that persists between paroxysms and can be associated with sensory impairment within the distribution of the glossopharyngeal nerve.

Treatment

Similar to TN, the first-line treatment of GPN is pharmacologic with many of the same agents and dosages described above, including carbamazepine or oxcarbazepine, gabapentin, pregabalin, and phenytoin.[97] Surgical options, including MVD and rhizotomy, are also available and were shown to be very effective. MVD, in particular, has shown in several studies to have long-term pain-free outcomes in upwards of 80% and usually greater than 90% of subjects treated[14,98–101] with a low rate of complications such dysphagia or hoarseness. Other treatment options for TN (described above) have also been performed in GPN in several case series and reports with good results, including radiofrequency ablation[102,103] and Gamma Knife ablation.[104–108]

SUMMARY

TN and GPN are painful conditions that, though rare, are often debilitating to those affected. Accurate diagnosis and treatment are crucial for improving patient outcomes. Medical therapy remains the first-line treatment of both, but surgical and radiosurgical modalities are often effective options for patients who remain refractory to medical treatment.

REFERENCES

1. Eboli P, Stone JL, Aydin S, et al. Historical characterization of trigeminal neuralgia. Neurosurgery 2009;64(6):1183–6.
2. Penman J. Trigeminal neuralgia. In: Vinken PJ, Bruyn GW, editors. Handbook of clinical neurlogy. Amsterdam: North-Holland Publishing Company; 1968. p. 296–322.
3. Katusic S, Beard CM, Bergstralh E, et al. Incidence and clinical features of trigeminal neuralgia, Rochester, Minnesota, 1945–1984. Ann Neurol 1990;27(1): 89–95.
4. Ashkenazi A, Levin M. Three common neuralgias. How to manage trigeminal, occipital, and postherpetic pain. Postgrad Med 2004;116(3):16–8, 31.
5. Rozen TD. Trigeminal neuralgia and glossopharyngeal neuralgia. Neurol Clin 2004;22(1):185–206.
6. Manzoni GC, Torelli P. Epidemiology of typical and atypical craniofacial neuralgias. Neurol Sci 2005;26(Suppl 2):s65–7.

7. Katusic S, Williams DB, Beard CM, et al. Incidence and clinical features of glossopharyngeal neuralgia, Rochester, Minnesota, 1945–1984. Neuroepidemiology 1991;10(5–6):266–75.

8. Koopman JS, Dieleman JP, Huygen FJ, et al. Incidence of facial pain in the general population. Pain 2009;147(1–3):122–7.

9. Dieleman JP, Kerklaan J, Huygen FJ, et al. Incidence rates and treatment of neuropathic pain conditions in the general population. Pain 2008;137(3):681–8.

10. Hall GC, Carroll D, Parry D, et al. Epidemiology and treatment of neuropathic pain: the UK primary care perspective. Pain 2006;122(1–2):156–62.

11. Hooge JP, Redekop WK. Trigeminal neuralgia in multiple sclerosis. Neurology 1995;45(7):1294–6.

12. Solaro C, Brichetto G, Amato MP, et al. The prevalence of pain in multiple sclerosis: a multicenter cross-sectional study. Neurology 2004;63(5):919–21.

13. Knuckey NW, Gubbay SS. Familial trigeminal and glossopharyngeal neuralgia. Clin Exp Neurol 1979;16:315–9.

14. Rushton JG, Stevens JC, Miller RH. Glossopharyngeal (vagoglossopharyngeal) neuralgia: a study of 217 cases. Arch Neurol 1981;38(4):201–5.

15. Pollack IF, Jannetta PJ, Bissonette DJ. Bilateral trigeminal neuralgia: a 14-year experience with microvascular decompression. J Neurosurg 1988;68(4):559–65.

16. Duff JM, Spinner RJ, Lindor NM, et al. Familial trigeminal neuralgia and contralateral hemifacial spasm. Neurology 1999;53(1):216–8.

17. Smyth P, Greenough G, Stommel E. Familial trigeminal neuralgia: case reports and review of the literature. Headache 2003;43(8):910–5.

18. Herzberg L. Familial trigeminal neuralgia. Arch Neurol 1980;37(5):285–6.

19. Castaner-Vendrelle E, Barraquer-Borda SL. Six members de la meme familie avec tic douloureux de trijemeau. Monatsschr Psychiatr Neurol 1949;118(2):77–80.

20. Fromm GH. Pathophysiology of trigeminal neuralgia. In: Fromm GH, Sessle BJ, editors. Trigeminal neuralgia: current concepts regarding pathogenesis and treatment. Boston: Butterworth-Heinemann; 1991. p. 105–30.

21. Devor M, Amir R, Rappaport ZH. Pathophysiology of trigeminal neuralgia: the ignition hypothesis. Clin J Pain 2002;18(1):4–13.

22. Obermann M, Rodriguez-Raecke R, Naegel S, et al. Gray matter volume reduction reflects chronic pain in trigeminal neuralgia. Neuroimage 2013;74:352–8.

23. Headache Classification Committee of the International Headache Society (IHS). The International Classification of Headache Disorders, 3rd edition (beta version). Cephalalgia 2013;33(9):629–808.

24. Headache Classification Subcommittee of the International Headache Society. The International Classification of Headache Disorders: 2nd edition. Cephalalgia 2004;24(Suppl 1):9–160.

25. Cruccu G, Gronseth G, Alksne J, et al. AAN-EFNS guidelines on trigeminal neuralgia management. Eur J Neurol 2008;15(10):1013–28.

26. Zeng Q, Zhou Q, Liu Z, et al. Preoperative detection of the neurovascular relationship in trigeminal neuralgia using three-dimensional fast imaging employing steady-state acquisition (FIESTA) and magnetic resonance angiography (MRA). J Clin Neurosci 2013;20(1):107–11.

27. Yoshino N, Akimoto H, Yamada I, et al. Trigeminal neuralgia: evaluation of neuralgic manifestation and site of neurovascular compression with 3D CISS MR imaging and MR angiography. Radiology 2003;228(2):539–45.

28. Meaney JF, Miles JB, Nixon TE, et al. Vascular contact with the fifth cranial nerve at the pons in patients with trigeminal neuralgia: detection with 3D FISP imaging. AJR Am J Roentgenol 1994;163(6):1447–52.

29. Niwa Y, Shiotani M, Karasawa H, et al. Identification of offending vessels in trigeminal neuralgia and hemifacial spasm using SPGR-MRI and 3D-TOF-MRA. Rinsho Shinkeigaku 1996;36(4):544–50 [in Japanese].

30. Peker S, Dincer A, Necmettin PM. Vascular compression of the trigeminal nerve is a frequent finding in asymptomatic individuals: 3-T MR imaging of 200 trigeminal nerves using 3D CISS sequences. Acta Neurochir (Wien) 2009;151(9):1081–8.

31. Burchiel KJ. A new classification for facial pain. Neurosurgery 2003;53(5): 1164–6.

32. Iannone A, Baker AB, Morrell F. Dilantin in the treatment of trigeminal neuralgia. Neurology 1958;8(2):126–8.

33. Jorns TP, Zakrzewska JM. Evidence-based approach to the medical management of trigeminal neuralgia. Br J Neurosurg 2007;21(3):253–61.

34. Blom S. Trigeminal neuralgia: its treatment with a new anticonvulsant drug (G-32883). Lancet 1962;1(7234):839–40.

35. Killian JM, Fromm GH. Carbamazepine in the treatment of neuralgia. Use of side effects. Arch Neurol 1968;19(2):129–36.

36. Nicol CF. A four year double-blind study of tegretol in facial pain. Headache 1969;9(1):54–7.

37. Rockliff BW, Davis EH. Controlled sequential trials of carbamazepine in trigeminal neuralgia. Arch Neurol 1966;15(2):129–36.

38. Campbell FG, Graham JG, Zilkha KJ. Clinical trial of carbazepine (tegretol) in trigeminal neuralgia. J Neurol Neurosurg Psychiatry 1966;29(3):265–7.

39. Wiffen PJ, McQuay HJ, Moore RA. Carbamazepine for acute and chronic pain. Cochrane Database Syst Rev 2005;(3):CD005451.

40. Taylor JC, Brauer S, Espir ML. Long-term treatment of trigeminal neuralgia with carbamazepine. Postgrad Med J 1981;57(663):16–8.

41. Gomez-Arguelles JM, Dorado R, Sepulveda JM, et al. Oxcarbazepine monotherapy in carbamazepine-unresponsive trigeminal neuralgia. J Clin Neurosci 2008;15(5):516–9.

42. Zakrzewska JM, Patsalos PN. Long-term cohort study comparing medical (oxcarbazepine) and surgical management of intractable trigeminal neuralgia. Pain 2002;95(3):259–66.

43. Canavero S, Bonicalzi V, Ferroli P, et al. Lamotrigine control of idiopathic trigeminal neuralgia. J Neurol Neurosurg Psychiatry 1995;59(6):646.

44. Zakrzewska JM, Chaudhry Z, Nurmikko TJ, et al. Lamotrigine (lamictal) in refractory trigeminal neuralgia: results from a double-blind placebo controlled crossover trial. Pain 1997;73(2):223–30.

45. Leandri M, Lundardi G, Inglese M, et al. Lamotrigine in trigeminal neuralgia secondary to multiple sclerosis. J Neurol 2000;247(7):556–8.

46. Fromm GH, Terrence CF, Chattha AS. Baclofen in the treatment of trigeminal neuralgia: double-blind study and long-term follow-up. Ann Neurol 1984;15(3): 240–4.

47. Tate R, Rubin LM, Krajewski KC. Treatment of refractory trigeminal neuralgia with intravenous phenytoin. Am J Health Syst Pharm 2011;68(21):2059–61.

48. Albert HH. Infusion therapy of acute trigeminal neuralgia using phenytoin i.v. MMW Munch Med Wochenschr 1978;120(15):529–30 [in German].

49. Cheshire WP. Fosphenytoin: an intravenous option for the management of acute trigeminal neuralgia crisis. J Pain Symptom Manage 2001;21(6):506–10.

50. Sist T, Filadora V, Miner M, et al. Gabapentin for idiopathic trigeminal neuralgia: report of two cases. Neurology 1997;48(5):1467.

51. Pandey CK, Singh N, Singh PK. Gabapentin for refractory idiopathic trigeminal neuralgia. J Indian Med Assoc 2008;106(2):124–5.

52. Khan OA. Gabapentin relieves trigeminal neuralgia in multiple sclerosis patients. Neurology 1998;51(2):611–4.

53. Solaro C, Messmer UM, Uccelli A, et al. Low-dose gabapentin combined with either lamotrigine or carbamazepine can be useful therapies for trigeminal neuralgia in multiple sclerosis. Eur Neurol 2000;44(1):45–8.

54. Cheshire WP Jr. Defining the role for gabapentin in the treatment of trigeminal neuralgia: a retrospective study. J Pain 2002;3(2):137–42.

55. Obermann M, Yoon MS, Sensen K, et al. Efficacy of pregabalin in the treatment of trigeminal neuralgia. Cephalalgia 2008;28(2):174–81.

56. Perez C, Navarro A, Saldana MT, et al. Patient-reported outcomes in subjects with painful trigeminal neuralgia receiving pregabalin: evidence from medical practice in primary care settings. Cephalalgia 2009;29(7):781–90.

57. Domingues RB, Kuster GW, Aquino CC. Treatment of trigeminal neuralgia with low doses of topiramate. Arq Neuropsiquiatr 2007;65(3B):792–4.

58. Zvartau-Hind M, Din MU, Gilani A, et al. Topiramate relieves refractory trigeminal neuralgia in MS patients. Neurology 2000;55(10):1587–8.

59. Benoliel R, Sharav Y, Eliav E. Painful posttraumatic trigeminal neuropathy: a case report of relief with topiramate. Cranio 2007;25(1):57–62.

60. Wang QP, Bai M. Topiramate versus carbamazepine for the treatment of classical trigeminal neuralgia: a meta-analysis. CNS Drugs 2011;25(10): 847–57.

61. Moran J, Neligan A. Treatment resistant trigeminal neuralgia relieved with oral sumatriptan: a case report. J Med Case Rep 2009;3:7229.

62. Shimohata K, Shimohata T, Motegi R, et al. Nasal sumatriptan as adjunctive therapy for idiopathic trigeminal neuralgia: report of three cases. Headache 2009; 49(5):768–70.

63. Kanai A, Saito M, Hoka S. Subcutaneous sumatriptan for refractory trigeminal neuralgia. Headache 2006;46(4):577–82.

64. Kanai A, Suzuki A, Osawa S, et al. Sumatriptan alleviates pain in patients with trigeminal neuralgia. Clin J Pain 2006;22(8):677–80.

65. Pollock BE. Surgical management of medically refractory trigeminal neuralgia. Curr Neurol Neurosci Rep 2012;12(2):125–31.

66. Jannetta PJ. Arterial compression of the trigeminal nerve at the pons in patients with trigeminal neuralgia. J Neurosurg 1967;26(Suppl 1):159–62.

67. Barker FG, Jannetta PJ, Bissonette DJ, et al. The long-term outcome of microvascular decompression for trigeminal neuralgia. N Engl J Med 1996;334(17): 1077–83.

68. Sindou M, Leston J, Decullier E, et al. Microvascular decompression for primary trigeminal neuralgia: long-term effectiveness and prognostic factors in a series of 362 consecutive patients with clear-cut neurovascular conflicts who underwent pure decompression. J Neurosurg 2007;107(6):1144–53.

69. Theodosopoulos PV, Marco E, Applebury C, et al. Predictive model for pain recurrence after posterior fossa surgery for trigeminal neuralgia. Arch Neurol 2002;59(8):1297–302.

70. Miller JP, Magill ST, Acar F, et al. Predictors of long-term success after microvascular decompression for trigeminal neuralgia. J Neurosurg 2009;110(4): 620–6.

71. Amador N, Pollock BE. Repeat posterior fossa exploration for patients with persistent or recurrent idiopathic trigeminal neuralgia. J Neurosurg 2008; 108(5):916–20.

72. Hartel F. Block anaesthesia and injection of the Gasserian ganglion and the trigeminal roots. Langenbecks Arch Klin Chir 1912;100:16.

73. Taha JM, Tew JM Jr, Buncher CR. A prospective 15-year follow up of 154 consecutive patients with trigeminal neuralgia treated by percutaneous stereotactic radiofrequency thermal rhizotomy. J Neurosurg 1995;83(6):989–93.

74. Kanpolat Y, Savas A, Bekar A, et al. Percutaneous controlled radiofrequency trigeminal rhizotomy for the treatment of idiopathic trigeminal neuralgia: 25-year experience with 1,600 patients. Neurosurgery 2001;48(3):524–32.

75. Kanpolat Y, Berk C, Savas A, et al. Percutaneous controlled radiofrequency rhizotomy in the management of patients with trigeminal neuralgia due to multiple sclerosis. Acta Neurochir (Wien) 2000;142(6):685–9.

76. Taha JM, Tew JM Jr. Comparison of surgical treatments for trigeminal neuralgia: reevaluation of radiofrequency rhizotomy. Neurosurgery 1996;38(5): 865–71.

77. Tronnier VM, Rasche D, Hamer J, et al. Treatment of idiopathic trigeminal neuralgia: comparison of long-term outcome after radiofrequency rhizotomy and microvascular decompression. Neurosurgery 2001;48(6):1261–7.

78. Hakanson S. Retrogasserian injection of glycerol in the treatment of trigeminal neuralgia and other facial pains. Neurosurgery 1982;10(2):300.

79. Pollock BE. Percutaneous retrogasserian glycerol rhizotomy for patients with idiopathic trigeminal neuralgia: a prospective analysis of factors related to pain relief. J Neurosurg 2005;102(2):223–8.

80. Linderoth B, Hakanson S. Paroxysmal facial pain in disseminated sclerosis treated by retrogasserian glycerol injection. Acta Neurol Scand 1989;80(4): 341–6.

81. Kouzounias K, Lind G, Schechtmann G, et al. Comparison of percutaneous balloon compression and glycerol rhizotomy for the treatment of trigeminal neuralgia. J Neurosurg 2010;113(3):486–92.

82. Kouzounias K, Schechtmann G, Lind G, et al. Factors that influence outcome of percutaneous balloon compression in the treatment of trigeminal neuralgia. Neurosurgery 2010;67(4):925–34.

83. Park SS, Lee MK, Kim JW, et al. Percutaneous balloon compression of trigeminal ganglion for the treatment of idiopathic trigeminal neuralgia: experience in 50 patients. J Korean Neurosurg Soc 2008;43(4):186–9.

84. Skirving DJ, Dan NG. A 20-year review of percutaneous balloon compression of the trigeminal ganglion. J Neurosurg 2001;94(6):913–7.

85. Pollock BE, Phuong LK, Gorman DA, et al. Stereotactic radiosurgery for idiopathic trigeminal neuralgia. J Neurosurg 2002;97(2):347–53.

86. Dhople AA, Adams JR, Maggio WW, et al. Long-term outcomes of Gamma Knife radiosurgery for classic trigeminal neuralgia: implications of treatment and critical review of the literature. Clinical article. J Neurosurg 2009; 111(2):351–8.

87. Regis J, Metellus P, Hayashi M, et al. Prospective controlled trial of gamma knife surgery for essential trigeminal neuralgia. J Neurosurg 2006;104(6):913–24.

88. Kondziolka D, Zorro O, Lobato-Polo J, et al. Gamma Knife stereotactic radiosurgery for idiopathic trigeminal neuralgia. J Neurosurg 2010;112(4):758–65.

89. Zorro O, Lobato-Polo J, Kano H, et al. Gamma knife radiosurgery for multiple sclerosis-related trigeminal neuralgia. Neurology 2009;73(14):1149–54.

90. Linskey ME, Ratanatharathorn V, Penagaricano J. A prospective cohort study of microvascular decompression and Gamma Knife surgery in patients with trigeminal neuralgia. J Neurosurg 2008;109(Suppl):160–72.

91. Pollock BE, Schoeberl KA. Prospective comparison of posterior fossa exploration and stereotactic radiosurgery dorsal root entry zone target as primary surgery for patients with idiopathic trigeminal neuralgia. Neurosurgery 2010;67(3): 633–8.

92. Villavicencio AT, Lim M, Burneikiene S, et al. Cyberknife radiosurgery for trigeminal neuralgia treatment: a preliminary multicenter experience. Neurosurgery 2008;62(3):647–55.

93. Lim M, Villavicencio AT, Burneikiene S, et al. CyberKnife radiosurgery for idiopathic trigeminal neuralgia. Neurosurg Focus 2005;18(5):E9.

94. Elias J, Kuniyoshi R, Carloni WV, et al. Glossopharyngeal neuralgia associated with cardiac syncope. Arq Bras Cardiol 2002;78(5):510–9.

95. Blumenfeld A, Nikolskaya G. Glossopharyngeal neuralgia. Curr Pain Headache Rep 2013;17(7):343.

96. Katusic S, Williams DB, Beard CM, et al. Epidemiology and clinical features of idiopathic trigeminal neuralgia and glossopharyngeal neuralgia: similarities and differences, Rochester, Minnesota, 1945-1984. Neuroepidemiology 1991; 10(5–6):276–81.

97. Fromm GH. Clinical pharmacology of drugs used to treat head and face pain. Neurol Clin 1990;8(1):143–51.

98. Ferroli P, Fioravanti A, Schiariti M, et al. Microvascular decompression for glossopharyngeal neuralgia: a long-term retrospectic review of the Milan-Bologna experience in 31 consecutive cases. Acta Neurochir (Wien) 2009;151(10): 1245–50.

99. Kandan SR, Khan S, Jeyaretna DS, et al. Neuralgia of the glossopharyngeal and vagal nerves: long-term outcome following surgical treatment and literature review. Br J Neurosurg 2010;24(4):441–6.

100. Patel A, Kassam A, Horowitz M, et al. Microvascular decompression in the management of glossopharyngeal neuralgia: analysis of 217 cases. Neurosurgery 2002;50(4):705–10.

101. Sampson JH, Grossi PM, Asaoka K, et al. Microvascular decompression for glossopharyngeal neuralgia: long-term effectiveness and complication avoidance. Neurosurgery 2004;54(4):884–9.

102. Pagura JR, Schnapp M, Passarelli P. Percutaneous radiofrequency glossopharyngeal rhizotomy for cancer pain. Appl Neurophysiol 1983;46(1–4):154–9.

103. Isamat F, Ferran E, Acebes JJ. Selective percutaneous thermocoagulation rhizotomy in essential glossopharyngeal neuralgia. J Neurosurg 1981;55(4):575–80.

104. O'Connor JK, Bidiwala S. Effectiveness and safety of Gamma Knife radiosurgery for glossopharyngeal neuralgia. Proc (Bayl Univ Med Cent) 2013;26(3):262–4.

105. Stanic S, Franklin SD, Pappas CT, et al. Gamma knife radiosurgery for recurrent glossopharyngeal neuralgia after microvascular decompression. Stereotact Funct Neurosurg 2012;90(3):188–91.

106. Stieber VW, Bourland JD, Ellis TL. Glossopharyngeal neuralgia treated with gamma knife surgery: treatment outcome and failure analysis. Case report. J Neurosurg 2005;102(Suppl):155–7.

107. Williams BJ, Schlesinger D, Sheehan J. Glossopharyngeal neuralgia treated with gamma knife radiosurgery. World Neurosurg 2010;73(4):413–7.

108. Yomo S, Arkha Y, Donnet A, et al. Gamma Knife surgery for glossopharyngeal neuralgia. J Neurosurg 2009;110(3):559–63.

Index

Note: Page numbers of article titles are in **boldface** type.

Neurol Clin 32 (2014) 553–567
http://dx.doi.org/10.1016/S0733-8619(14)00011-5
0733-8619/14/$ – see front matter © 2014 Elsevier Inc. All rights reserved.

neurologic.theclinics.com

Moving?

Make sure your subscription moves with you!

To notify us of your new address, find your **Clinics Account Number** (located on your mailing label above your name), and contact customer service at:

Email: journalscustomerservice-usa@elsevier.com

800-654-2452 (subscribers in the U.S. & Canada)
314-447-8871 (subscribers outside of the U.S. & Canada)

Fax number: 314-447-8029

**Elsevier Health Sciences Division
Subscription Customer Service
3251 Riverport Lane
Maryland Heights, MO 63043**

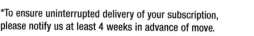

Printed and bound by CPI Group (UK) Ltd, Croydon, CR0 4YY

07/10/2024

01040499-0011